ILLUSTRATED

Anatomy OF THE
Head and Neck

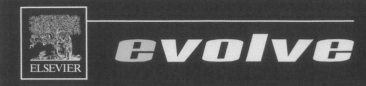

ELSEVIER

evolve

To access your Student Resources, visit:

http://evolve.elsevier.com/Fehrenbach/headneck/

Evolve® Student Learning Resources for *Fehrenbach/Herring: Illustrated Anatomy of the Head and Neck,* **Third Edition,** offer the following features:

Student Resources

- **Supplemental Study Considerations**
  The Supplemental Study Considerations provide the student with additional areas of study, expanding upon the material found in the book. A variety of topics are discussed, including laryngeal cancer, hormone replacement therapy (HRT), acromegaly, botulinum toxin and facial muscles, thyroid malignancy, and the blood-brain barrier.

- **Interactive Head and Neck Review Cases**
  This excellent review tool provides case studies, which include a patient history, a clinical photo, and a series of multiple choice questions. After answering the questions, students can submit their answers to see what they got right and what they got wrong.

- **Discussion Questions**
  Discussion Questions are provided for each chapter. They can be used to stimulate classroom discussion as wel as for group or self-study and review.

- **Crossword Puzzles and Word Searches**
  Crossword Puzzles and Word Searches are provided for each chapter. These are an excellent way for students to test their knowledge of head and neck terminology.

- **Update Section**
  Content Updates will be posted periodically to help keep students informed of new and exciting developments in the field as well as address additional concepts and information that may not be covered in the text.

ILLUSTRATED

Anatomy OF THE
Head and Neck

THIRD EDITION

MARGARET J. FEHRENBACH, RDH, MS
Oral Biologist and Dental Hygienist
Adjunct Faculty Position, Marquette University, Milwaukee, Wisconsin
Educational Consultant and Private Practice, Seattle, Washington

SUSAN W. HERRING, PhD
Professor of Orthodontics and Oral Biology, School of Dentistry
Adjunct Professor of Biological Structure, School of Medicine and Biology
School of Arts and Sciences
University of Washington
Seattle, Washington

Illustrated by

PAT THOMAS, CMI
Certified Medical Illustrator, AMI
Oak Park, Illinois

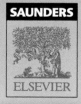

SAUNDERS

ELSEVIER

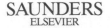

11830 Westline Industrial Drive
St. Louis, Missouri 63146

ILLUSTRATED ANATOMY OF THE HEAD AND NECK ISBN-13: 978-1-4160-3403-2
Copyright © 2007, 2002, 1996 by Saunders, an imprint of Elsevier Inc. ISBN-10: 1-4160-3403-X

Previous editions copyrighted 2002, 1996

Library of Congress Cataloging-in-Publication Data

Fehrenbach, Margaret J.
    Illustrated anatomy of the head and neck/Margaret J. Fehrenbach, Susan W. Herring;
illustrated by Pat Thomas.
        p. cm.
    Includes bibliographical references and index.
    ISBN-13: 978-1-4160-3403-2   ISBN-10: 1-4160-3403-X (alk. paper)
        1. Head–Anatomy.   2. Neck–Anatomy. I. Herring, Susan W. II. Thomas, Pat, CMI.
III. Title.

QM535F44 2006
611'.91–dc22   2006046298

ISBN-13: 978-1-4160-3403-2
ISBN-10: 1-4160-3403-X

Senior Editor: John Dolan
Developmental Editor: Courtney Sprehe
Publishing Services Manager: Pat Joiner
Project Manager: Jennifer Clark
Designer: Jyotika Shroff

Printed in Canada

Last digit is the print number: 9 8 7 6 5 4 3 2

Preface

OVERVIEW

To meet the needs of today's dental professional, the third edition of *Illustrated Anatomy of the Head and Neck* offers more than just basic information on head and neck anatomy. Special emphasis is placed on the specific anatomy of the temporomandibular joint, which will help the dental professional to better understand the disorders associated with this joint. The textbook also includes a chapter on the anatomical basis of local anesthesia for pain control and a chapter on the spread of dental infection.

FEATURES

To facilitate the learning process, the chapters of the textbook are divided into anatomical systems of study, culminating in the regional study of fascia and spaces and the spread of dental infection. Each chapter begins with an outline, learning objectives, and a list of key terms with a pronunciation guide. This pronunciation guide is based on *Dorland's Medical Dictionary,* 30th edition, Philadelphia, 2003, Saunders.

Each chapter features organized text and includes a pronunciation guide for each anatomical structure. The anatomical terms follow those outlined in the internationally approved official body of anatomical nomenclature, *Nomina Anatomica,* 6th edition, New York, 1989, Churchill Livingstone. High-quality, full-color original illustrations and clinical photographs are included throughout the text and help to clarify essential concepts. All chapter topics have been chosen to be relevant to the present needs of the dental professional and to build on former topics.

Each chapter features two different types of highlighted terms: terms that appear in **bold/red** and terms that appear in **bold/black**. The terms appearing in **bold and red** are key terms and appear on the key terms list at the beginning of the chapter. The terms that appear in **bold and black** are anatomical terms that are important to the material being discussed in the chapter (and are therefore emphasized), but they do not appear on the key terms list at the beginning of the chapter. All highlighted terms can be found in the glossary.

Tables that easily summarize important information appear throughout the text. Within each chapter, there may be cross-references to other chapters, which will allow the reader to review or investigate interrelated subjects. Identification exercises and review questions are included for each chapter and are great tools for both the classroom and self-study.

At the end of the text is the glossary of key and anatomical terms (conveniently located in one place for easy access) and two appendices, which feature a bibliography and a review of the procedures for performing extraoral and intraoral examinations.

This textbook is coordinated with the *Illustrated Dental Embryology, Histology, and Anatomy,* 2nd edition by Mary Bath-Balogh and Margaret J. Fehrenbach and can be considered a companion textbook to complete the curriculum in oral biology.

NEW TO THIS EDITION

The important anatomy-related chapters on the temporomandibular joint, local anesthesia, and spread of dental infection have been significantly revised. Twenty-four full-color flashcards are now included in the back of the text. The cards are perforated for easy removal from the text and are an excellent study tool for students who want to test their knowledge of head and neck anatomy.

A new *Evolve* website is a key addition to the third edition. The *Evolve* site provides a variety of resources for both instructors and students. For instructors there are an image collection, classroom activities, a PowerPoint presentations, answers to the review questions found in the text, a 200-question test bank, and an updates section. For students, there are supplemental study considerations, crossword puzzles, word searches, discussion questions for each chapter, and an updates section.

As authors, we have tried to make the text easy to understand as well as interesting to read. We hope that it challenges the reader to incorporate the information presented into clinical situations.

Margaret J. Fehrenbach, RDH, MS
Susan W. Herring, PhD

Acknowledgments

We would like to thank Heidi Schlei, RDH, MS, Instructor, Dental Hygiene Program, Waukesha County Technical College, Pewaukee, Wisconsin and Lori Drummer, RDH, MEd, Assistant Professor, Department of Dental Hygiene, College of DuPage, Glen Ellyn, Illinois. We would also like to thank Doreen Naughton, RDH, BS, Dental Hygiene Health Services, Seattle, and Dental Public Health Sciences Department, University of Washington Dental School, Seattle, for her assistance. Finally, we would like to thank Publisher Penny Rudolph, Senior Editor John Dolan, Developmental Editor Courtney Sprehe, Project Manager Jennifer Clark, and the staff of Elsevier for making the new edition possible.

Margaret J. Fehrenbach, RDH, MS
Susan W. Herring, PhD

Contents

CHAPTER 7: GLANDULAR TISSUE, 168

CHAPTER 8: NERVOUS SYSTEM, 182

CHAPTER 9: ANATOMY OF LOCAL ANESTHESIA, 216

CHAPTER 10: LYMPHATIC SYSTEM, 249

CHAPTER 11: FASCIA AND SPACES, 272

CHAPTER 12: SPREAD OF DENTAL INFECTION, 295

APPENDIX A: BIBLIOGRAPHY, 306

APPENDIX B: PROCEDURE FOR PERFORMING EXTRAORAL AND INTRAORAL EXAMINATIONS, 307

GLOSSARY OF KEY TERMS AND ANATOMICAL STRUCTURES, 310

INDEX, 325

FLASHCARDS

CHAPTER 1

Introduction to Head and Neck Anatomy

OUTLINE

- Clinical Applications
- Anatomical Nomenclature
- Normal Anatomical Variation

LEARNING OBJECTIVES

After studying this chapter, the reader should be able to do the following:

1. Define and pronounce all the key terms and anatomical terms in this chapter.
2. Discuss the clinical applications of the study of head and neck anatomy by dental professionals.
3. Apply the correct anatomical nomenclature during the study of head and neck anatomy.
4. Discuss normal anatomical variation and how it applies to different structures of the head and neck.
5. Correctly complete the review questions and activities for this chapter.

KEY TERMS

Anatomical Nomenclature (an-ah-**tom**-ik-al **no**-men-**kla**-cher) System of names of anatomical structures.

Anatomical Position Position in which the body is erect, with arms at the sides, palms and toes directed forward, and eyes looking forward.

Anterior Front of an area of the body.

Apex (**ay**-peks) Pointed end of a conical structure.

Contralateral (kon-trah-**lat**-er-il) Structures on the opposite side of the body.

Deep Structures located inward, away from the body surface.

Distal (**dis**-tl) Area that is farther away from the median plane of the body.

Dorsal (**dor**-sal) Back of an area of the body.

External Outer side of the wall of a hollow structure.

Frontal Plane Plane created by an imaginary line that divides the body at any level into anterior and posterior portions.

Frontal Section Section of the body through any frontal plane.

Horizontal Plane Plane created by an imaginary line that divides the body at any level into superior and inferior portions.

Inferior Area that faces away from the head and toward the feet of the body.

Internal Inner side of the wall of a hollow structure.

Ipsilateral (ip-see-**lat**-er-il) Structures on the same side of the body.

Lateral Area that is farther away from the median plane of the body or structure.

Medial (**me**-dee-il) Area that is closer to the median plane of the body or structure.

Median (**me**-dee-an) Structure at the median plane.

Median Plane Plane created by an imaginary line that divides the body into right and left halves.

(Continued)

KEY TERMS (continued)

Midsagittal Section (mid-**saj**-i-tl) Section of the body through the median plane.
Posterior Back of an area of the body.
Proximal (**prok**-si-mil) Area closer to the median plane of the body.
Sagittal Plane (**saj**-i-tl) Any plane of the body created by an imaginary plane parallel with the median plane.

Superficial Structures located toward the surface of the body.
Superior Area that faces toward the head of the body, away from the feet.
Transverse Section (trans-**vers**) Section of the body through any horizontal plane.
Ventral (**ven**-tral) Front of an area of the body.

CLINICAL APPLICATIONS

The dental professional must have a thorough knowledge of head and neck anatomy when performing patient examination procedures, both extraoral and intraoral (Figure 1-1). Knowledge of normal anatomy will help determine whether any abnormalities or lesions exist and possibly indicate the etiology and amount of involvement. This knowledge will also provide a basis for the description of the lesion and its location for record-keeping purposes.

Head and neck anatomy is also useful when performing dental radiology procedures. Landmarks are used by the dental professional in the placement of the films, and knowledge of anatomy is important in the mounting and analysis of the films.

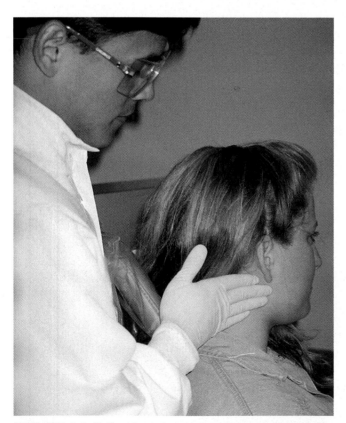

FIGURE 1-1 Both extraoral and intraoral examination of the patient are based on knowledge of head and neck anatomy.

A patient may also present features of a temporomandibular joint disorder. A dental professional must have knowledge of the normal anatomy of the joint in order to understand the various disorders associated with it.

More specifically, the administration of local anesthesia is based on landmarks of the head and neck. The knowledge of anatomy will assist treatment planning of local anesthesia by the dental professional for the reduction of pain during various dental procedures. This knowledge will also allow for the correct placement of the syringe, potentially avoiding complications.

During the examination of the patient, the dental professional may also note the presence of a dental infection. It is important to know the source of the infection as well as the areas to which it could spread by way of certain anatomical features of the head and neck. Knowledge of the anatomy will supply the background for understanding the spread of dental infection.

ANATOMICAL NOMENCLATURE

Before beginning the study of head and neck anatomy, the dental professional may need to review the basic **anatomical nomenclature,** which is the system of names of anatomical structures. This review will allow for the easy application of these terms to the head and neck area.

The nomenclature of anatomy is based on the body being in **anatomical position** (Figure 1-2). In anatomical position, the body is standing erect. The arms are at the sides with the palms and toes directed forward and the eyes looking forward. This position is assumed even when the body may be supine (on the back) or prone (on the front).

When studying the body in anatomical position, certain terms are used to refer to areas in relationship to other areas (Figure 1-3). The front of an area in relationship to the entire body is its **anterior** portion. The back of an area is its **posterior** portion. The **ventral** portion is directed toward the anterior and is the opposite of the **dorsal** portion when considering the entire body.

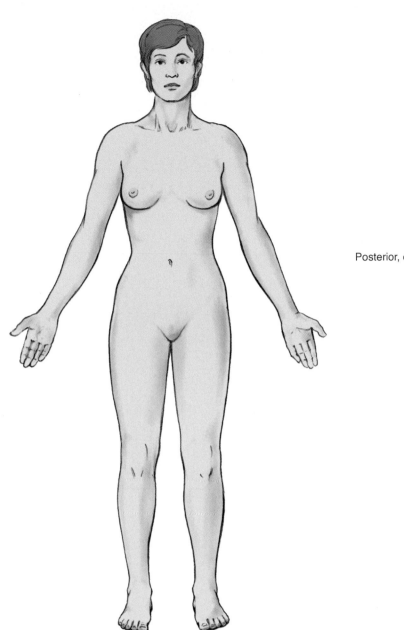

FIGURE 1-2 Body in anatomical position.

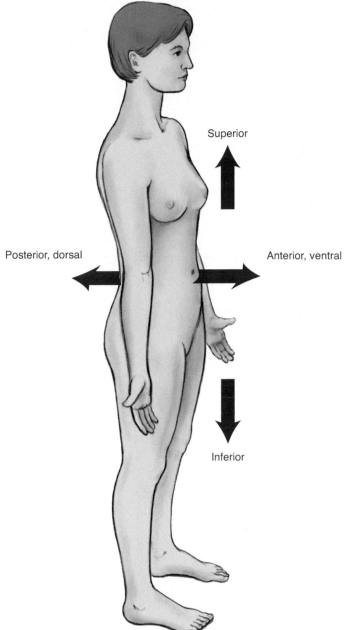

FIGURE 1-3 Body in anatomical position with the anterior (or ventral), posterior (or dorsal), superior, and inferior areas noted.

Other terms can be used to refer to areas in relationship to other areas of the body. An area that faces toward the head and away from the feet is its **superior** portion. An area that faces away from the head and toward the feet is its **inferior** portion. As an example, the face is on the anterior side of the head, and the hair is superior and posterior to the face. The **apex** or tip is the pointed end of a conical structure such as the tongue apex or tip.

The body in anatomical position can be divided by planes or flat surfaces (Figure 1-4). The **median plane** or midsagittal plane is created by an imaginary line dividing the body into right and left halves. On the surface of the body, these halves are generally symmetrical in structure, yet the same symmetry does not apply to all internal structures.

Other planes can be created by different imaginary lines. A **sagittal plane** is any plane created by an imaginary plane parallel to the median plane. A **frontal plane** or coronal plane is created by an imaginary line dividing the body at any level into anterior and posterior portions. A **horizontal plane** is created by an

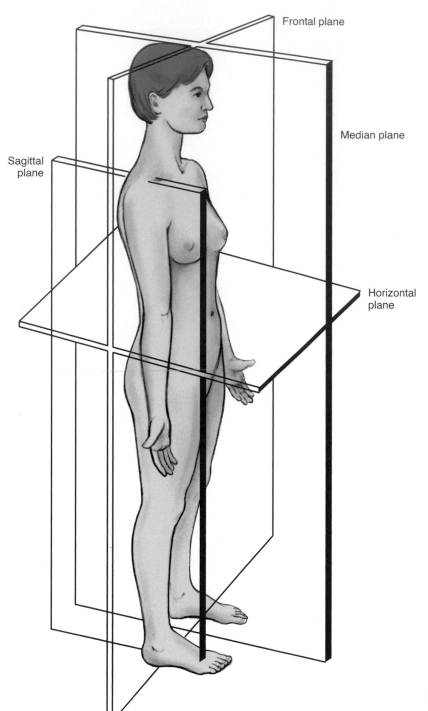

FIGURE 1-4 Body in anatomical position with the median, sagittal, horizontal, and frontal planes noted.

imaginary line dividing the body at any level into superior and inferior portions and is perpendicular to the median plane.

Portions of the body in anatomical position can also be described in relationship to these planes (Figure 1-5). A structure located at the median plane (e.g., the nose) is considered **median.** An area closer to the median plane of the body or structure is considered **medial.** An area farther from the median plane of the body or structure is considered **lateral.** For example, the eyes are medial to the ears, and the ears are lateral to the eyes.

Terms can be used to describe the relationship of portions of the body in anatomical position. An area closer to the median plane is considered by anatomists to be **proximal,** and an area farther from the median plane is **distal.** For example, in the upper limb the shoulder is proximal and the fingers are distal.

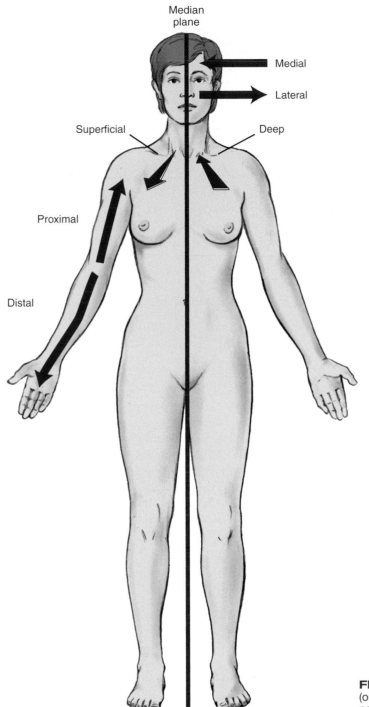

Median
plane

Medial

Lateral

Superficial

Deep

Proximal

Distal

FIGURE 1-5 Body in anatomical position with the medial (or proximal), lateral (or distal), and superficial (or deep) areas noted.

Additional terms can be used to describe relationships between structures. Structures on the same side of the body are considered **ipsilateral.** Structures on the opposite side of the body are considered **contralateral.** For example, the right leg is ipsilateral to the right arm but contralateral to the left arm.

Certain terms can be used to give information about the depth of a structure in relationship to the surface of the body. The structures located toward the surface of the body are **superficial.** The structures located

inward, away from the body surface, are **deep.** For example, the skin is superficial, and the bones are deep.

Terms also can be used to give information about location in hollow structures such as the braincase of the skull. The inner side of the wall of a hollow structure is referred to as **internal.** The outer side of the wall of a hollow structure is **external.**

The body or portions of it in anatomical position can also be cut or divided into sections along various planes in order to study the specific anatomy of a

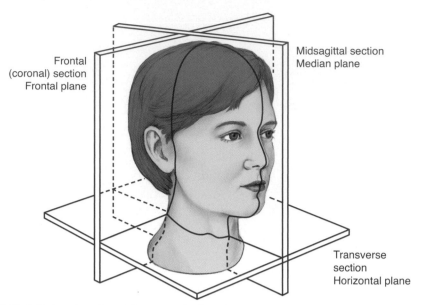

Frontal
(coronal) section
Frontal plane

Midsagittal section
Median plane

Transverse
section
Horizontal plane

FIGURE 1-6 Head and neck in anatomical position showing the midsagittal, transverse, and frontal sections.

region (Figure 1-6). The **midsagittal section** or median section is a cut through the median plane. The **frontal section** or coronal section is a cut through any frontal plane. The **transverse section** or horizontal section is a cut through a horizontal plane.

NORMAL ANATOMICAL VARIATION

When studying anatomy, the dental professional must understand that there can be anatomical variations of head and neck structures that are still within normal limits. The number of bones and muscles in the head and neck is usually constant, but specific details of these structures can vary from patient to patient. Bones may have different sizes of processes. Muscles may differ in size and details of their attachments. Joints, vessels, nerves, glands, lymph nodes, and fascial planes and spaces of an individual can vary in size, location, and even presence. The most common variations of the head and neck that affect dental treatment are discussed in this text.

Identification Exercises

Identify the structures on the following diagrams by filling in each blank with the correct anatomical term. You can check your answers by looking back at the figure indicated in parentheses for each identification diagram.

1. (Figure 1-3)

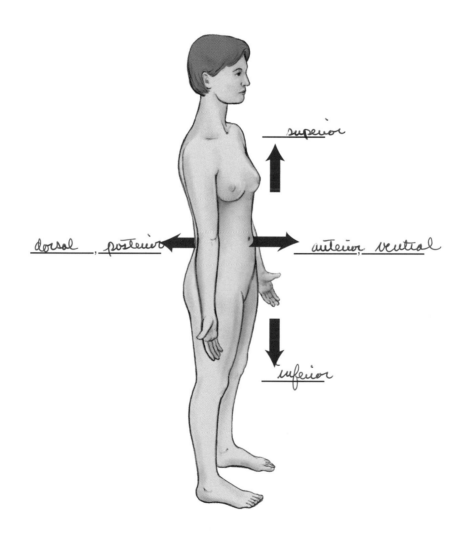

2. (Figure 1-4)

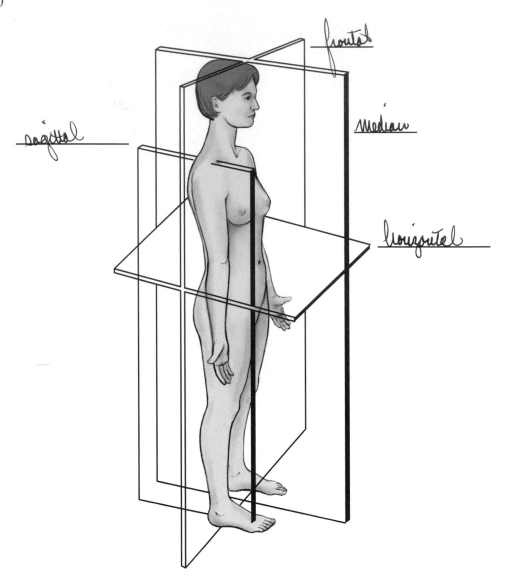

3. (Figure 1-5)

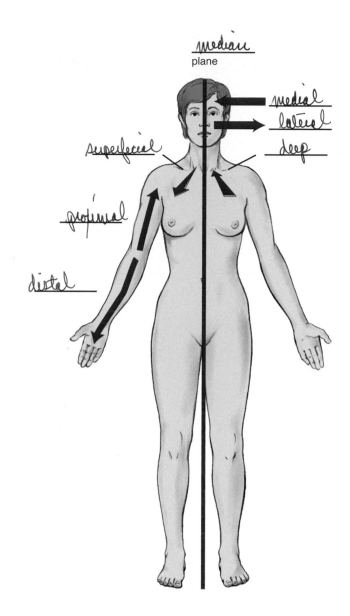

median plane

medial
lateral
deep
superficial
proximal
distal

4. (Figure 1-6)

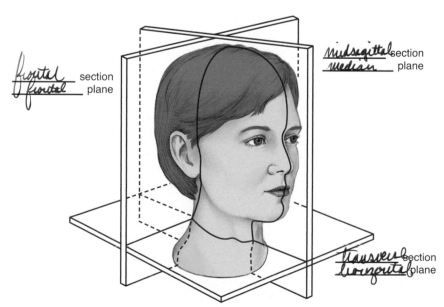

frontal section plane

midsagittal section
median plane

transverse section
horizontal plane

■ REVIEW QUESTIONS

1. Which of the following divides the body in anatomical position into right and left halves?
   A. Horizontal plane
   B. Median plane
   C. Coronal plane
   D. Frontal plane

2. Which of the following is used to describe an area of the body that is farther from the median plane?
   A. Proximal
   B. Lateral
   C. Medial
   D. Ipsilateral
   E. Contralateral

3. Structures on the same side of the body are considered:
   A. Proximal
   B. Lateral
   C. Medial
   D. Ipsilateral
   E. Contralateral

4. An area of the body in anatomical position that faces toward the head is considered:
   A. Inferior
   B. Superior
   C. Proximal
   D. Distal
   E. Dorsal

5. Through which plane of the body in anatomical position is a midsagittal section taken?
   A. Horizontal plane
   B. Median plane
   C. Coronal plane
   D. Frontal plane

6. Which of the following statements concerning anatomical position is correct?
   A. Body is erect with eyes looking forward.
   B. Arms are at sides with palms directed backward.
   C. Arms are behind the head with toes directed forward.
   D. Body is supine with eyes closed.

7. Which of the following sections is a horizontal section?
   A. Midsagittal section
   B. Transverse section
   C. Frontal section
   D. Median section

8. Structures that are located inward, away from the body surface, are considered:
   A. Distal
   B. Superficial
   C. Deep
   D. Contralateral
   E. External

9. Which plane divides any portion of the body into anterior and posterior portions?
   A. Sagittal
   B. Horizontal
   C. Frontal
   D. Median

10. Which of the following is a correct statement concerning human anatomy?
    A. The apex of a conical structure is the flat base.
    B. The two halves of the body are completely symmetrical.
    C. The external surface is the inner wall of a hollow structure.
    D. Joints, vessels, nerves, glands, and nodes vary in size.

11. Which is correct?
    A. The ears are medial to the nose.
    B. The ears are lateral to the nose.
    C. The ears are medial to the eyes.
    D. The mouth is lateral to the nose.

12. *Proximal* refers to:
    A. A body part that is closer to the medial plane of the body than another part
    B. A body part that is farther from the medial plane of the body than another part
    C. A body part that is farther from the point of attachment to the body than another part
    D. A body part that is closer to the point of attachment to the body than another part

13. The median plane will divide the right arm and the:
   A. Right leg
   B. Brain
   C. Nose
   D. Left leg

14. A frontal plane will bisect the:
   A. Nose
   B. Mouth
   C. Arms
   D. Eyes

15. If a transverse plane occurs through the navel, which of the following is true?
   A. The chest and ears will be on different portions.
   B. The chest and knees will be on the same portion.
   C. The feet and knees will be on different portions.
   D. The thighs and feet will be on the same portion.

Surface Anatomy

LEARNING OBJECTIVES

After studying this chapter, the reader should be able to do the following:

1. Define and pronounce all the key terms and anatomical terms in this chapter.
2. Discuss the anatomical considerations for patient examination and dental radiology of the head and neck region.
3. Locate and identify the regions and associated surface landmarks of the head and neck on a diagram and a patient.
4. Correctly complete the review questions and activities for this chapter.
5. Integrate the knowledge of surface anatomy into the clinical practice of patient examination and dental radiology of the head and neck regions.

KEY TERMS

Buccal (buk-al) Structures closest to the inner cheek.
Facial Structures closest to the facial surface.
Golden These guidelines can be used to consider the facial view of the anterior teeth or the vertical dimensions of the face to create a pleasing proportion.

Labial (lay-be-al) Structures closest to the lips.
Lingual (ling-gwal) Structures closest to the tongue.
Palatal (pal-ah-tal) Structures closest to the palate.
Vertical Dimension of the Face The face divided into thirds.

SURFACE ANATOMY

The dental professional must be thoroughly familiar with the surface anatomy of the head and neck in order to examine patients. The features of the surface provide essential landmarks for many of the deeper anatomical structures. Thus the examination of these accessible surface features by visualization and palpation can give information about the health of deeper tissues (see Appendix B). Any changes in these surface features must be recorded by the dental professional.

Many radiographs taken by the dental professional also use surface landmarks. Portions of the eye, nose, and ear are used for this purpose. This use of landmarks allows for easy film placement and consistency in taking radiographs.

A certain amount of variation in surface features is within a normal range. However, a change in a surface feature in a given person may signal a condition of clinical significance. Thus it is not the variations among individuals that should be noted but the changes in a particular individual.

The study of anatomy of the head and neck begins with the division of the surface into regions. Within each region are certain surface landmarks. Practice finding these landmarks in each region on yourself to improve the skills of examination.

REGIONS OF THE HEAD

The **regions of the head** include the frontal, parietal, occipital, temporal, orbital, nasal, infraorbital, zygomatic, buccal, oral, and mental regions (Figure 2-1). These regions are all noted during an overall evaluation of the face, head, and neck. During an extraoral examination, the patient is seated upright and relaxed, and the symmetry and coloration of the surface is noted.

The superficial to deep relationships of the head are relatively simple over most of its posterior and superior surfaces but are more difficult in the region of the face. The underlying bony structure of the head is covered in Chapter 3. The underlying muscles of the head are covered in Chapter 4. The underlying glandular tissue such as the salivary and lacrimal glands and thyroid gland is covered in Chapter 7. Lymph nodes that are located throughout the tissues of the head are covered in Chapter 10.

Frontal Region

The **frontal region** of the head includes the forehead and the area superior to the eyes (Figure 2-2). Just inferior to each eyebrow is the **supraorbital ridge** (soo-prah-**or**-bit-al) or superciliary ridge. The smooth elevated area between the eyebrows is the **glabella** (glah-**bell**-ah), which tends to be flat in children and

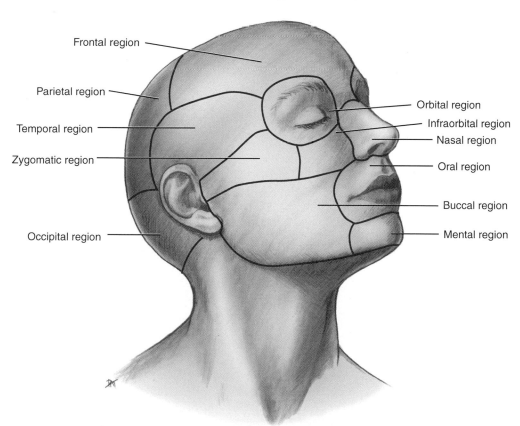

FIGURE 2-1 Regions of the head: frontal, parietal, occipital, temporal, orbital, nasal, infraorbital, zygomatic, buccal, oral, and mental.

Frontal region
Parietal region
Temporal region
Zygomatic region
Occipital region

Orbital region
Infraorbital region
Nasal region
Oral region
Buccal region
Mental region

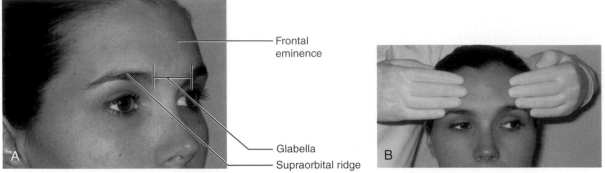

FIGURE 2-2 Frontal view of the head with the landmarks of the frontal region noted **(A)** and palpation of the forehead during an extraoral examination **(B).**

adult females and to form a rounded prominence in adult males. The prominence of the forehead, the **frontal eminence** (**em**-i-nins), is also evident. The frontal eminence is typically more pronounced in children and adult females, and the supraorbital ridge is more prominent in adult males. Stand near the patient to visually inspect the forehead and bilaterally palpate during an extraoral examination.

Parietal and Occipital Regions

The **parietal region** (pah-**ri**-it-al) and **occipital region** (ok-**sip**-it-al) of the head are covered by the scalp. The **scalp** consists of layers of soft tissue overlying the bones of the braincase. Large areas of the scalp may be covered by hair. Trying to survey these areas during an extraoral examination is important because many lesions may be hidden visually from the clinician as well as the patient. During an extraoral examination, stand near the patient to visually inspect the entire scalp by moving the hair, especially around the hairline, starting from one ear and proceeding to the other ear (Figure 2-3).

Temporal Region

Within the **temporal region** (**tem**-poh-ral) of the head, the external ear is a prominent feature (Figure 2-4). The external ear is composed of an **auricle** (**aw**-ri-kl) or oval flap of the ear and the **external acoustic meatus** (ah-**koos**-tik me-**ate**-us). The auricle collects sound waves. The external acoustic meatus is a tube through which sound waves are transmitted to the middle ear within the skull.

The superior and posterior free margin of the auricle is the **helix** (**heel**-iks), which ends inferiorly at the **lobule** (**lob**-yule), the fleshy protuberance of the earlobe. The upper apex of the helix is typically level with the eyebrows and the glabella, and the lobule is approximately at the level of the apex of the nose.

The portion of the auricle anterior to the external acoustic meatus is a smaller flap of tissue called the

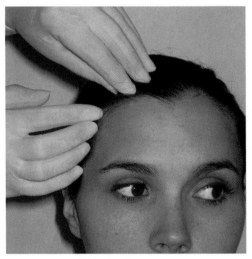

FIGURE 2-3 Visual inspection of the entire scalp during an extraoral examination.

tragus (**tra**-gus). The tragus, as well as the rest of the auricle, is flexible when palpated due to its underlying cartilage. The other flap of tissue opposite the tragus is the **antitragus** (an-tie-**tra**-gus). Between the tragus and antitragus is a deep notch, the **intertragic notch** (in-ter-**tra**-gic). The external acoustic meatus and tragus are important landmarks to use when taking extraoral radiographs and performing local anesthesia on a patient. During an extraoral examination, each external ear, as well as the scalp and face around each ear, is visually inspected and manually palpated (Figure 2-5).

Orbital Region

In the **orbital region** (**or**-bit-al) of the head, the eyeball and all its supporting structures are contained in the bony socket called the **orbit** (**or**-bit) (Figure 2-6). The eyes are usually near the midpoint of the vertical height of the head. The width of each eye is typically the same as the distance between the eyes. On the eyeball is the white area or **sclera** (**skler**-ah) with its central area of coloration, the circular **iris** (**eye**-ris). The

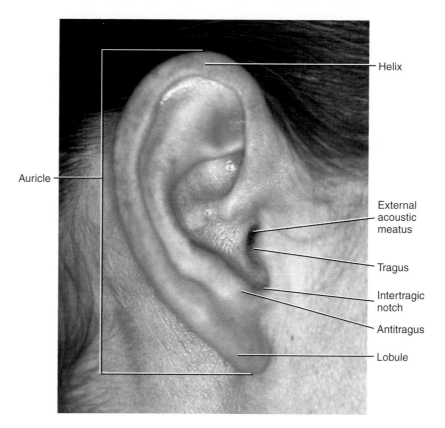

Helix

Auricle

External acoustic meatus

Tragus

Intertragic notch

Antitragus

Lobule

FIGURE 2-4 Lateral view of the right external ear with its landmarks within the temporal region noted.

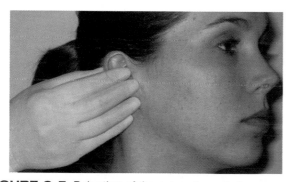

FIGURE 2-5 Palpation of the external ear during an extraoral examination.

opening in the center of the iris is the **pupil** (**pew**-pil), which appears black and changes size as the iris responds to changing light conditions.

Two movable **eyelids,** upper and lower, cover and protect each eyeball. Behind each upper eyelid and within the orbit is the **lacrimal gland** (**lak**-ri-mal), which produces lacrimal fluid or tears.

The **conjunctiva** (kon-junk-**ti**-vah) is the delicate and thin membrane lining the inside of the eyelids and the front of the eyeball. The outer corner where the upper and lower eyelids meet is called the **lateral canthus** (plural, **canthi**) (**kan**-this, **kan**-thy) or outer canthus.

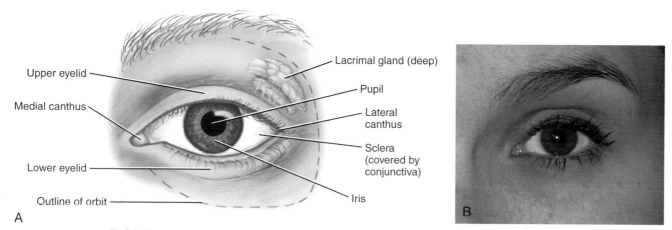

Upper eyelid

Medial canthus

Lower eyelid

Outline of orbit

Lacrimal gland (deep)

Pupil

Lateral canthus

Sclera (covered by conjunctiva)

Iris

A

B

FIGURE 2-6 Frontal view of the left eye with the landmarks of the orbital region noted **(A)** and visualization of the eye during an extraoral examination **(B).**

The inner angle of the eye is called the **medial canthus** or inner canthus. These canthi are important landmarks to use when taking extraoral radiographs. During an extraoral examination, the orbital region including the eyes is examined by standing near the patient and visually inspecting the eyes and their movements and responses.

Nasal Region

The main feature of the **nasal region** (**nay**-zil) of the head is the external nose (Figure 2-7). The **root of the nose** is located between the eyes. Inferior to the glabella is a midpoint landmark of the nasal region that corresponds with the junction between the underlying bones, the **nasion** (**nay**-ze-on). Inferior to the nasion is the bony structure that forms the **bridge of the nose.** The tip or **apex of the nose** is flexible when palpated because it is formed from cartilage.

Inferior to the apex on each side of the nose is a nostril or **naris** (plural, **nares**) (**nay**-ris, **nay**-rees). The nares are separated by the midline **nasal septum** (**nay**-zil **sep**-tum). The nares are bounded laterally by winglike cartilaginous structures, the **ala** (plural, **alae**) (**a**-lah, **a**-lay) of the nose. The width between the alae should be about the same width as one eye or the space between the eyes. The nasion and the alae of the nose are important landmarks to use when taking extraoral radiographs. Standing near the patient, the external nose is visually inspected and palpated during an extraoral examination, by starting at the root of the nose and proceeding to its apex (Figure 2-8).

Infraorbital, Zygomatic, and Buccal Regions

The infraorbital, zygomatic, and buccal regions of the head are all located on the facial aspect (Figure 2-9). The **infraorbital region** (in-frah-**or**-bit-al) of the head is

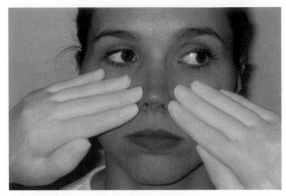
FIGURE 2-8 Palpation of the external nose during an extraoral examination.

located inferior to the orbital region and lateral to the nasal region. Farther laterally is the **zygomatic region** (zy-go-**mat**-ik), which overlies the cheekbone, the **zygomatic arch.** The zygomatic arch extends from just inferior to the lateral margin of the eye toward the upper portion of the ear.

Inferior to the zygomatic arch, and just anterior to the ear, is the **temporomandibular joint** (tem-poh-ro-man-**dib**-you-lar). This is where the upper skull forms a joint with the lower jaw. The movements of the joint can be felt when opening and closing the mouth or moving the lower jaw to the right or left. One way to feel the lower jaw moving at the temporomandibular joint is to gently place a finger into the outer portion of the external acoustic meatus.

The **buccal region** of the head is composed of the soft tissues of the cheek. The **cheek** forms the side of the face and is a broad area of the face among the nose, mouth, and ear. Most of the upper cheek is fleshy and is mainly formed by a mass of fat and muscles. One of these is the strong **masseter muscle (mass**-et-er), which is felt when a patient clenches the teeth together. The sharp angle of the lower jaw inferior to the ear's lobule is termed the **angle of the mandible.** During an extraoral examination, the infraorbital, zygomatic, and buccal regions, as well as the temporomandibular joint, are examined by standing near the patient, and visually inspecting and palpating bilaterally (see Figures 5-7 and 5-8).

The face is sometimes thought of as divided into thirds, and this perspective is called the **vertical dimension of the face.** A discussion of vertical dimension allows a comparison of the three portions of the face for functional and aesthetic purposes using the **Golden Proportions,** a set of guidelines. Loss of height in the lower third, which contains the teeth and jaws, can occur in certain circumstances.

Oral Region

The **oral region** of the head has many structures within it such as the lips, oral cavity, palate, tongue, floor of

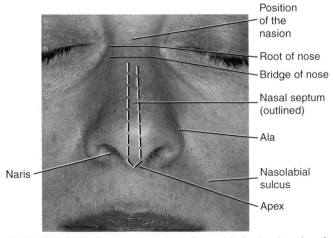

Position of the nasion

Root of nose

Bridge of nose

Nasal septum (outlined)

Ala

Nasolabial sulcus

Naris

Apex

FIGURE 2-7 Frontal view of the face with the landmarks of the nasal region noted.

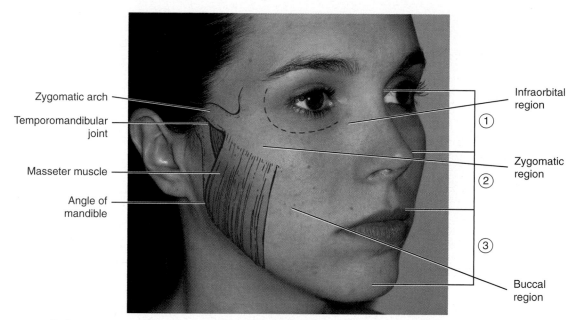

Zygomatic arch

Temporomandibular joint

Masseter muscle

Angle of mandible

Infraorbital region

①

Zygomatic region

②

③

Buccal region

FIGURE 2-9 Landmarks of the zygomatic and buccal regions are noted. Also noted is the vertical dimension of the face, where the face is divided into thirds, which allows a comparison of the three portions of the face for functional and aesthetic purposes using the Golden Proportions.

the mouth, and portions of the throat. The lips are the gateway of the oral region, and each lip's **vermilion zone** (ver-**mil**-yon) has a darker appearance than the surrounding skin (Figure 2-10). The lips are outlined from the surrounding skin by a transition zone, the **vermilion border.** The width of the lips at rest should be about the same distance as that between the irises of the eyes.

On the midline of the upper lip, extending downward from the nasal septum, is a vertical groove called the **philtrum** (**fil**-trum). The philtrum terminates in a thicker area or **tubercle of the upper lip** (**too**-ber-kl). The upper and lower lips meet at each corner of the mouth or **labial commissure** (**kom**-i-shoor). The groove running upward between the labial commissure and the ala of the nose is called the **nasolabial sulcus** (nay-zo-**lay**-be-al **sul**-kus) (see Figure 2-7). The lower lip extends to the horizontal **labiomental groove** (lay-bee-

o-**ment**-il), which separates the lower lip from the chin in the mental region. The lips are bidigitally palpated during an intraoral examination, as well as visually inspected in a systematic manner, from one commissure to the other.

ORAL CAVITY

The inside of the mouth is known as the **oral cavity.** The jaws are within the oral cavity and deep to the lips (Figure 2-11). Underlying the upper lip is the upper jaw or **maxilla** (mak-**sil**-ah). The bone underlying the lower lip is the lower jaw or **mandible** (**man**-di-bl).

Many areas in the oral cavity are termed or identified by their relationship to the tongue, palate, cheek, facial surface, or lips. Those structures closest to the tongue are termed **lingual.** Those structures closest to the palate are termed **palatal.** Those structures closest to the facial surface or lips are termed **facial** or **labial.**

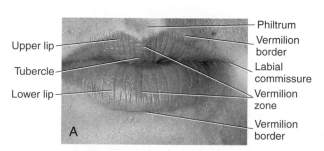

Upper lip

Tubercle

Lower lip

Philtrum

Vermilion border

Labial commissure

Vermilion zone

Vermilion border

A

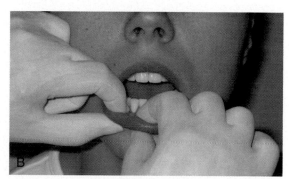

B

FIGURE 2-10 Frontal view of the lips within the oral region **(A)** and bidigital palpation of the lips during an intraoral examination **(B).**

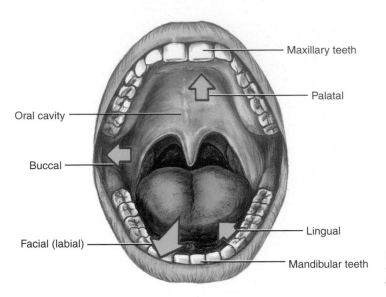

Oral cavity

Buccal

Facial (labial)

Maxillary teeth

Palatal

Lingual

Mandibular teeth

FIGURE 2-11 The oral cavity and jaws with the designation of the terms *lingual, palatal, buccal, facial,* and *labial* within the oral cavity.

Those structures closest to the inner cheek are also considered **buccal.**

The oral cavity is lined by a mucous membrane or **mucosa** (mu-**ko**-sah) (Figure 2-12). The inner portions of the lips are lined by a pink and thick **labial mucosa.** The labial mucosa is continuous with the equally pink and thick **buccal mucosa** that lines the inner cheek.

The buccal mucosa covers a dense pad of inner tissue, the **buccal fat pad.** To visually examine the labial mucosa during an intraoral examination, ask the patient to open the mouth slightly. Pull the lips away from the teeth. Then gently pull the buccal mucosa slightly away from the teeth so as to bidigitally palpate, using circular compression.

Further landmarks can be noted in the oral cavity. On the inner portion of the buccal mucosa, just opposite the maxillary second molar, is a small elevation of tissue called the **parotid papilla** (pah-**rot**-id pah-**pil**-ah),

which contains the duct opening from the parotid salivary gland. During an intraoral examination, the area is direct and the flow of saliva from each duct is observed. An elevation on the posterior aspects of the maxilla is the **maxillary tuberosity** (**mak**-sil-lare-ee too-beh-**ros**-i-tee).

The upper and lower spaces between the cheeks, lips, and gums are the maxillary and mandibular **vestibules** (**ves**-ti-bules). Deep within each vestibule, the pink and thick labial or buccal mucosa meets the redder and thinner **alveolar mucosa** (al-**ve**-o-lar) at the **mucobuccal fold** (mu-ko-**buk**-al). The **labial frenum** (**free**-num) or frenulum is a fold of tissue located at the midline between the labial mucosa and the alveolar mucosa of the maxilla and mandible (Figure 2-13).

Teeth of the oral cavity are located within the upper and lower jaws of the oral cavity. The teeth of the maxilla are the **maxillary teeth,** and the teeth of the

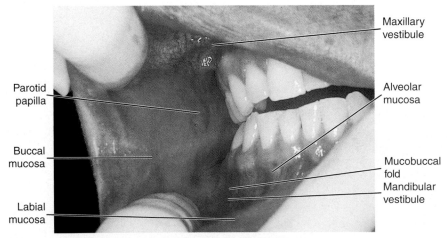

Parotid
papilla

Buccal
mucosa

Labial
mucosa

Maxillary
vestibule

Alveolar
mucosa

Mucobuccal
fold

Mandibular
vestibule

FIGURE 2-12 View of the buccal and labial mucosa of the oral cavity with landmarks noted while being palpated during an intraoral examination.

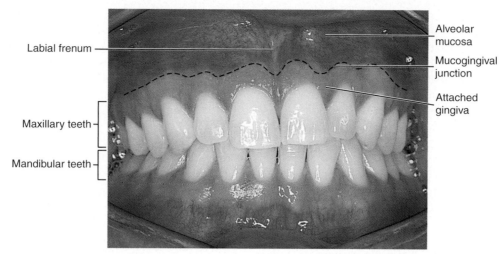

Labial frenum

Maxillary teeth

Mandibular teeth

Alveolar mucosa

Mucogingival junction

Attached gingiva

FIGURE 2-13 Frontal view of the oral cavity with its landmarks noted.

mandible are the **mandibular teeth** (man-**dib**-you-lar). The maxillary anterior teeth should overlap the mandibular anterior teeth, and posteriorly, the maxillary buccal cusps should overlap the mandibular buccal cusps. Both dental arches in the adult have permanent teeth that include the **incisors** (in-**sigh**-zers), **canines** (**kay**-nines), **premolars** (pre-**mo**-lers), and **molars** (**mo**-lers).

Surrounding the maxillary and mandibular teeth are the gums or **gingiva** (jin-**ji**-vah), composed of a firm, pink mucosa (Figure 2-14; see also Figure 2-13). The gingiva that tightly adheres to the bone around the roots of the teeth is the **attached gingiva.** The attached gingiva may have areas of pigmentation. The line of demarcation between the firmer and pinker attached gingiva and the movable and redder alveolar mucosa is the scallop-shaped **mucogingival junction** (mu-ko-**jin**-ji-val).

At the gingival margin of each tooth is the nonattached or **marginal gingiva.** The inner surface of the marginal gingiva faces a space or **sulcus** (plural, **sulci**) (**sul**-kus, **sul**-ky). The gingiva between the teeth is

an extension of attached gingiva and is called the **interdental gingiva** (in-ter-**den**-tal) or interdental papilla. During an intraoral examination, the buccal and labial mucosal tissues are retracted enough to visually inspect and bidigitally palpate the vestibular area, using circular compression, including the gingival tissues.

PALATE

The roof of the mouth or **palate** (**pal**-it) has two portions: an anterior portion and a posterior portion (Figure 2-15). The firmer, whiter, anterior portion is called the **hard palate.** A midline ridge of tissue on the hard palate is the **median palatine raphe** (**pal**-ah-tine **ra**-fe). A small bulge of tissue at the most anterior portion of the hard palate, lingual to the anterior teeth, is the **incisive papilla** (in-**sy**-ziv pah-**pil**-ah). Directly posterior to this papilla are **palatine rugae** (**ru**-ge), which are firm, irregular ridges of tissue.

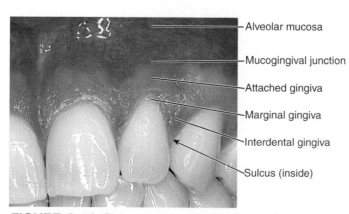

Alveolar mucosa

Mucogingival junction

Attached gingiva

Marginal gingiva

Interdental gingiva

Sulcus (inside)

FIGURE 2-14 Close-up view of the gingiva and its associated landmarks.

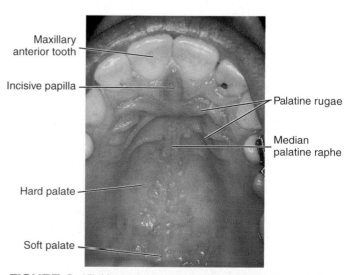

Maxillary anterior tooth

Incisive papilla

Hard palate

Soft palate

Palatine rugae

Median palatine raphe

FIGURE 2-15 View of the palate with its landmarks noted.

The yellower and looser posterior portion of the palate is called the **soft palate** (see Figures 2-15 and 2-21). It is the smaller part of the total palate because it only comprises 15% of the palate. A midline muscular structure, the **uvula of the palate** (**u**-vu-lah), hangs from the posterior margin of the soft palate. The **pterygomandibular fold** (teh-ri-go-man-**dib**-yule-lar) is a fold of tissue that extends from the junction of hard and soft palates down to the mandible, just behind the most distal mandibular tooth, and stretches when the patient opens the mouth wider. This fold covers a deeper fibrous structure and separates the cheek from the throat. Just distal to the last tooth of the mandible is a dense pad of tissue, the **retromolar pad** (re-tro-**moh**-ler). During an intraoral examination, have the patient tilt their head back slightly and extend the tongue to visually inspect the soft palate. The palate is viewed using a mouth mirror to intensify the light source (see Chapter 4). Then, the mouth mirror is gently placed (mirror side down) on the middle of the tongue and the patient is asked to say *"ah"*. As this is done, the uvula is visually inspected. Then, the hard and soft palates are compressed with the first or second finger of one hand, avoiding circular compression to prevent initiating the gag reflex.

TONGUE

The **tongue** is a prominent feature of the oral region (Figure 2-16). The posterior third is the **base of the tongue** or pharyngeal portion. The base of the tongue attaches to the floor of the mouth. The base of the tongue does not lie within the oral cavity but within the oral portion of the throat. The anterior two thirds of the tongue is termed the **body of the tongue** or oral portion and lies within the oral cavity. The tip of the tongue is the **apex of the tongue.** Certain surfaces

of the tongue have small elevated structures of specialized mucosa called **lingual papillae** (pah-**pil**-ay), some of which are associated with taste buds.

The side or **lateral surface of the tongue** is noted for its vertical ridges of lingual papillae called **foliate lingual papillae** (**fo**-le-ate), some of which contain taste buds. These lingual papillae are more prominent in children.

The top surface or **dorsal surface of the tongue** (Figure 2-17) has a midline depression, the **median lingual sulcus,** corresponding with the position of a midline fibrous structure deeper in the tongue. In the tongue, *dorsal* and *posterior* are not equivalent terms, nor are *ventral* and *anterior* the same. Instead, they are four different locations. This is because the tongue of humans still has the same orientation as the tongue of four-footed animals, in which *anterior* and *posterior* mean toward the nose and tail, respectively, and *dorsal* and *ventral* refer to the back and belly, respectively. Upright posture is the reason that *dorsal* and *posterior* have become synonyms in the rest of the body.

The dorsal surface of the tongue also has many lingual papillae. The slender, threadlike lingual papillae are the **filiform lingual papillae** (**fil**-i-form), which give the dorsal surface its velvety texture. The red mushroom-shaped dots are called **fungiform lingual papillae** (**fun**-ji-form). These lingual papillae are more numerous on the apex and contain taste buds.

Farther posteriorly on the dorsal surface of the tongue and more difficult to see clinically is a V-shaped groove, the **sulcus terminalis** (**ter**-mi-nal-is). The sulcus terminalis separates the base from the body of the tongue. Where the sulcus terminalis points backward toward the throat is a small, pitlike depression called the **foramen cecum** (for-**ay**-men **se**-kum). The

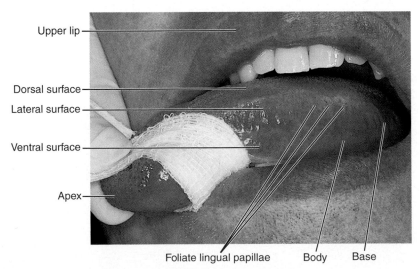

Upper lip

Dorsal surface

Lateral surface

Ventral surface

Apex

Foliate lingual papillae   Body   Base

FIGURE 2-16 The lateral view of the tongue with its portions and landmarks noted while undergoing an extraoral examination.

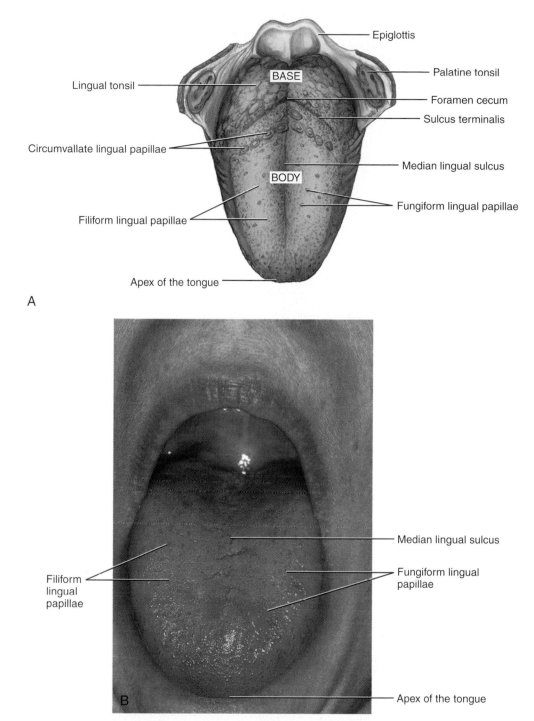

FIGURE 2-17 Dorsal view of the tongue with its landmarks noted **(A)** and its more anterior landmarks noted clinically **(B)**.

circumvallate lingual papillae (serk-um-**val**-ate), which are 10 to 14 in number, line up along the anterior side of the sulcus terminalis on the body. These large mushroom-shaped lingual papillae have taste buds. Even farther posteriorly on the dorsal surface of the tongue base is an irregular mass of tonsillar tissue, the **lingual tonsil** (**ton**-sil).

The underside or ventral surface of the tongue is noted for its visible large blood vessels, the deep **lingual veins,** that run close to the surface (Figure 2-18). Lateral to each deep lingual vein is the **plica fimbriata** (plural, **plicae fimbriatae**) (**pli**-kah fim-bree-**ay**-tah, **pli**-kay fim-bree-**ay**-tay), a fold with fringelike projections. Again, the term used for the underside of the tongue, *ventral*, referred to four-footed animals in anatomical position.

To examine the dorsal and lateral surfaces of the tongue, have the patient gently extend the tongue

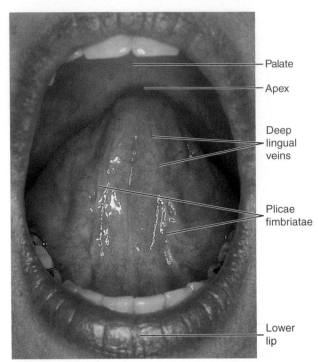

FIGURE 2-18 Ventral surface of the tongue with its landmarks noted.

while a gauze square is wrapped around the anterior third of the tongue in order to obtain a firm grasp (see Figure 2-16). The dorsal surface is digitally palpated. Then, the tongue is turned slightly on its side to visually inspect and bidigitally palpate its base and lateral borders. To examine the ventral surface, have the patient lift the tongue; visually inspect and digitally palpate the surface.

FLOOR OF THE MOUTH

The floor of the mouth is located inferior to the ventral surface of the tongue (Figure 2-19; see also Chapter 7

for palpation of area). The **lingual frenum** (**free**-num) or frenulum is a midline fold of tissue between the ventral surface of the tongue and the floor of the mouth.

A ridge of tissue also exists on each side of the floor of the mouth, the **sublingual fold** (sub-**ling**-gwal) or plica sublingualis. Together these folds are arranged in a V-shaped configuration from the lingual frenum to the base of the tongue. The sublingual folds contain duct openings from the sublingual salivary gland. The small papilla or **sublingual caruncle** (**kar**-unk-el) at the anterior end of each sublingual fold contains the duct openings from both the submandibular and sublingual salivary glands.

Visually inspect the mucosa of the floor of the mouth and check the lingual frenum. Use the mouth mirror to facilitate lighting. Bimanually palpate the sublingual area by placing an index finger intraorally and the fingertips of the opposite hand extraorally under the chin, compressing the tissue between the fingers. Check the lingual frenum. Dry the sublingual caruncle with gauze and observe the saliva flow from the duct.

PHARYNX

The oral cavity also provides the entrance into the throat or **pharynx** (**far**-inks). The pharynx is a muscular tube that serves both the respiratory and digestive systems. The pharynx consists of three portions: the nasopharynx, the oropharynx, and the laryngopharynx (Figure 2-20). Portions of the nasopharynx and oropharynx are visible in an intraoral examination when examining the palatal area with the patient saying "ah." The **laryngopharynx** (lah-ring-gah-**far**-inks) is more inferior, close to the laryngeal opening, and thus is not visible in an intraoral examination.

The portion of the pharynx that is superior to the level of the soft palate is the **nasopharynx** (nay-zo-**far**-inks). The nasopharynx is continuous with the nasal

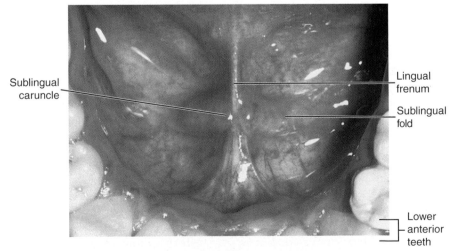

FIGURE 2-19 View of the floor of the mouth with its landmarks noted.

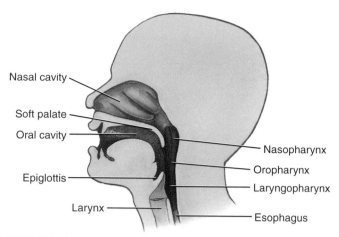

Nasal cavity

Soft palate

Oral cavity

Nasopharynx

Oropharynx

Laryngopharynx

Epiglottis

Larynx

Esophagus

FIGURE 2-20 Midsagittal section of the head and neck illustrating portions of the pharynx.

to cover the entrance to the larynx, preventing food and liquid from entering the trachea and then entering the lungs.

The opening from the oral region into the oropharynx is the **fauces** (**faw**-seez) or the faucial isthmus. The fauces are formed laterally by the **anterior faucial pillar** (**faw**-shawl **pil**-er) and the **posterior faucial pillar.** Older terms for these structures that border the fauces are the *tonsillar pillars* or *palatal arches*. Tonsillar tissue, the **palatine tonsils** (**pal**-ah-tine), is located between these pillars or folds of tissue created by underlying muscles. The palatine tonsils are the tonsillar tissue that patients call their "tonsils."

Mental Region

The chin is the major feature of the **mental region** (**ment**-il) of the head (Figure 2-22). The prominence of the chin is called the **mental protuberance** (pro-**too**-ber-ins). The mental protuberance is often more pronounced in adult males. The **labiomental groove** (lay-bee-o-**ment**-il), a horizontal groove between the lower lip and the chin mentioned in the description of the oral region, should be approximately midway between the apex of the nose and the chin and level with the angle of the mandible. Also present on the chin in some individuals is a midline depression or dimple that marks the underlying bony fusion of the

cavity. The portion of the pharynx that is between the soft palate and the opening of the larynx is the **oropharynx** (or-o-**far**-inks) (Figure 2-21; see also Chapter 4 for more information on the muscles of the pharnyx). Behind the base of the tongue and in front of the oropharynx is the **epiglottis** (ep-ih-**glah**-tis), a flap of cartilage. At rest, the epiglottis is upright and allows air to pass through the larynx and into the rest of the respiratory system. During swallowing, it folds back

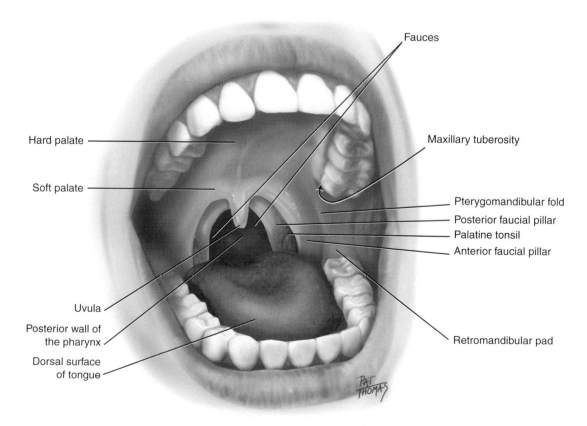

Fauces

Hard palate

Maxillary tuberosity

Soft palate

Pterygomandibular fold

Posterior faucial pillar

Palatine tonsil

Anterior faucial pillar

Uvula

Posterior wall of the pharynx

Retromandibular pad

Dorsal surface of tongue

FIGURE 2-21 Oral view of the oropharynx and oral cavity with its landmarks noted.

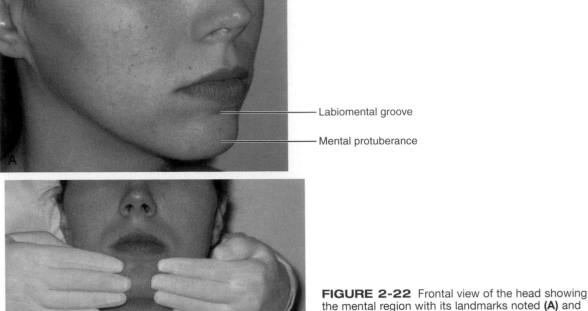

FIGURE 2-22 Frontal view of the head showing the mental region with its landmarks noted **(A)** and palpation of the mental region during an intraoral examination **(B).**

lower jaw. The mental region is visually inspected and bilaterally palpated during an extraoral examination.

REGIONS OF THE NECK

The neck extends from the skull and mandible down to the clavicles and sternum. The **regions of the neck** can be divided into different cervical triangles on the basis of the large bones and muscles in the area (Figure 2-23). Chapters 3 and 4 further describe these bones and muscles, respectively, with their cervical triangles as well as their extraoral examination (see Appendix B). Structures deep to the surface of these cervical triangles are also discussed in other chapters.

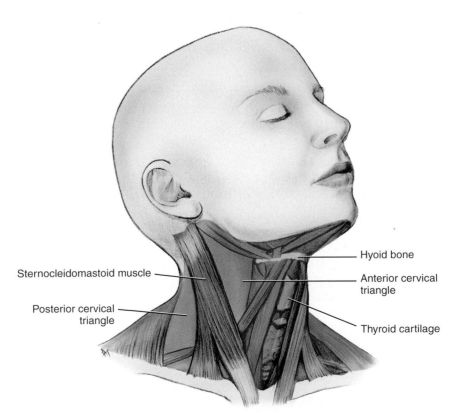

FIGURE 2-23 Regions of the neck: the anterior cervical triangle and posterior cervical triangle.

The large strap muscle, the **sternocleidomastoid muscle** (stir-no-kli-do-**mass**-toid), divides each side of the neck diagonally into an **anterior cervical triangle** (**ser**-vi-kal) and **posterior cervical triangle.** The anterior region of the neck corresponds with the two anterior cervical triangles, which are separated by a midline. The lateral region of the neck, posterior to the sternocleidomastoid muscle, is considered the posterior cervical triangle on each side.

At the anterior midline, the prominence of the larynx, the **thyroid cartilage** (**thy**-roid), is visible as the "Adam's apple," especially in adult males (Figure 2-24). The vocal cords or ligaments are attached to the posterior surface of the thyroid cartilage.

The **hyoid bone** (**hi**-oid) is also located in the anterior midline, superior to the thyroid cartilage. Many muscles attach to the hyoid bone. The hyoid bone can be effectively palpated by feeling inferior to and medial to the angles of the mandible. Do not confuse the hyoid bone with the inferiorly placed thyroid cartilage when palpating the neck.

The anterior cervical triangle can be further subdivided into smaller triangular regions by muscles in the area that are not as prominent as the sternocleidomastoid muscle (Figure 2-25). For example, the superior portion of each anterior cervical triangle is demarcated by portions of the digastric muscle (both bellies) and the mandible, forming a **submandibular**

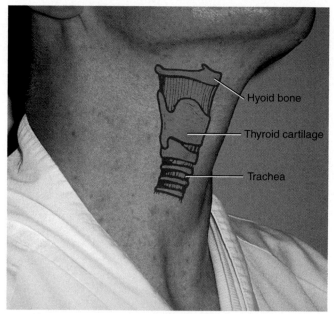

FIGURE 2-24 Lateral view of the anterior cervical triangle of the neck, highlighting its skeletal landmarks.

- Hyoid bone
- Thyroid cartilage
- Trachea

triangle (sub-man-**dib**-you-lar). The inferior portion of each anterior cervical triangle is further subdivided by the omohyoid muscle into a **carotid triangle** (kah-**rot**-id) superior to it and a **muscular triangle** inferior to it. A midline **submental triangle** (sub-**men**-tal) is also

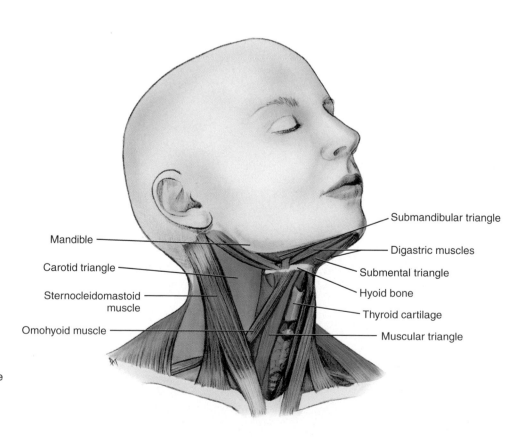

- Submandibular triangle
- Digastric muscles
- Submental triangle
- Hyoid bone
- Thyroid cartilage
- Muscular triangle
- Mandible
- Carotid triangle
- Sternocleidomastoid muscle
- Omohyoid muscle

FIGURE 2-25 Divisions of the anterior cervical triangle: submandibular, submental, carotid, and muscular.

formed by portions of the digastric muscle (right and left anterior bellies) and the hyoid bone.

Each posterior cervical triangle can also be further subdivided into smaller triangular regions by muscles in the area (Figure 2-26). The omohyoid muscle divides the posterior cervical triangle into the **occipital triangle** (ok-**sip**-it-al) superior to it and the **subclavian triangle** (sub-**klay**-vee-an) inferior to it on each side.

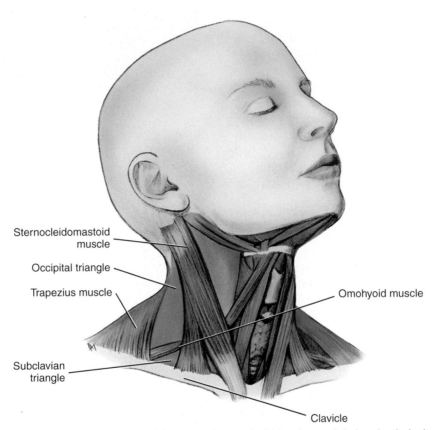

Sternocleidomastoid muscle

Occipital triangle

Trapezius muscle

Omohyoid muscle

Subclavian triangle

Clavicle

FIGURE 2-26 Divisions of the posterior cervical triangle: occipital and subclavian.

Identification Exercises

Identify the structures on the following diagrams by filling in each blank with the correct anatomical term. You can check your answers by looking back at the figure indicated in parentheses for each identification diagram.

1. (Figures 2-1, 2-2, 2-4, and 2-9)

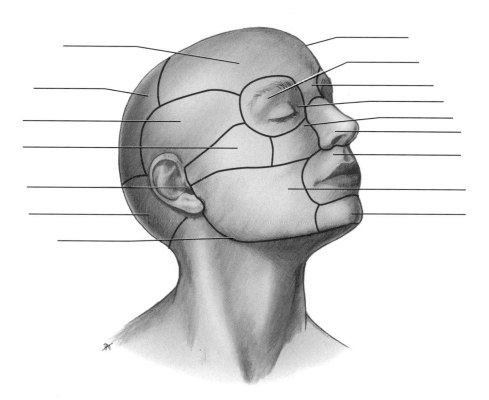

2. (Figure 2-6, *A*)

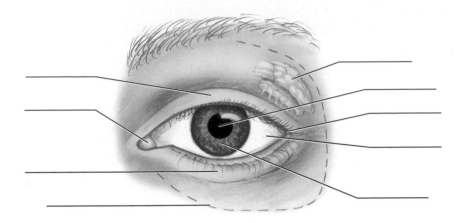

3. (Figure 2-11)

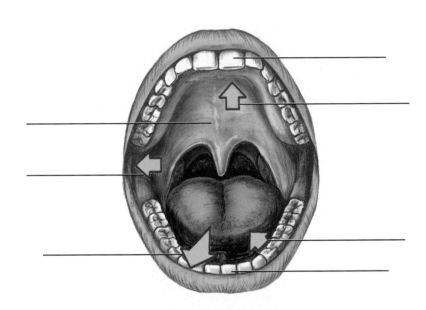

4. (Figure 2-17, *A*)

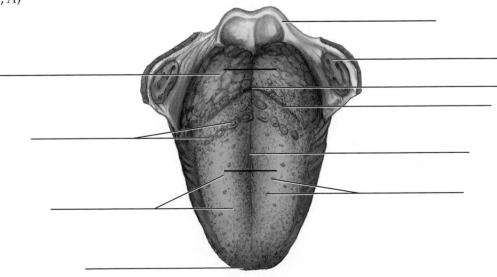

5. (Figure 2-20)

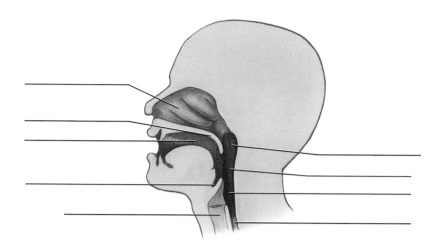

6. (Figure 2-21)

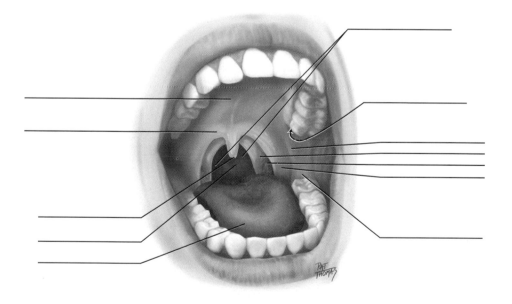

7. (Figure 2-23)

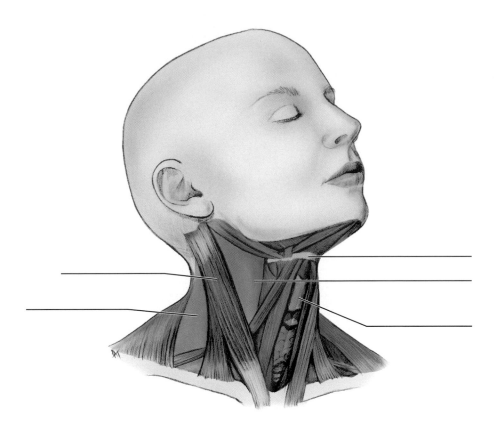

8. (Figure 2-25)

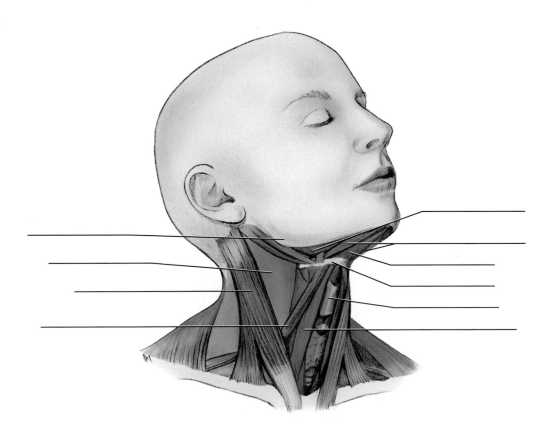

9. (Figure 2-26)

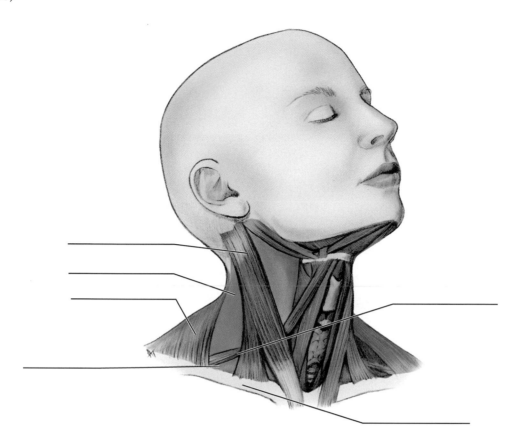

■ REVIEW QUESTIONS

1. Those structures in the oral region that are closest to the tongue are called:
   A. Buccal
   B. Facial
   C. Lingual
   D. Pharyngeal
   E. Palatal

2. Which of the following terms is used to describe the smooth, elevated area between the eyebrows in the frontal region?
   A. Supraorbital ridge
   B. Medial canthus
   C. Glabella
   D. Alae
   E. Auricle

3. In which region of the head and neck is the tragus located?
   A. Frontal region
   B. Nasal region
   C. Temporal region
   D. Anterior cervical triangle
   E. Submandibular triangle

4. The tissue at the junction between the labial or buccal mucosa and the alveolar mucosa is the:
   A. Mucogingival junction
   B. Mucobuccal fold
   C. Vermilion border
   D. Labial frenum
   E. Labiomental groove

5. Into which cervical triangles does the sternocleido-mastoid muscle divide the neck?
   A. Superior and inferior
   B. Medial and lateral
   C. Anterior and posterior
   D. Proximal and distal

6. The parietal and occipital regions are covered by the:
   A. Temporal region
   B. Layers of scalp
   C. Eyelids
   D. External acoustic meatus

7. Which of the following statements concerning the location of the medial canthus is correct when comparing it with the lateral canthus?
   A. It is nearer to the nose.
   B. It is nearer to the ear.
   C. It is where the upper and lower eyelid meet.
   D. It is where the upper and lower lip meet.

8. Which of the following structures extends from just inferior to the lateral margin of the eye toward the ear?
   A. Pterygomandibular fold
   B. Zygomatic arch
   C. Sulcus terminalis
   D. Sternocleidomastoid muscle

9. The opening from the oral region into the oropharynx is the:
   A. Fauces
   B. Palatine tonsils
   C. Pterygomandibular fold
   D. Nasopharynx

10. Which of the following terms is given to the small papilla at the anterior end of each sublingual fold?
    A. Lingual frenum
    B. Plica fimbriata
    C. Foliate papillae
    D. Sublingual caruncle
    E. Incisive papilla

11. Which of the following structures is the opening in the center of the iris?
    A. Sclera
    B. Pupil
    C. Orbit
    D. Iris

12. Which of the following structures is located between the tragus and the antitragus?
    A. Orbit of the eye
    B. Intertragic notch
    C. Angle of the mandible
    D. Helix of the ear
    E. Labial commissure

13. Which of the following structures separates the lower lip from the chin?
A. Vermilion border
B. Tubercle of upper lip
C. Labial commissure
D. Labiomental groove
E. Nasolabial sulcus

14. Which of the following structures is located on the dorsal surface of the tongue?
A. Labiomental groove
B. Mucobuccal fold
C. Median lingual sulcus
D. Pterygomandibular fold
E. Median palatine raphe

15. Which of the following structures is located directly posterior to the incisive papilla?
A. Palatine rugae
B. Mucogingival junction
C. Vermilion zone
D. Labial frenum

Skeletal System

OUTLINE

- Overview of the Skeletal System
  - Bony Prominences
  - Bony Depressions
  - Bony Openings
  - Skeletal Articulations
- Bones of the Head and Neck
  - Skull Views
  - Cranial Bones
  - Facial Bones
  - Paranasal Sinuses
  - Fossae of the Skull
  - Bones of the Neck
- Abnormalities of Bone

LEARNING OBJECTIVES

After studying this chapter, the reader should be able to do the following:

1. Define and pronounce all the key terms and anatomical terms in this chapter.
2. Locate and identify the bones of the head and neck and their landmarks on a diagram, skull, and patient.
3. Describe in detail the various portions and landmarks of the maxilla and mandible.
4. Discuss certain abnormalities of bone.
5. Correctly complete the review questions and activities for this chapter.
6. Integrate the knowledge about the skeletal system into the overall study of the head and neck anatomy and clinical dental practice.

KEY TERMS

Aperture (ap-er-cher) Opening or orifice in bone.
Arch Prominent bridgelike bony structure.
Articulation (ar-tik-you-lay-shin) Area where the bones are joined to each other.

Bones Mineralized structures of the body that protect internal soft tissues and serve as the biomechanical basis for movement.

(Continued)

KEY TERMS (continued)

Canal Opening in bone that is long, narrow, and tubelike.

Condyle (**kon**-dyl) Oval bony prominence typically located at articulations.

Cornu (**kor**-nu) Small hornlike prominence.

Crest Roughened border or ridge on the bone surface.

Eminence (**em**-i-nins) Tubercle or rounded elevation on a bony surface.

Fissure (**fish**-er) Opening in bone that is narrow and cleftlike.

Foramen/foramina (fo-**ray**-men, fo-ram-i-nah) Short, windowlike opening in bone.

Fossa/fossae (**fos**-ah, **fos**-ay) Depression on a bony surface.

Head Rounded surface projecting from a bone by a neck.

Incisura (in-si-**su**-rah) Indentation or notch at the edge of the bone.

Joint Site of a junction or union between two or more bones.

Line Straight, small ridge of bone.

Meatus (**me**-ate-us) Opening or canal in the bone.

Notch Indentation at the edge of a bone.

Ostium/ostia (**os**-tee-um, **os**-tee-ah) Small opening in bone.

Perforation (per-fo-**ray**-shun) Abnormal hole in a hollow organ, such as in the wall of a sinus.

Plate Flat structure of bone.

Primary sinusitis (sy-nu-**si**-tis) Inflammation of the sinus.

Process General term for any prominence on a bony surface.

Secondary sinusitis (sy-nu-**si**-tis) Inflammation of the sinus related to another source.

Spine Abrupt, small prominence of bone.

Sulcus/sulci (**sul**-kus, **sul**-ky) Shallow depression or groove such as that on the bony surface.

Suture (**su**-cher) Generally immovable articulation in which bones are joined by fibrous tissue.

Tubercle (**too**-ber-kl) Eminence or small, rounded elevation on the bony surface.

Tuberosity (too-beh-**ros**-i-tee) Large, often rough prominence on the surface of bone.

OVERVIEW OF THE SKELETAL SYSTEM

The **bones** of the skeletal system are mineralized structures in the body. Bones protect the internal soft tissues. Bones also serve as the biomechanical basis for movement of the body along with muscles, tendons, and ligaments. Bones are also a consideration in the spread of dental infection (see Chapter 12).

The prominences and depressions on the bony surface are landmarks for the attachments of associated muscles, tendons, and ligaments. The openings in the bone are also landmarks where various nerves and blood vessels enter or exit. Areas of the bones that are not prominences or depressions, such as a **plate,** which is a flat, bony structure, can also be demarcated.

Bony Prominences

A general term for any prominence on a bony surface is a **process.** One specific type of prominence located on the bony surface is a **condyle,** a relatively large, convex prominence usually involved in joints. A rounded surface projecting from a bone by a neck is a **head.** Another large, often rough prominence is a **tuberosity.** Tuberosities are typically attachment areas for muscles or tendons. An **arch** is shaped like a bridge with a bowlike outline. A **cornu** is a hornlike prominence.

Other prominences of the bone include epicondyles, tubercles, crests, lines, and spines. These primarily serve as muscle and ligament attachments. A **tubercle** or **eminence** is a rounded elevation on the bony surface. A **crest** is a prominent, often roughened border or ridge. A **line** is a straight, small ridge. An abrupt prominence of the bone that may be a blunt or sharply pointed projection is a **spine.**

Bony Depressions

One type of depression on the bony surface is an **incisura** or **notch,** an indentation at the edge of the bone. Another depression on a bony surface is a **sulcus** (plural, **sulci**), which is a shallow depression or groove that usually marks the course of an artery or nerve. A generally deeper depression on a bony surface is a **fossa** (plural, **fossae**). Fossae can be portions of joints, be attachment areas for muscles, or have other functions.

Bony Openings

The bone can have openings such as a foramen or canal. A **foramen** (plural, **foramina**) is a short window-like opening in the bone. A **canal** is a longer, narrow tubelike opening in the bone. A **meatus** is a type of canal. Another opening in a bone is a **fissure,** which is a narrow cleftlike opening. A small opening, especially as an entrance into a hollow organ or canal, is an **ostium** (plural, **ostia**). Another opening or orifice is an **aperture.**

Skeletal Articulations

An **articulation** is an area of the skeleton where the bones are joined to each other. An articulation of the bones can be either a movable or an immovable type of joint. A **suture** is the union of bones joined by fibrous tissue. Sutures appear on the dry skull as jagged lines. Sutures are considered to be generally immovable but may provide mechanical protection from the force of a blow by moving slightly to absorb the force. Sutures are the most flexible in infants. Much of the early growth of the skull occurs at the sutural edges of the cranial bones.

BONES OF THE HEAD AND NECK

The bones of the head and neck serve as a base during palpation of the soft tissues in the area. The bones also serve as markers when identifying the location of soft tissue lesions. These bones are also examined externally during a head and neck examination by a dental professional because they may be affected by a disease process. A dental professional must not only locate each of the head and neck bones but also recognize any abnormalities in the bony surface structure (discussed later).

In order to recognize any bony abnormalities, the dental professional must know the normal anatomy of the bones of the head and neck. The knowledge of the normal anatomy includes locating the surface bony prominences, depressions, and articulations. It also includes the openings in these bones and the blood vessels and nerves that travel through those openings. For effective study of the bones of the head and neck, it is helpful to use photographs and illustrations of these bones as well as the skull model and palpation of a patient.

Bones and their associated surface tissues also serve as landmarks when taking dental radiographs (see Chapter 2), before administering a local anesthetic injection (see Chapter 9), and in understanding the spread of dental infections (see Chapter 12).

Skull

The **skull** of a patient has 22 bones, not including the small bones of the middle ear (Table 3-1). The bones of the skull or braincase can be divided into the **cranium** (**kray**-nee-um) (the portion housing the brain) with its **cranial bones** (**kray**-nee-al) and the **face** with its **facial bones.** The bones of the skull, whether facial or cranial, can be single or paired. These bones create the facial features, are involved in the temporomandibular joints, and participate with growth in the formation of dentition. Many anatomists use the alternative terms "neurocranium" for the cranial bones because they enclose the brain and "viscerocranium" for the facial bones.

Growth takes place in all bones of the skull. Growth of the upper face occurs at the sutures between the maxillary bones and other bones as well as at the bony surfaces. Growth in the lower face takes place at the bony surfaces of the mandible and at the head of its condyle. Inadequate or disproportionate growth of the upper face and mandible may leave inadequate room for the developing dentition and cause other occlusal problems. This failure of growth can be addressed by orthodontic treatment and possibly endocrine therapy and surgery.

All skull bones are immovable, except the mandible with its temporomandibular joint. The articulation of many of the bones in the skull is by sutures (Table 3-2). The skull also has a movable articulation with the bony vertebral column in the neck area.

TABLE 3-1

CRANIAL AND FACIAL BONES*

Cranial Bones		Facial Bones	
Occipital bone	Single	Vomer	Single
Frontal bone	Single	Lacrimal bones	Paired
Parietal bones	Paired	Nasal bones	Paired
Temporal bones	Paired	Inferior nasal conchae	Paired
Sphenoid bone	Single	Zygomatic bones	Paired
Ethmoid bone	Single	Maxillary bones	Paired
		Mandible	Single

*Note that there are single and paired bones. Also note that the palatine bones are paired bones of the skull that are not strictly considered facial bones.

TABLE 3-2

SUTURES OF THE SKULL AND THEIR BONY ARTICULATIONS

Suture	Bony Articulations
Coronal suture	Frontal and parietal bones
Sagittal suture	Parietal bones
Lambdoidal suture	Occipital and parietal bones
Squamosal suture	Temporal and parietal bones
Temporozygomatic suture	Zygomatic and temporal bones
Median palatine suture	Palatine bones
Transverse palatine suture	Maxillae and palatine bones

Many skull bones have openings for important nerves and blood vessels of the head and neck (Table 3-3). Skull bones also have many associated processes that are involved in important structures of the face and head (Table 3-4). This chapter may also be reviewed after reading the chapters on the vascular and nervous systems (Chapters 6 and 8), as well as the chapters on the muscles of the head and neck (Chapter 4) and temporomandibular joint (Chapter 5).

Studying the skull is made easier by first looking at its various views: the superior, anterior, lateral, and inferior views. Then the skull should be studied by looking at its individual bones and their various landmarks: the cranial bones, facial bones, and neck bones. The features of the skull bones such as the fossae and paranasal sinuses should then be studied. This chapter follows this format of study.

SUPERIOR VIEW OF THE SKULL

When the skull is viewed from above, four cranial bones are visible (Figure 3-1). At the front of the skull is the single **frontal bone** (**frunt**-il). At the sides are the paired **parietal bones** (pah-**ri**-it-al). At the back of the skull is the single **occipital bone** (ok-**sip**-it-al). This main division of the cranial bones of the skull is discussed later.

Sutures on Superior View

Three sutures among these four skull bones are also visible on the superior view (Figure 3-2; see Table 3-2). The suture extending across the skull, between the frontal and parietal bones, is the **coronal suture** (kor-**oh**-nahl). A second suture, the **sagittal suture** (**saj**-i-tel), extends from the front to the back of the skull, between the paired parietal bones. These two sutures generally form a right angle with each other. The third suture, located between the single occipital bone and the paired parietal bones, is the **lambdoidal suture** (lam-**doid**-al). Among the skull sutures, the lambdoidal suture is by far more serrated-looking than either the coronal or the sagittal sutures.

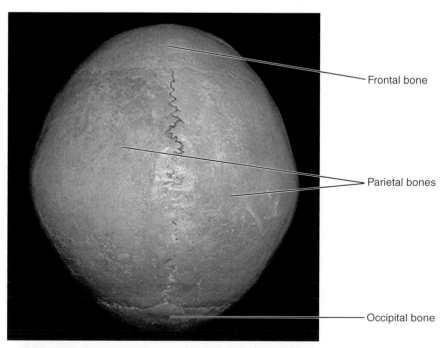

Frontal bone

Parietal bones

Occipital bone

FIGURE 3-1 Superior view of the bones of the skull.

TABLE 3-3

BONY OPENINGS IN THE SKULL AND THEIR ASSOCIATED NERVES AND BLOOD VESSELS

Bony Opening	Location	Nerves and Blood Vessels
Carotid canal	Temporal bone	Internal carotid artery
Cribriform plate with foramina	Ethmoid bone	Olfactory nerves
External acoustic meatus	Temporal bone	Opening to tympanic cavity
Foramen lacerum	Sphenoid, occipital, and temporal bones	Cartilage
Foramen magnum	Occipital bone	Spinal cord, vertebral arteries, and eleventh cranial nerve
Foramen ovale	Sphenoid bone	Mandibular division of the fifth cranial nerve
Foramen rotundum	Sphenoid bone	Fifth cranial nerve
Foramen spinosum	Sphenoid bone	Middle meningeal artery
Greater palatine foramen	Palatine bone	Greater palatine nerve and vessels
Hypoglossal canal	Occipital bone	Twelfth cranial nerve
Incisive foramen	Maxilla	Nasopalatine nerve and branches of the sphenopalatine artery
Inferior orbital fissure	Sphenoid bone and maxilla	Infraorbital and zygomatic nerves, infraorbital artery, and ophthalmic vein
Infraorbital foramen and canal	Maxilla	Infraorbital nerve and vessels
Internal acoustic meatus	Temporal bone	Seventh and eighth cranial nerves
Jugular foramen	Occipital and temporal bones	Internal jugular vein and ninth, tenth, and eleventh cranial nerves
Lesser palatine foramen	Palatine bone	Lesser palatine nerve and vessels
Mandibular foramen	Mandible	Inferior alveolar nerve and vessels
Mental foramen	Mandible	Mental nerve and vessels
Optic canal and foramen	Sphenoid bone	Optic nerve and ophthalmic artery
Petrotympanic fissure	Temporal bone	Chorda tympani nerve
Pterygoid canal	Sphenoid bone	Area nerves and vessels
Stylomastoid foramen	Temporal bone	Seventh cranial nerve
Superior orbital fissure	Sphenoid bone	Third, fourth, and sixth cranial nerves and ophthalmic nerve and vein

TABLE 3-4

PROCESSES AND ASSOCIATED STRUCTURES OF THE SKULL BONES

Processes of Skull	Skull Bones	Associated Structures
Alveolar process	Mandible	Contains roots of mandibular teeth
Alveolar process	Maxilla	Contains roots of maxillary teeth
Coronoid process	Mandible	Portion of ramus
Frontal process	Maxilla	Forms medial infraorbital rim
Frontal process	Zygomatic bone	Forms anterior lateral orbital wall
Lesser wing	Sphenoid bone	Anterior process to sphenoid bone body
Greater wing	Sphenoid bone	Posterolateral process to sphenoid bone body
Mastoid process	Temporal bone	Composed of mastoid air cells
Maxillary process	Zygomatic bone	Forms infraorbital rim and portion of anterior lateral orbital wall
Palatine process	Maxilla	Forms anterior hard palate
Postglenoid process	Temporal bone	Posterior to temporomandibular joint
Pterygoid process	Sphenoid bone	Consists of medial and lateral pterygoid plates
Styloid process	Temporal bone	Serves as attachment for muscles and ligaments
Temporal process	Zygomatic bone	Portion of zygomatic arch
Zygomatic process	Frontal bone	Lateral to orbit
Zygomatic process	Maxilla	Forms lateral portion of infraorbital rim
Zygomatic process	Temporal bone	Portion of zygomatic arch

ANTERIOR VIEW OF THE SKULL

When the skull is viewed from the front, certain bones of the skull (or portions of these bones) are visible (Figure 3-3). These bones include the single frontal, ethmoid, vomer, and sphenoid bones and the mandible as well as the paired lacrimal, nasal, inferior nasal conchal, zygomatic, and maxillary bones.

Facial Bones on Anterior View.

The facial bones visible on the anterior view of the skull include the **lacrimal bone** (lak-ri-mal), **nasal bone** (nay-zil), **vomer** (vo-mer), **inferior nasal concha** (nay-zil kong-kah, plural, **conchae** [kong-kee]), **zygomatic bone** (zy-go-mat-ik), **maxilla** (mak-sil-ah), and **mandible** (man-di-bl) (Figure 3-4). The **palatine bones** (pal-ah-tine) are not visible on this view and are not strictly considered facial bones by anatomists, but for

ease of learning, they are included under the heading of facial bones. This main division of the facial bones of the skull is discussed later.

Orbit and Associated Structures.

The **orbit** (or-bit) or eye cavity, which contains and protects the eyeballs, is a prominent feature of the anterior view (Figure 3-5). Many skull bones form the walls and apex of each of the orbits (Table 3-5). The larger **orbital walls** (or-bit-al) are composed of the orbital plates of the frontal bone (making the roof or superior wall), ethmoid bone (forming the greatest portion of the medial wall), lacrimal bone (at the anterior medial corner of the orbit and the orbital surfaces of the maxilla [floor or inferior wall]), and zygomatic bone (anterior portion of the lateral wall). The orbital surface of the greater wing of the sphenoid

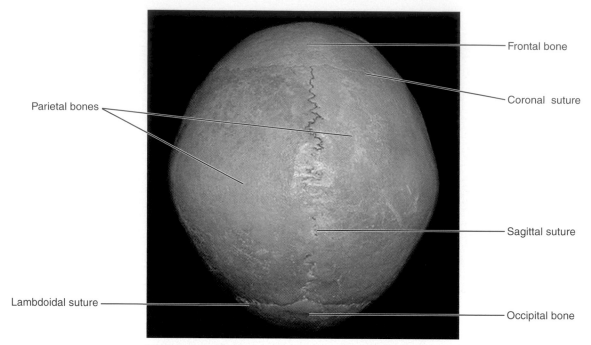

Frontal bone

Coronal suture

Parietal bones

Sagittal suture

Lambdoidal suture

Occipital bone

FIGURE 3-2 Superior view of the skull and its suture lines.

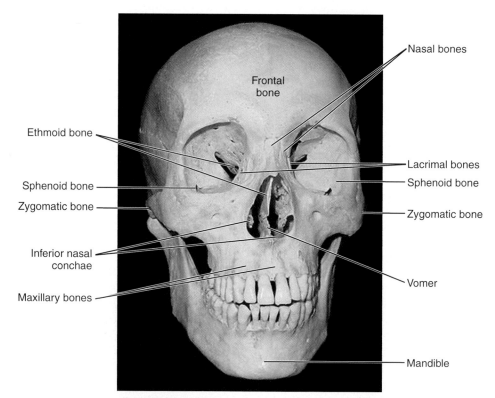

Nasal bones

Frontal bone

Ethmoid bone

Lacrimal bones

Sphenoid bone

Sphenoid bone

Zygomatic bone

Zygomatic bone

Inferior nasal conchae

Vomer

Maxillary bones

Mandible

FIGURE 3-3 Anterior view of the bones of the skull.

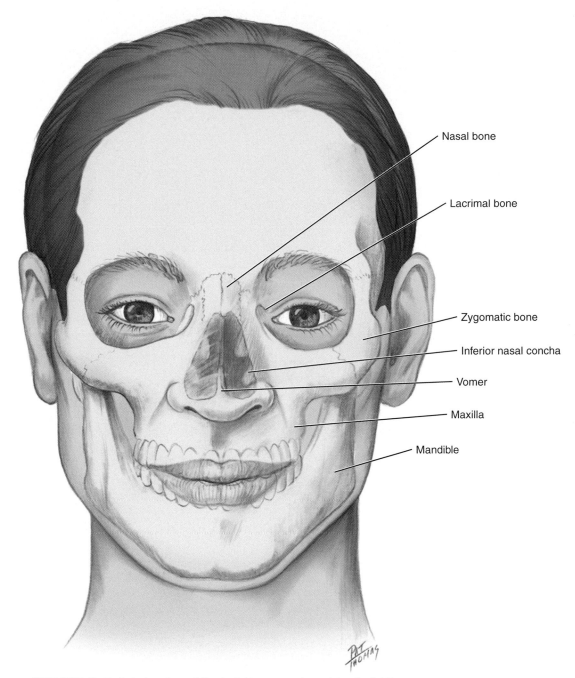

Nasal bone

Lacrimal bone

Zygomatic bone

Inferior nasal concha

Vomer

Maxilla

Mandible

FIGURE 3-4 Anterior view of the facial bones and overlying facial tissues.

bone is also included (the posterior portion of the lateral wall).

The **orbital apex** or the deepest portion of the orbit is composed of the lesser wing of the sphenoid bone (forming the base) and the palatine bone (a small inferior portion) (Figure 3-6; see Table 3-5). The round opening in the orbital apex is the **optic canal** (op-tik), which lies between the two roots of the lesser wing of the sphenoid bone (see Table 3-3). The second cranial or optic nerve passes through the optic canal to reach the eyeball. The ophthalmic artery also extends through the canal to reach the eye.

Two orbital fissures are noted on the anterior aspect: the superior orbital fissure and inferior orbital fissure (Figure 3-7; see Table 3-3). Lateral to the optic canal is the curved and slitlike **superior orbital fissure,** between the greater and lesser wings of the sphenoid bone. Like the optic canal, the superior orbital fissure connects the orbit with the cranial cavity. The third cranial or oculomotor nerve, the fourth cranial or trochlear nerve, the sixth cranial or abducent nerve, and the ophthalmic nerve (from the fifth cranial or trigeminal nerve) and vein travel through this fissure.

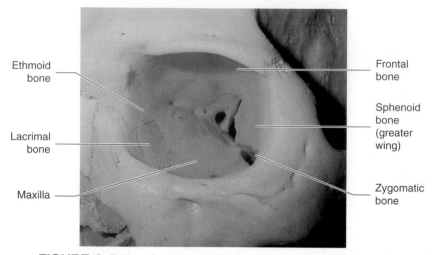

Ethmoid bone

Lacrimal bone

Maxilla

Frontal bone

Sphenoid bone (greater wing)

Zygomatic bone

FIGURE 3-5 Anterior view of the left orbit of the skull and its walls.

TABLE 3-5

BONES OF THE SKULL THAT FORM THE ORBIT

Portion of Orbit	Skull Bones
Roof or superior wall	Frontal bone
Medial wall	Ethmoid and lacrimal bones
Lateral wall	Zygomatic and sphenoid bones
Apex or base	Sphenoid and palatine bones*

*Note that the maxilla, a facial bone, completes the apex or base portion of the orbit.

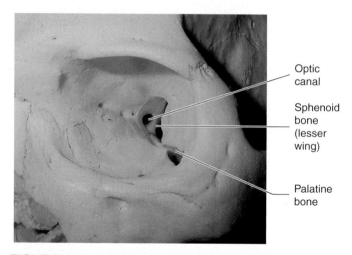

Optic canal

Sphenoid bone (lesser wing)

Palatine bone

FIGURE 3-6 Anterior view of the left orbit and the orbital apex.

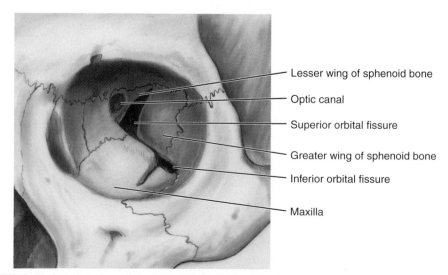

Lesser wing of sphenoid bone

Optic canal

Superior orbital fissure

Greater wing of sphenoid bone

Inferior orbital fissure

Maxilla

FIGURE 3-7 Anterior view of the left orbit and the orbital fissures.

The **inferior orbital fissure** can also be seen between the greater wing of the sphenoid bone and the maxilla. The inferior orbital fissure connects the orbit with the infratemporal and pterygopalatine fossae (discussed later). The infraorbital and zygomatic nerves, branches of the maxillary nerve, and infraorbital artery enter the orbit through this fissure. The inferior ophthalmic vein travels through this fissure to join the pterygoid plexus of veins.

Nasal Cavity and Associated Structures.

The **nasal cavity** (**nay**-zil) can also be viewed from the anterior aspect (Figure 3-8; see also Figure 3-56 and Chapter 2). The **nasion** (**nay**-ze-on), a midpoint landmark, is located at the junction of the frontal and nasal bones. The anterior opening of the nasal cavity, the **piriform aperture** (**pir**-i-form), is large and triangular. The **bridge of the nose** is formed from the paired nasal bones. The lateral boundaries of the nasal cavity are formed by the maxillae.

Each lateral wall of the nasal cavity has three projecting structures that extend inward from the maxilla, which are called the **nasal conchae** (**kong**-kay). These are the superior, middle, and inferior nasal conchae. Each extends like a scroll into the nasal cavity. The superior nasal concha and middle nasal concha are formed from the ethmoid bone. The inferior nasal concha is a separate facial bone. Deep to each concha is a groove known as a **nasal meatus** (me-**ate**-us). Each meatus has

openings through which the paranasal sinuses or nasolacrimal duct communicates with the nasal cavity.

The vertical partition of the nasal cavity, the **nasal septum** (**sep**-tum), divides the nasal cavity into two portions (Figure 3-9). Although it is frequently deflected slightly to the left or right, in general the septum is aligned perpendicularly. Anteriorly, the nasal septum is formed by both the nasal septal cartilage inferiorly and the perpendicular plate of the ethmoid bone superiorly. The posterior portions of the nasal septum are formed by the vomer.

EXTERNAL LATERAL VIEW OF THE SKULL

When viewed from the side, the external skull shows both cranial bones and facial bones. A division between the cranial bones and facial bones can be reinforced by making an imaginary diagonal line that passes downward and backward from the supraorbital ridge of the frontal bone to the tip of the mastoid process of the temporal bone (Figure 3-10). These two main divisions of the bones of the skull are discussed later.

On the lateral external surface of the skull are two separate parallel ridges or **temporal lines** (**tem**-poh-ral), crossing both the frontal and parietal bones (Figure 3-11; see Figure 3-1). The superior ridge is the superior temporal line. The inferior ridge or inferior temporal line is the superior boundary of the

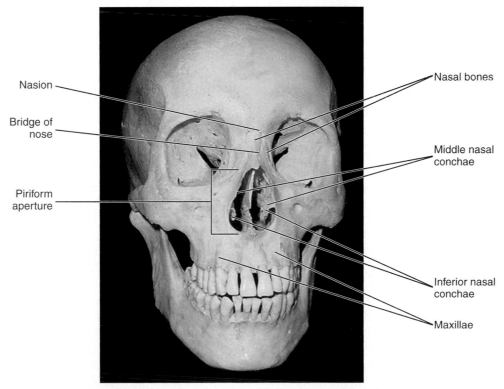

FIGURE 3-8 Anterior view of the skull and the nasal cavity.

Labels on figure: Nasion; Bridge of nose; Piriform aperture; Nasal bones; Middle nasal conchae; Inferior nasal conchae; Maxillae

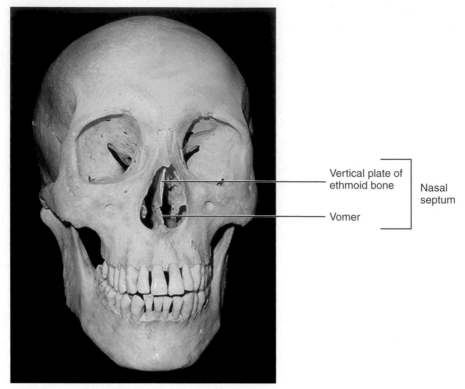

FIGURE 3-9 Anterior view of the skull and the nasal septum.

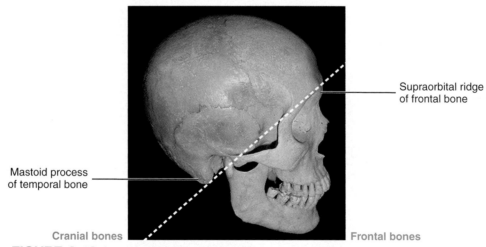

FIGURE 3-10 Lateral view of the skull and an imaginary diagonal line separating the cranial bones and facial bones.

temporal fossa and where the fan-shaped temporalis muscle attaches.

Cranial Bones on External Lateral View.
The cranium is easily seen from the lateral view, including the cranial bones: the occipital , frontal, parietal, temporal, **sphenoid** (**sfe**-noid), and **ethmoid** bones (**eth**-moid). This main division of the bones of the skull is discussed later.

Also present on the lateral view of the cranium are the associated sutures (Figure 3-12; see Table 3-2).

These sutures include the **coronal suture** (kor-**oh**-nahl), an articulation between the frontal and parietal bones, and the lambdoidal suture, an articulation between the parietal and occipital bones. Also present is the arched **squamosal suture** (**skway**-mus-al), between the temporal and parietal bones.

Fossae on External Lateral View.
The **temporal fossa** is easily seen on the lateral aspect of the skull (Figure 3-13). The temporal fossa is formed by several bones of the skull and contains the body of

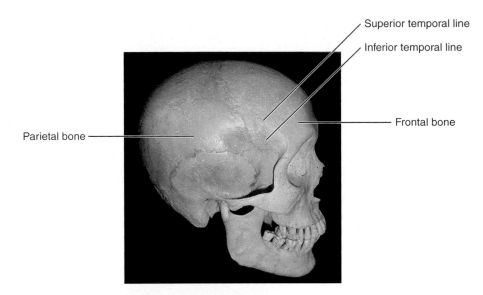

Superior temporal line
Inferior temporal line
Frontal bone
Parietal bone

FIGURE 3-11 Lateral view of the skull and superior and inferior temporal lines.

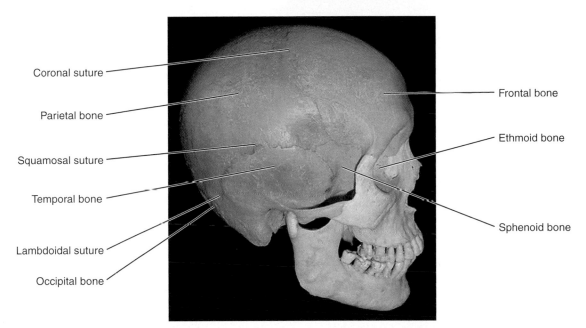

Coronal suture
Parietal bone
Squamosal suture
Temporal bone
Lambdoidal suture
Occipital bone
Frontal bone
Ethmoid bone
Sphenoid bone

FIGURE 3-12 Lateral view of the cranial bones and their suture lines.

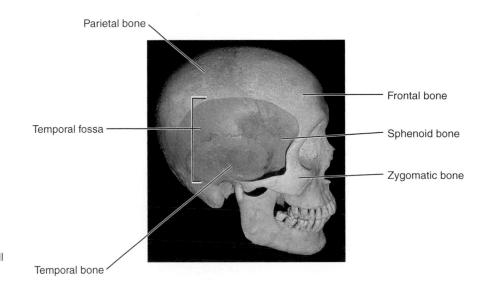

Parietal bone
Temporal fossa
Frontal bone
Sphenoid bone
Zygomatic bone
Temporal bone

FIGURE 3-13 Lateral view of the skull and temporal fossa.

the temporalis muscle. Inferior to the temporal fossa is the **infratemporal fossa** (in-frah-**tem**-poh-ral). Deep to the infratemporal fossa and more difficult to see is the **pterygopalatine fossa** (**teh**-ri-go-**pal**-ah-tine). The temporal, infratemporal, and pterygopalatine fossae are discussed later and contain many important head and neck structures.

Zygomatic Arch and Temporomandibular Joint on External Lateral View.

Farther inferior on the lateral aspect are many important bony landmarks (Figure 3-14). The **zygomatic arch** or cheekbone is visible, formed by the union of the broad temporal process of the zygomatic bone and the slender zygomatic process of the temporal bone (see Table 3-4). The suture between these two bones is the **temporozygomatic suture** (tem-por-oh-zi-go-**mat**-ik). The zygomatic arch serves as the origin for the masseter muscle.

The **temporomandibular joint** (tem-poh-ro-man-**dib**-you-lar) is also noted and is a movable articulation between the temporal bone and the mandible. A **joint** is a site of a junction or union between two or more bones. The specifics of this joint are discussed in Chapter 5. Further landmarks of these bones are discussed later.

INFERIOR VIEW OF THE EXTERNAL SURFACE OF THE SKULL

Most of the structures of the inferior aspect of the skull surface are more easily viewed on the skull model if the mandible is temporarily removed. The maxillary, zygomatic, vomer, temporal, sphenoid, occipital, and palatine bones are visible on this inferior view of the skull's external surface (Figure 3-15).

Hard Palate and Associated Structures.

At the anterior portion of the skull's inferior aspect is the **hard palate** (**pal**-it), bordered by the **alveolar process of the maxilla** (al-ve-o-lar) with its **maxillary teeth** (**mak**-sil-lare-ee) (Figure 3-16; see Table 3-4). The hard palate is formed by the two palatine processes of the maxillae and the two horizontal plates of the palatine bones.

Two prominent sutures are present on the hard palate (see Table 3-2). One suture is the **median palatine suture,** a midline articulation between the two palatine processes of the maxillae anteriorly and the two horizontal plates of the palatine bones posteriorly. The other suture is the **transverse palatine suture,** an articulation between the two palatine processes of the maxillae and the two horizontal plates of the palatine bones.

The hard palate forms the floor of the nasal cavity as well as the roof of the mouth. The posterior edge of the hard palate forms the inferior border of two funnel-shaped cavities, the **posterior nasal apertures** or **choanae** (ko-a-nay). The superior border of each aperture is formed by the vomer and the sphenoid bone. The posterior edge of the vomer forms the medial border of the posterior nasal apertures. The posterior nasal apertures are the posterior openings of the nasal cavity.

Near the superior border of each posterior nasal aperture is a small canal, the **pterygoid canal** (teh-ri-goid) (see Table 3-3). The pterygoid canal extends to open into the **pterygopalatine fossa** and carries the

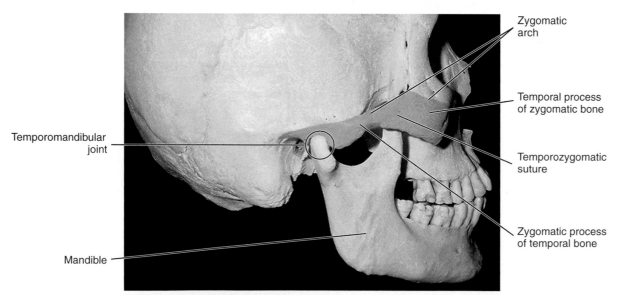

FIGURE 3-14 Lateral view of the skull showing the zygomatic arch and the temporomandibular joint.

Zygomatic arch

Temporal process of zygomatic bone

Temporozygomatic suture

Zygomatic process of temporal bone

Temporomandibular joint

Mandible

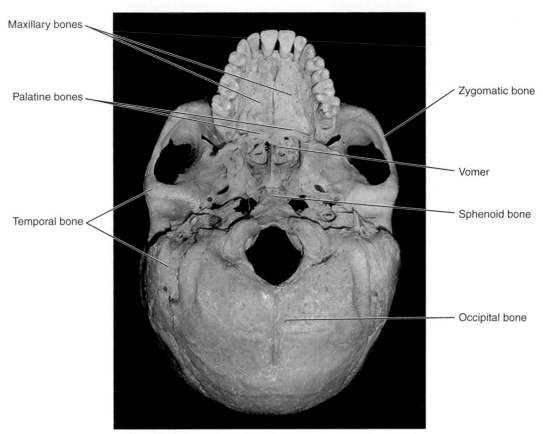

Maxillary bones

Palatine bones

Temporal bone

Zygomatic bone

Vomer

Sphenoid bone

Occipital bone

FIGURE 3-15 Inferior view of the external surface of the skull.

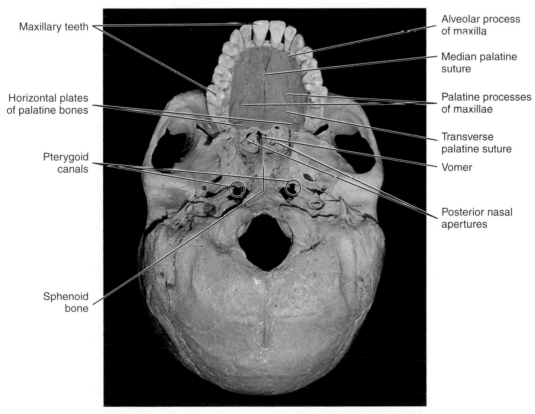

Maxillary teeth

Horizontal plates
of palatine bones

Pterygoid
canals

Sphenoid
bone

Alveolar process
of maxilla

Median palatine
suture

Palatine processes
of maxillae

Transverse
palatine suture

Vomer

Posterior nasal
apertures

FIGURE 3-16 External surface of the skull with the hard palate highlighted.

pterygoid nerve and blood vessels (the fossa is discussed later).

Middle Portion of the External Skull Surface.

The middle portion of the inferior aspect of the external skull surface has many important surface prominences and depressions on the sphenoid bone (Figure 3-17). The lateral borders of the posterior nasal apertures are formed on each side by the **pterygoid process** of the sphenoid bone (see Table 3-4).

Each pterygoid process consists of a thin **medial pterygoid plate** and a flattened **lateral pterygoid plate.** The depression between the medial and lateral plates is called the **pterygoid fossa.** At the inferior portion of the medial plate of the pterygoid process is a thin curved process, the **hamulus** (**ha**-mu-lis). The sphenoid bone and its landmarks are discussed later.

Foramina of the External Skull Surface.

The underside of the skull has a large number of foramina (Figure 3-18; see Table 3-3). These openings provide entrances and exits for the arteries and veins that supply the brain and facial tissues (see Chapter 6). They also allow the cranial nerves to pass to and from the brain (see Chapter 8).

The larger anterior oval opening on the sphenoid bone is the **foramen ovale** (o-**va**-lee) for the mandibular division of the fifth cranial or trigeminal nerve. The smaller and more posterior opening is the **foramen spinosum** (**spine**-o-sum), which carries the middle meningeal artery into the cranial cavity. The foramen spinosum receives its name from the nearby **spine of the sphenoid bone,** which is at the posterior extremity of the sphenoid bone.

Also on the external surface of the skull is the large, irregularly shaped **foramen lacerum** (lah-**ser**-um), which in life is filled with cartilage. Posterolateral to the foramen lacerum is a round opening in the petrous portion of the temporal bone, the **carotid canal** (kah-**rot**-id). The carotid canal carries the internal carotid artery and sympathetic carotid plexus. A pointed bony projection, the **styloid process** (**sty**-loid), is visible lateral and posterior to the carotid canal (see Table 3-4). Immediately posterior to the styloid process is the **stylomastoid foramen** (sty-lo-**mas**-toid), an opening through which the seventh cranial or facial nerve exits from the skull to the face.

The **jugular foramen** (**jug**-you-lar), just medial to the styloid process, is more easily seen if the skull model is tilted to one side. The jugular foramen is the

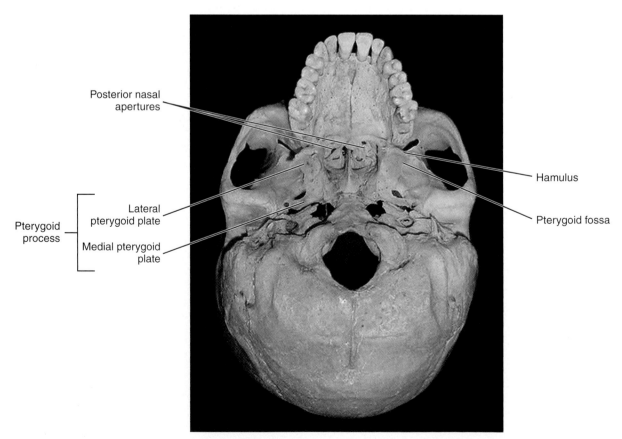

FIGURE 3-17 Structures on the middle portion of the external skull surface.

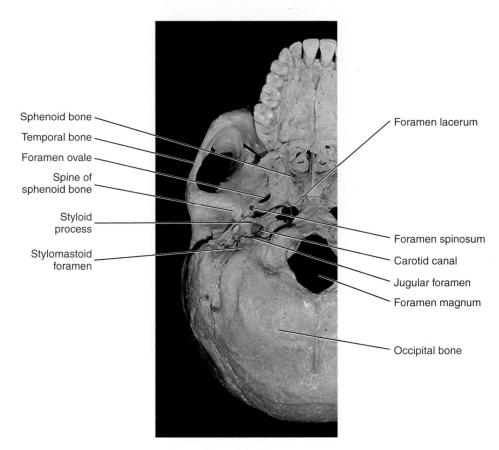

FIGURE 3-18 Foramina and associated structures of the external skull surface.

opening through which pass the internal jugular vein and three cranial nerves: the ninth cranial or glossopharyngeal nerve, tenth cranial or vagus nerve, and eleventh cranial or accessory nerve.

The largest opening on the inferior view is the **foramen magnum** (**mag**-num) of the occipital bone, through which the spinal cord, vertebral arteries, and eleventh cranial or accessory nerve pass.

SUPERIOR VIEW OF THE INTERNAL SURFACE OF THE SKULL

The internal surface of the skull is viewed by carefully removing the top half of the skull model. The frontal, ethmoid, sphenoid, temporal, occipital, and parietal bones are visible from this view of the internal surface of the skull (Figure 3-19).

Foramina of the Internal Skull Surface.

Also present are the inside openings of the optic canal, superior orbital fissure, foramen ovale, foramen spinosum, foramen lacerum, jugular foramen, and foramen magnum, as discussed before when viewing the external skull surface (see Figure 3-19; see Table 3-3). Additionally, many other foramina are present on the internal surface of the skull. The perforated **cribriform plate** (**krib**-ri-form), with foramina for the first cranial or olfactory nerve, and the **foramen rotundum** (row-**tun**-dum) for the maxillary division of the fifth cranial or trigeminal nerve are also seen from this view.

Finally, also present are the **hypoglossal canal** (hi-poh-**gloss**-al) for the twelfth cranial or hypoglossal nerve and the **internal acoustic meatus** (ah-**koos**-tik) for the seventh cranial or facial nerve and the eighth cranial or vestibulocochlear nerve.

Cranial Bones

The cranium is formed from the cranial bones. The cranial bones include the single occipital, frontal, sphenoid, and ethmoid bones and the paired parietal and temporal bones (Figure 3-20).

OCCIPITAL BONE

The occipital bone is a single cranial bone located in the most posterior portion of the skull (Figure 3-21). The occipital bone articulates with the parietal, temporal, and sphenoid bones of the skull. The occipital bone also articulates with the first cervical vertebra

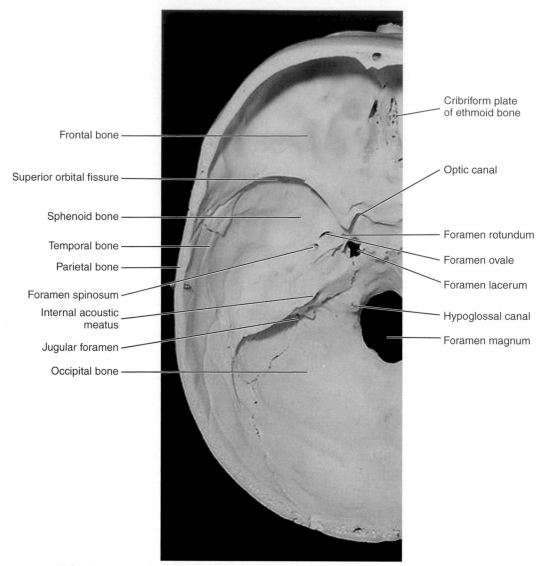

Frontal bone

Superior orbital fissure

Sphenoid bone

Temporal bone

Parietal bone

Foramen spinosum

Internal acoustic meatus

Jugular foramen

Occipital bone

Cribriform plate of ethmoid bone

Optic canal

Foramen rotundum

Foramen ovale

Foramen lacerum

Hypoglossal canal

Foramen magnum

FIGURE 3-19 Superior view of the internal surface of the skull showing foramina.

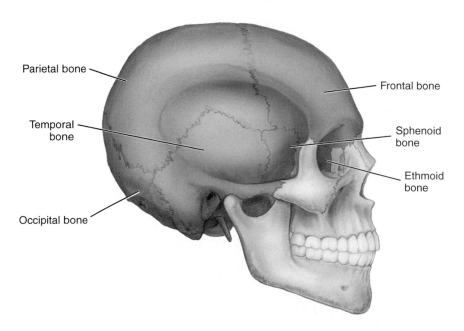

Parietal bone

Temporal bone

Occipital bone

Frontal bone

Sphenoid bone

Ethmoid bone

FIGURE 3-20 Lateral view of the skull and the cranial bones.

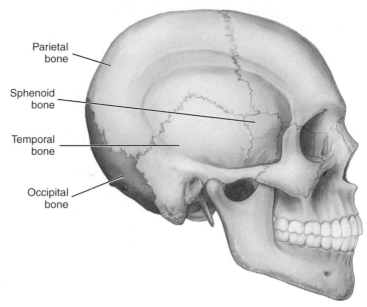

Parietal bone

Sphenoid bone

Temporal bone

Occipital bone

FIGURE 3-21 Lateral view of the skull with the occipital bone and its bony articulations.

(the atlas). The occipital bone can easily be studied from an inferior view of its external surface.

Inferior View of External Surface of the Occipital Bone.
On the external surface of the occipital bone from an inferior view, it can be seen that the foramen magnum is completely formed by this bone (Figure 3-22; see Table 3-3). Lateral and anterior to the foramen magnum are the paired **occipital condyles,** curved and smooth projections. The occipital condyles have a movable articulation with the atlas, the first cervical vertebra of the vertebral column (discussed later). On the stout **basilar portion** (**bas**-i-lar), a four-sided plate anterior to the foramen magnum, is a midline projection, the **pharyngeal tubercle** (fah-**rin**-je-al).

When tilting the skull model, the openings anterior and lateral to the foramen magnum are visible on the inferior view of the occipital bone (see Table 3-3). These openings are the paired hypoglossal canals (see Figure 3-22, *arrow*). The twelfth cranial or hypoglossal nerve is transmitted through the hypoglossal canals. The **jugular notch of the occipital bone,** the medial portion of the two bones that form the jugular foramen, is also present (a portion of the temporal bone is part of the other).

FRONTAL BONE
The frontal bone is a single cranial bone that forms both the forehead and the superior portion of the orbits (Figure 3-23). The frontal bone articulates with the parietal bones, sphenoid bone, lacrimal bones, nasal bones, ethmoid bone, zygomatic bones, and maxillae. The frontal bone's portion of the superior temporal line and inferior temporal line is visible when the bone

is viewed from the lateral aspect. Internally, the frontal bone contains the paired paranasal sinuses, the **frontal sinuses** (discussed later). The frontal bone can also be studied from anterior and inferior views.

Anterior View of Frontal Bone.
On the anterior aspect (Figure 3-24), certain landmarks are visible on the frontal bone (see Chapter 2). The orbital plates of the frontal bone create the superior wall or orbital roof. The curved elevations over the superior portion of the orbit are the **supraorbital ridges** (soo-prah-**or**-bit-al), subjacent to the eyebrows. The supraorbital ridges are more prominent in adult males. The **supraorbital notch** is located on the medial portion of the supraorbital ridge and is where the supraorbital artery and nerve travel from the orbit to the forehead. The supraorbital notch is located about 1 inch from the midline and can produce soreness when palpated with pressure.

Between the supraorbital ridges is the **glabella** (glah-**bell**-ah), the smooth elevated area between the eyebrows, which tends to be flat in children and adult females and forms a rounded prominence in adult males. The prominence of the forehead, the **frontal eminence** (**em**-i-nins), is also evident. The frontal eminence is typically more pronounced in children and adult females. Lateral to the orbit is a projection, the orbital surface of the **zygomatic process of the frontal bone** (see Table 3-4).

Inferior View of Frontal Bone.
From the inferior view of the frontal bone, each **lacrimal fossa** (**lak**-ri-mal) is visible (Figure 3-25). The lacrimal fossa is located just inside the lateral portion of the supraorbital ridge. This fossa contains the

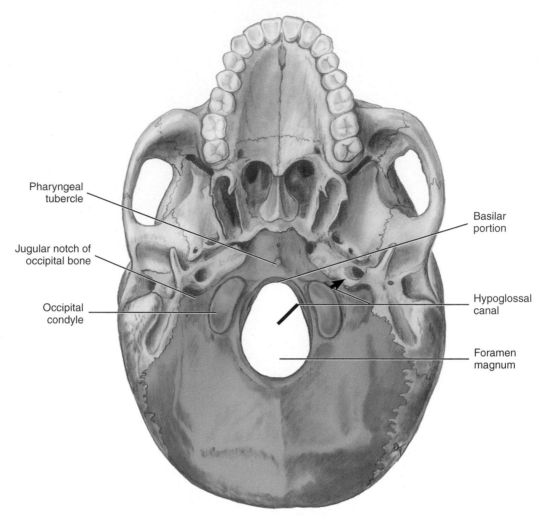

Pharyngeal
tubercle

Jugular notch of
occipital bone

Occipital
condyle

Basilar
portion

Hypoglossal
canal

Foramen
magnum

FIGURE 3-22 Inferior view of the external surface of the skull with the occipital bone highlighted.

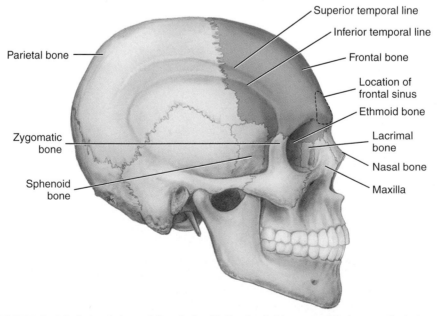

Parietal bone

Zygomatic
bone

Sphenoid
bone

Superior temporal line

Inferior temporal line

Frontal bone

Location of
frontal sinus

Ethmoid bone

Lacrimal
bone

Nasal bone

Maxilla

FIGURE 3-23 Lateral view of the skull with the frontal bone and its bony articulations.

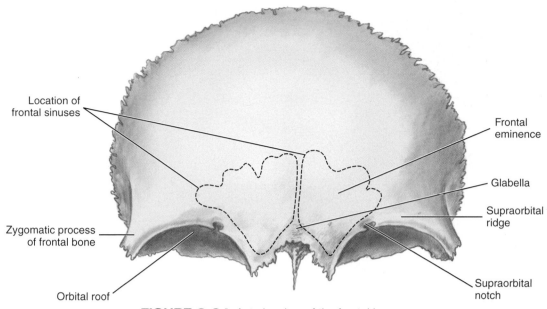

FIGURE 3-24 Anterior view of the frontal bone.

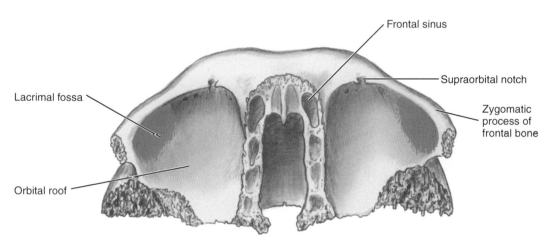

FIGURE 3-25 Inferior view of the frontal bone with the lacrimal fossa highlighted.

lacrimal gland, which produces lacrimal fluid or tears (see Chapter 7). After lubricating the eye, the lacrimal fluid empties into the nasal cavity through the naso-lacrimal duct.

PARIETAL BONES

The parietal bones are paired cranial bones and articulate with each other at the sagittal suture (Figure 3-26; see Table 3-2). The parietal bones also articulate with the occipital, frontal, temporal, and sphenoid bones.

TEMPORAL BONES

The **temporal bones** are paired cranial bones that form the lateral walls of the skull (Figure 3-27). Each temporal bone articulates with one zygomatic and one parietal bone, the occipital and sphenoid bones, and the mandible. Each temporal bone is composed of three portions: the squamous, tympanic, and petrous portions.

Portions of Temporal Bone.

The portions of the temporal bone can be viewed from the lateral aspect of the skull (Figure 3-28). The large, fan-shaped, flat portion on each of the temporal bones is the **squamous portion of the temporal bone (skwa-**mus). The second portion is the small, irregularly shaped **tympanic portion of the temporal bone** (tim-**pan**-ik), which is associated with the ear canal. The third portion is the **petrous portion of the temporal bone (pet-**rus), which is inferiorly located and helps form the cranial floor.

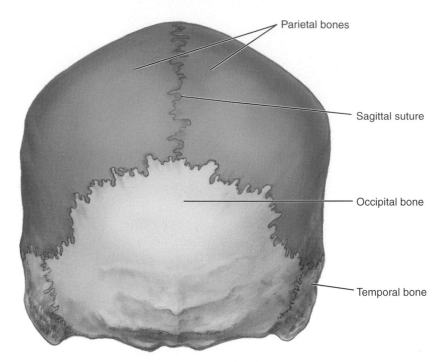

FIGURE 3-26 Posterior view of the skull with the parietal bone and some of its bony articulations.

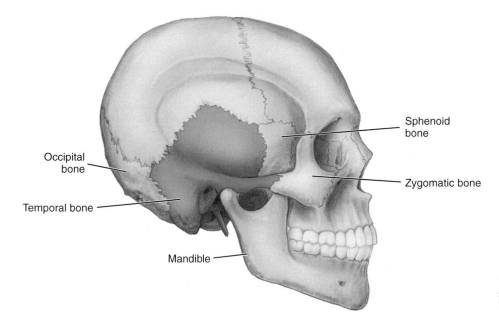

FIGURE 3-27 Lateral view of the skull with the temporal bone and its bony articulations.

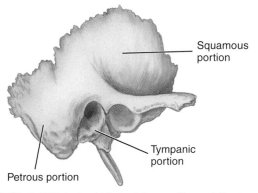

FIGURE 3-28 Lateral view of the portions of the temporal bone: squamous portion, tympanic portion, and petrous portion.

Squamous Portion of Temporal Bone.

In addition to helping form the braincase, the squamous portion of the temporal bone forms the zygomatic process of the temporal bone, which forms a portion of the zygomatic arch (Figure 3-29; see Table 3-4). This portion of the temporal bone also forms the cranial portion of the temporomandibular joint. This joint is discussed in detail in Chapter 5. On the inferior surface of the zygomatic process of the temporal bone is the **articular fossa** (ar-**tik**-you-ler).

Anterior to the articular fossa is the **articular eminence,** and posterior is the **postglenoid process** (post-**gle**-noid) (see Table 3-4). The articular fossa and

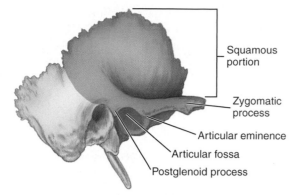

FIGURE 3-29 Lateral view of the temporal bone with the squamous portion highlighted.

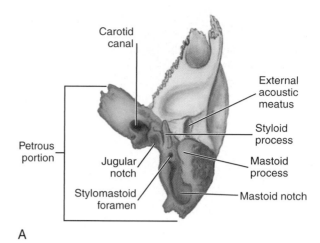

A

eminence are portions of the temporal bone that articulate with the mandible at the temporomandibular joint.

Tympanic Portion of Temporal Bone.

The tympanic portion of the temporal bone forms most of the **external acoustic meatus** (ah-**koos**-tik), a short canal leading to the tympanic cavity, located posterior to the articular fossa (Figure 3-30; see Table 3-3). Also, posterior to the articular fossa, the tympanic portion is separated from the petrosal portion by a fissure, the **petrotympanic fissure** (pe-troh-tim-**pan**-ik), through which the chorda tympani nerve emerges.

Petrous Portion of Temporal Bone.

On the inferior aspect of the petrous portion of the temporal bone, posterior to the external acoustic meatus, is a large roughened projection, the **mastoid process** (**mass**-toid) (Figure 3-31; see Table 3-4). The mastoid process is composed of air spaces or **mastoid air cells** that communicate with the middle ear cavity. The mastoid process also serves as the site for attachment of the large muscles of the neck such as the sternocleidomastoid muscle.

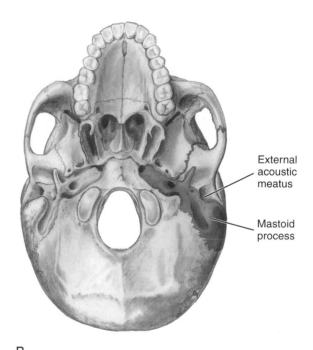

B

FIGURE 3-31 A, Inferior view of the temporal bone with the petrous portion highlighted. **B,** Location of the petrous portion of the temporal bone demonstrated on an inferior view of the skull.

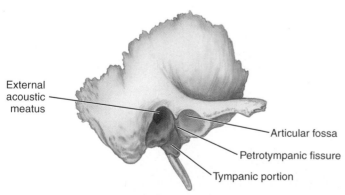

FIGURE 3-30 Lateral view of the temporal bone with the tympanic portion highlighted.

Medial to the mastoid process is the **mastoid notch** (see Figure 3-31). Inferior and medial to the external acoustic meatus is a long, pointed bony projection, the **styloid process** (**sty**-loid), a structure that serves for the attachment of tongue and pharyngeal muscles and ligaments (see Table 3-4). The **stylomastoid foramen** carries the seventh cranial or facial nerve and is named for its location between the styloid process and mastoid process (see Table 3-3). The large circular aperature of the **carotid canal** is also noted, which ascends at first vertically, and then, making a bend, runs horizontally forward and medialward; it transmits into the cranium the internal carotid artery, and the carotid plexus of nerves. When the skull model is tilted, the **jugular notch of the temporal bone** is visible (see Table 3-3), which is the lateral portion of the two bones that form the jugular foramen (the other bone is the occipital bone).

On the intracranial surface is the internal acoustic meatus, which carries the eighth cranial or vestibulo-cochlear nerve and the seventh cranial or facial nerve (see Figure 3-21; see Table 3-3). Both of these cranial nerves enter the skull from the brain. The vestibulo-cochlear nerve remains inside the petrous portion of the temporal bone, which houses the inner ear. In contrast, the facial nerve takes a convoluted path through the bone, eventually emerging at the stylo-mastoid foramen.

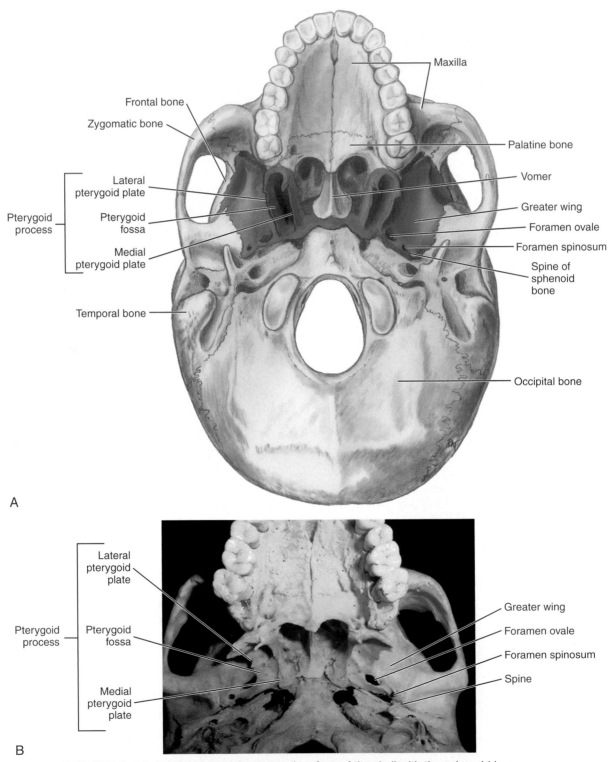

FIGURE 3-32 Inferior view of the external surface of the skull with the sphenoid bone highlighted **(A)** and close-up view of the sphenoid bone **(B).**

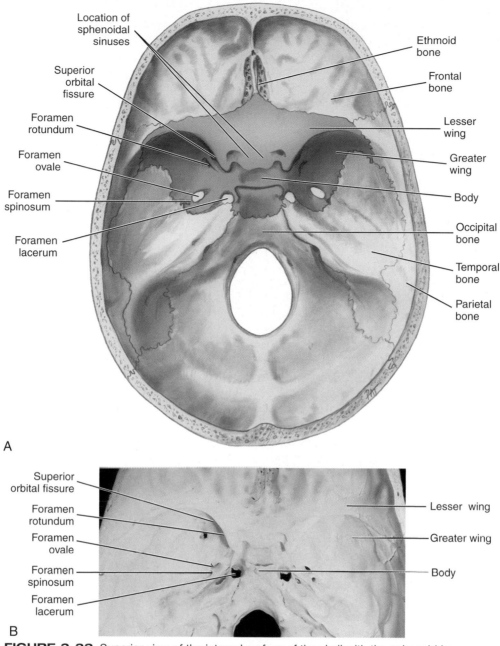

FIGURE 3-33 Superior view of the internal surface of the skull with the sphenoid bone highlighted **(A)** and close-up view of the sphenoid bone **(B).**

SPHENOID BONE

The next cranial bone of the skull to be considered is the single sphenoid bone (Figures 3-32 and 3-33). The sphenoid is a midline bone that articulates with the frontal, parietal, ethmoid, temporal, zygomatic, maxillary, palatine, vomer, and occipital bones. The sphenoid runs through the midsagittal section and helps to connect the cranial skeleton to the facial skeleton. It somewhat resembles a bat with its wings extended.

This bone is complex, with some portions of it encountered in almost every significant area of the skull. It has a number of features and projections, which allow it to be seen from various views of the skull. Thus it is one of the more difficult bones to describe and visualize. The sphenoid bone has important foramina and different portions: the body and its processes.

Foramina of the Sphenoid Bone.

Many foramina or fissures are located in the sphenoid, such as the superior orbital fissure, foramen ovale, foramen rotundum, and foramen spinosum, which carry important nerves and blood vessels of the head and neck (see Figures 3-32 and 3-33; see Table 3-3).

Body of the Sphenoid Bone.

The middle portion of the sphenoid is the **body of the sphenoid bone,** which articulates on its anterior surface with the ethmoid bone (see Figures 3-32 and 3-33). The body of the sphenoid bone articulates posteriorly with the basilar portion of the occipital bone. The body contains the paired paranasal sinuses, the **sphenoidal sinuses** (discussed later).

Processes of the Sphenoid Bone.

The body of the sphenoid bone has three paired processes that arise from it: the lesser wing, greater wing, and pterygoid process (Figure 3-34; see Figures 32-32 and 32-33 and Table 3-4). The anterior process is the **lesser wing of the sphenoid bone,** which comprises up the base of the orbital apex. The posterolateral process is the **greater wing of the sphenoid bone.**

Inferior to the greater wing of the sphenoid bone is the pterygoid process, an area for the attachment of some of the muscles of mastication. The pterygoid process consists of two plates, the flattened lateral pterygoid plate and thinner medial pterygoid plate, with the pterygoid fossa between them. The hamulus, a thin curved process, is the inferior termination of the medial pterygoid plate.

A sharp, pointed area, the **spine of the sphenoid bone,** is located at the posterior corner of each greater wing of the sphenoid bone. Each greater wing is divided into two smaller surfaces by the **infratemporal crest,** the temporal and infratemporal surfaces.

ETHMOID BONE

The ethmoid bone is a single midline cranial bone of the skull that runs through the midsagittal plane and aids to connect the cranial skeleton to the facial skeleton similar to the sphenoid bone. (Figure 3-35). The ethmoid articulates with the frontal, sphenoid, lacrimal, and maxillary bones and adjoins the vomer at its inferior and posterior border. If the sphenoid is the most difficult cranial bone to describe and visualize, the ethmoid is the second most difficult. It has a number of features and projections, but unlike the sphenoid it cannot be seen from various views of the skull.

Plates of the Ethmoid Bone and Associated Structures.

The ethmoid has two unpaired plates, the midline vertical **perpendicular plate** (per-pen-**dik**-you-lar) and the horizontal cribriform plate, which it crosses. The perpendicular plate is easily seen in the nasal cavity and aids the vomer and nasal septal cartilage in forming the nasal septum (see Figure 3-35). The cribriform plate, visible from the inside of the cranial cavity and present on the superior aspect of the bone, is perforated by foramina to allow the passage of olfactory nerves for the sense of smell (Figures 3-36 and 3-37).

The **ethmoidal sinuses** or ethmoid air cells are a variable number of small cavities in the lateral mass of the ethmoid (discussed later). A vertical midline

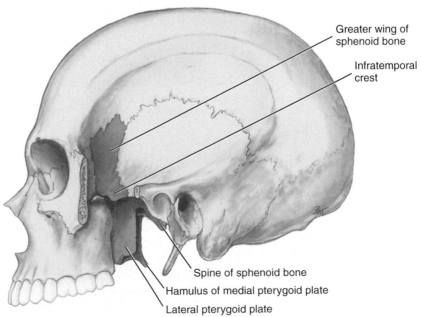

Greater wing of sphenoid bone

Infratemporal crest

Spine of sphenoid bone

Hamulus of medial pterygoid plate

Lateral pterygoid plate

FIGURE 3-34 Cutaway view of the lateral aspect of the upper portion of the skull with the sphenoid bone highlighted.

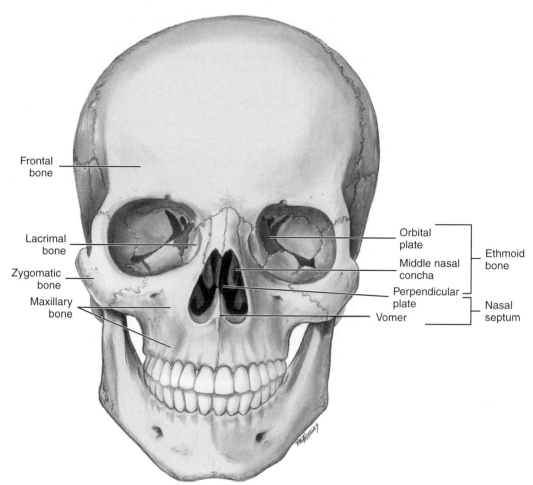

Frontal
bone

Lacrimal
bone

Zygomatic
bone

Maxillary
bone

Orbital
plate

Middle nasal
concha

Perpendicular
plate

Vomer

Ethmoid
bone

Nasal
septum

FIGURE 3-35 Anterior view of the skull with the ethmoid bone highlighted.

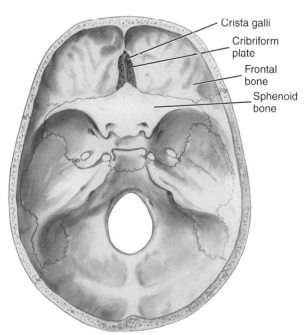

Crista galli

Cribriform
plate

Frontal
bone

Sphenoid
bone

FIGURE 3-36 Superior view of the internal surface of the skull with the ethmoid bone highlighted.

continuation of the perpendicular plate into the cranial cavity is the **crista galli** (**kris**-tah **gal**-lee). The crista galli serves as an attachment for layers covering the brain.

Nasal Conchae and Associated Structures.
The lateral portions of the ethmoid form the **superior nasal conchae** (**kong**-kee) and **middle nasal conchae** in the nasal cavity and the paired orbital plates (Figure 3-38; see Figure 3-37). The **orbital plate of the ethmoid bone** forms the medial orbital wall. Between the orbital plate and the conchae are the **ethmoidal sinuses,** which consist of air-filled spaces (discussed later).

Facial Bones

The facial bones create the facial features and serve as a base for dentition. The facial bones include the single vomer and mandible and the paired lacrimal, nasal, inferior nasal conchal, zygomatic, and maxillary bones (see Figure 3-4). For ease of learning, the palatine bones are considered under the heading of facial bones, but they are not strictly considered facial bones.

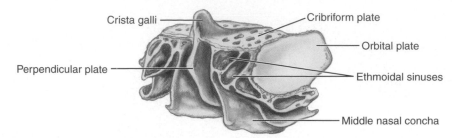

FIGURE 3-37 Oblique anterior view of the ethmoid bone with its perpendicular, cribriform, and orbital plates.

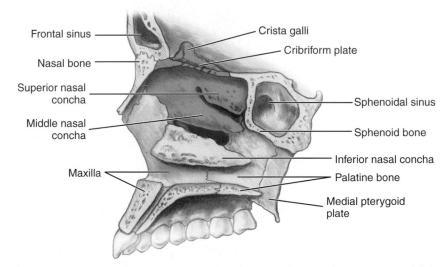

FIGURE 3-38 Lateral wall of the right nasal cavity with the ethmoid bone highlighted.

Many bones of the face are shared by two or more soft tissue components of the face. For example, the frontal bone forms both the forehead and the areas around the eyes. This is important to remember because an abnormality in one facial bone often involves many soft tissue components (discussed later).

VOMER

The vomer is a single midline facial bone of the skull that forms the posterior portion of the nasal septum. It is located in the midsagittal plane inside the nasal cavity. The articulations of the vomer are easily seen on a lateral view of the bone (Figure 3-39). The vomer articulates with the ethmoid bone on its antero-superior border, the nasal cartilage anteriorly, the palatine bones and maxillae inferiorly, and the sphenoid bone on its posterosuperior border. The postero-inferior border is free of any bony articulation. The vomer has no muscle attachments.

LACRIMAL BONES, NASAL BONES, AND INFERIOR NASAL CONCHAE

The paired lacrimal bones are irregular, thin plates of bone that form a small portion of the anterior medial wall of the orbit (Figure 3-40). The lacrimal bones are the smallest and most fragile of the facial bones. Each lacrimal bone articulates with the ethmoid, frontal, and maxillary bones. The **nasolacrimal duct** (nay-so-lak-rim-al) is formed at the junction of the lacrimal and maxillary bones. Lacrimal fluid or tears from the lacrimal gland are drained through this duct into the inferior nasal meatus (see Chapter 7).

The nasal bones are paired facial bones that form the bridge of the nose, articulating with each other in the midline superior to the piriform aperture. The nasal bones fit between the frontal processes of the maxillae and thus articulate with the frontal bone superiorly and the maxillae laterally (see Figure 3-40).

The inferior nasal conchae are paired facial bones that project from the maxilla to form a portion of

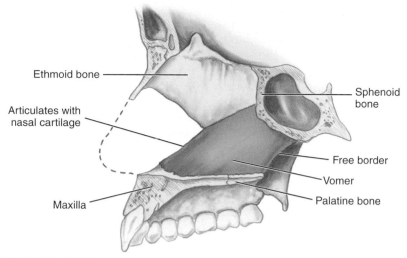

Ethmoid bone

Articulates with
nasal cartilage

Maxilla

Sphenoid
bone

Free border

Vomer

Palatine bone

FIGURE 3-39 Medial wall of the left nasal cavity with the vomer highlighted (outline of nasal cartilage).

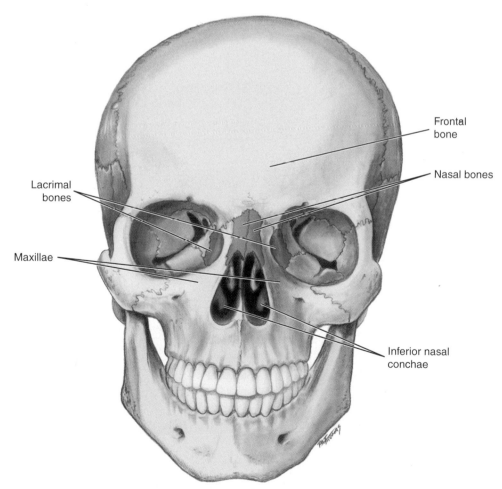

Lacrimal
bones

Maxillae

Frontal
bone

Nasal bones

Inferior nasal
conchae

FIGURE 3-40 Anterior view of the skull with the nasal bones, lacrimal bones, and inferior nasal conchae highlighted.

the lateral walls of the nasal cavity (see Figure 3-40). Unlike the superior and middle nasal conchae that also project from the maxillae, the inferior nasal conchae are separate facial bones. Each inferior nasal concha is composed of fragile, thin, spongy bone curved onto itself like a scroll. By projecting into the nasal cavity, the medial surface of these bones assists in increasing the surface area within the cavity and thus increases the amount of mucous membrane and olfactory nerve endings exposed to inhaled odors. These bones articulate with the ethmoid, lacrimal, palatine, and maxillary bones. The inferior nasal conchae do not have any muscle attachments.

ZYGOMATIC BONES

The zygomatic bones are paired facial bones of the skull that form the cheekbones or malar surfaces (Figures 3-41 and 3-42). The zygomatic bones articulate with the frontal, temporal, sphenoid, and maxillary bones. Each zygomatic bone has a diamond shape composed of three processes with similarly named associated bony articulations: the frontal, temporal, and maxillary processes.

Processes of the Zygomatic Bone.
Each process of the zygomatic bone forms important structures of the skull (see Figures 3-41 and 3-42 and Table 3-4). The orbital surface of the **frontal process of the zygomatic bone** forms the anterior lateral orbital wall. The **temporal process of the zygomatic bone** forms the zygomatic arch, together with the zygomatic process of the temporal bone. The orbital surface of the **maxillary process of the zygomatic bone** forms a portion of the **infraorbital rim** (in-frah-or-bit-al) and a small portion of the anterior portion of the lateral orbital wall.

PALATINE BONES

The palatine bones are paired bones of the skull that are not strictly considered facial bones, but they are considered under this heading for ease of learning. Each palatine bone consists of two plates, the horizontal and vertical plates.

Plates of the Palatine Bone.
Both the horizontal and vertical plates can be seen from a posterior view of a palatine bone (Figure 3-43).

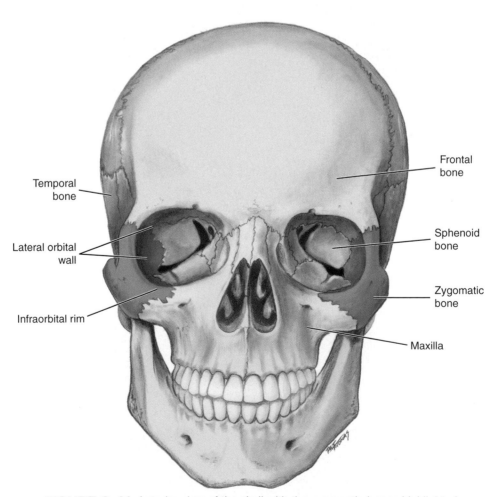

FIGURE 3-41 Anterior view of the skull with the zygomatic bones highlighted.

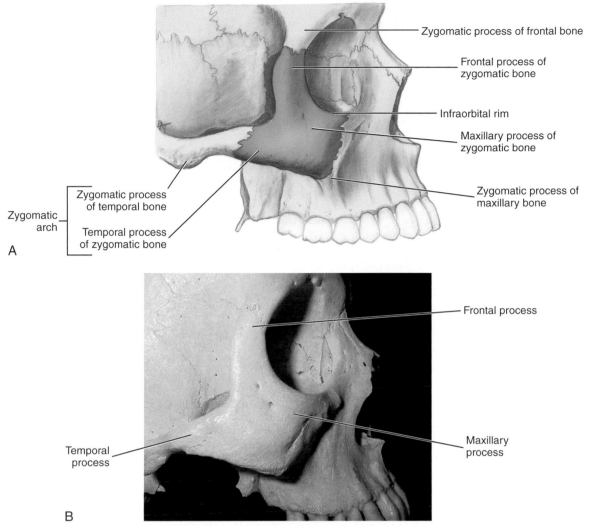

Zygomatic process of frontal bone

Frontal process of zygomatic bone

Infraorbital rim

Maxillary process of zygomatic bone

Zygomatic process of maxillary bone

Zygomatic process of temporal bone

Temporal process of zygomatic bone

Zygomatic arch

A

Frontal process

Maxillary process

Temporal process

B

FIGURE 3-42 Lateral view of the upper portion of the skull with the zygomatic bone highlighted **(A)** and close-up view of the zygomatic bone **(B).**

The **horizontal plates of the palatine bones** form the posterior portion of the hard palate. The **vertical plates of the palatine bones** form a portion of the lateral walls of the nasal cavity, and each plate contributes a small lip of bone to the orbital apex.

Suture of the Palatine Bones.
The palatine bones serve as a link between the maxillae and the sphenoid bone with which they articulate, as well as with each other. The two horizontal plates articulate with each other at the posterior portion of the median palatine suture (Figure 3-44; see Table 3-2).

Foramina of the Palatine Bones.
Two important foramina in the palatine bones, the greater and lesser palatine foramina (see Figure 3-44 and Table 3-3), transmit nerves and blood vessels to this region. The **greater palatine foramen** is located in the posterolateral region of each of the palatine bones, usually at the apex of the maxillary third molar. The greater palatine foramen transmits the greater palatine nerve and blood vessels and is a landmark for the administration of the greater palatine local anesthetic block.

A smaller opening nearby, the **lesser palatine foramen,** transmits the lesser palatine nerve and blood vessels to the soft palate and tonsils. Both foramina are openings of the pterygopalatine canal that carries the descending palatine nerves and blood vessels from the pterygopalatine fossa to the palate.

MAXILLA
The upper jaw or maxilla consists of two maxillary bones or **maxillae** (mak-**sil**-lay) that are fused together at the intermaxillary suture (Figure 3-45). The maxillae articulate with the frontal, lacrimal, nasal, inferior nasal conchal, vomer, sphenoid, ethmoid, palatine,

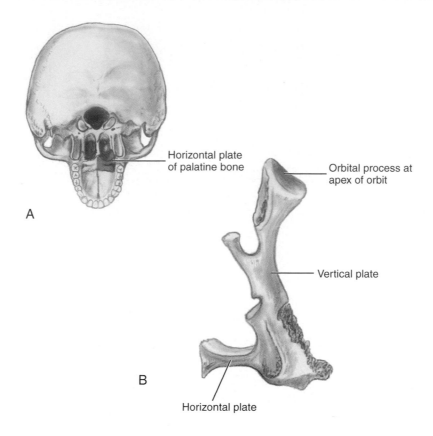

FIGURE 3-43 Posterior view of the right palatine bone with its location demonstrated on a posterior-inferior view of the skull.

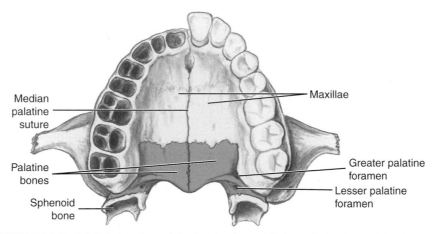

FIGURE 3-44 Inferior view of the hard palate with the palatine bones highlighted.

and zygomatic bones. Each maxilla includes a body and four processes: the frontal, zygomatic, palatine, and alveolar processes.

The **body of the maxilla** has orbital, nasal, infra-temporal, and facial surfaces. The bodies contain air-filled spaces or paranasal sinuses, the **maxillary sinuses** (discussed later). The maxilla can be studied from its three views: the anterior, lateral, and inferior views.

Anterior View of the Maxilla.

The **frontal process of the maxilla** articulates with the frontal bone and forms the medial orbital rim with the lacrimal bone on its anterior surface (Figures 3-46 and 3-47; see Figure 3-45 and Table 3-4). Each maxilla's orbital surface is separated from the sphenoid bone by the **inferior orbital fissure** (see Figure 3-7 and Table 3-3). The inferior orbital fissure carries the infraorbital and zygomatic nerves, infraorbital artery, and inferior

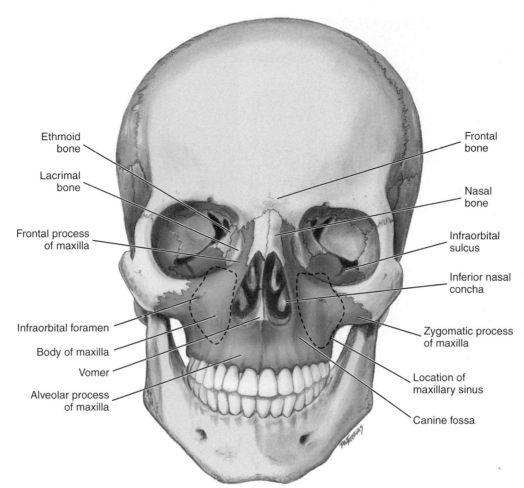

FIGURE 3-45 Anterior view of the skull with the maxilla and its bony articulations *(articulation of the maxilla with the pterygoid process of the sphenoid bone and palatine bones cannot be seen in this view).*

ophthalmic vein. The groove in the floor of the orbital surface is the **infraorbital sulcus.**

The infraorbital sulcus becomes the **infraorbital canal** and then terminates on the facial surface of the maxilla as the **infraorbital foramen** (see Table 3-3). It is located approximately 2 cm inferior to the midpoint of the lower margin of the orbit, in a vertical line with the supraorbital and notch, which is superior to it. This foramen transmits the infraorbital nerve and blood vessels. The infraorbital foramen is a landmark for the administration of the infraorbital local anesthetic block. Palpation of the infraorbital foramen will cause soreness on a patient. Inferior to the infraorbital foramen is an elongated depression, the **canine fossa** (**kay**-nine). The canine fossa is just posterosuperior to the roots of the maxillary canine teeth.

Each tooth of the maxillary arch is covered by a prominent facial ridge of bone, a portion of the alveolar process of the maxilla (see Table 3-4). The facial ridge over the maxillary canine, the **canine eminence,** is especially prominent, making it a landmark for the administration of the anterior superior alveolar local anesthetic block. The maxillary bone over the facial surface of the maxillary teeth is less dense than the mandible over similar teeth. This allows a greater incidence of clinically adequate local anesthesia for the maxillary teeth when the agent is administered as a local infiltration (see Chapter 9).

Lateral View of the Maxilla.

The **zygomatic process of the maxilla** articulates with the zygomatic bone laterally, completing the **infraorbital rim** (see Figures 3-46 and 3-47 and Table 3-4). Some of the landmarks noted in the anterior view of the maxilla are also present.

Inferior View of the Maxillae.

On the inferior surface, each **palatine process of the maxilla** articulates with the other to form the anterior, major portion of the hard palate (Figure 3-48; see Figure 3-46 and Table 3-4). The suture between these two palatine processes of the maxillae is the anterior portion of the median palatine suture (see Table 3-2). In the patient, this is covered by the median palatine raphe, a midline fibrous band of tissue.

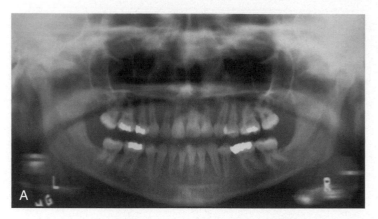

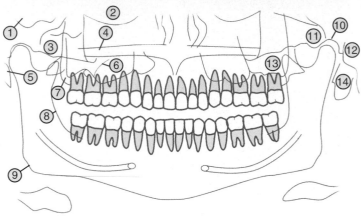

① Middle cranial fossa	⑧ External oblique line
② Orbit	⑨ Angle of mandible
③ Zygomatic arch	⑩ Glenoid fossa
④ Palate	⑪ Articular eminence
⑤ Styloid process	⑫ Vertebra
⑥ Septa in maxillary sinus	⑬ Maxillary sinus
⑦ Maxillary tuberosity	⑭ Ear lobe

FIGURE 3-46 A, Panoramic radiograph. **B,** Panoramic anatomy of the midface. (**A,** From Bath-Balogh M, Fehrenbach MJ: *Illustrated dental embryology, histology, and anatomy*, ed 6, St. Louis, 2006, Saunders. **B,** Modified from Olson SS: *Dental radiography laboratory manual,* Philadelphia, 1995, WB Saunders.)

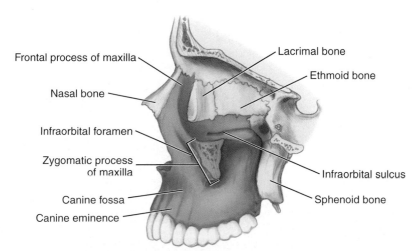

Frontal process of maxilla

Nasal bone

Infraorbital foramen

Zygomatic process of maxilla

Canine fossa

Canine eminence

Lacrimal bone

Ethmoid bone

Infraorbital sulcus

Sphenoid bone

FIGURE 3-47 Cutaway view of the lateral aspect of the skull with the maxilla highlighted.

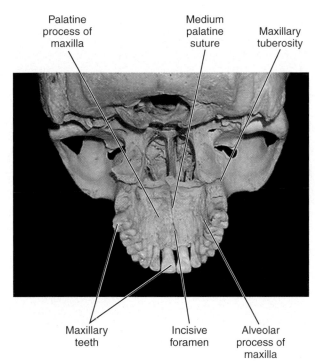

Palatine process of maxilla

Medium palatine suture

Maxillary tuberosity

Maxillary teeth

Incisive foramen

Alveolar process of maxilla

FIGURE 3-48 Posteroinferior view of the maxillae and hard palate.

In the anterior midline portion of the palatine process, just posterior to the maxillary central incisors, is the **incisive foramen** (in-sy-ziv) (see Table 3-3). This foramen carries the branches of the right and left nasopalatine nerves and blood vessels from the nasal cavity to the palate. The incisive foramen is a landmark for the administration of the nasopalatine local anesthetic block. The soft tissue that bulges over the incisive foramen in the patient is called the **incisive papilla.**

The alveolar process of the maxilla usually contains the roots of the maxillary teeth (see Figures 3-46 and 3-48 and Table 3-4). The alveolar process of the maxilla can become resorbed in a patient who is completely edentulous in the maxillary arch (resorption occurs to a lesser extent in partially edentulous cases), possibly leading to problems with the maxillary sinuses (discussed later). The body of the maxilla is not resorbed with tooth loss, but its walls may become thinner in this case.

The density of the maxillary bone in an area determines the route that a dental infection takes with abscess and fistula formation (see Chapter 12). Finally, the differences in alveolar process density determine the easiest and most convenient areas of bony fracture used during tooth extraction. Thus the maxillary teeth are mechanically easier to remove by fracturing the thinner facial surface rather than the thicker lingual surface.

On the posterior portion of the body of the maxilla is a rounded, roughened elevation, the **maxillary tuberosity,** just posterior to the most distal molar of the maxillary dentition (see Figures 3-46 to 3-48). The superolateral portion of the maxillary tuberosity is perforated by one or more **posterior superior alveolar foramina,** where the posterior superior alveolar nerve and blood vessel branches enter the bone from the back. The maxillary tuberosity is a landmark for the administration of the posterior superior alveolar local anesthetic block.

MANDIBLE

The lower jaw, or mandible, is a single facial bone that is the only freely movable bone of the skull (Figures 3-49 and 3-50). This bone is also the largest and strongest facial bone. The mandible has a movable

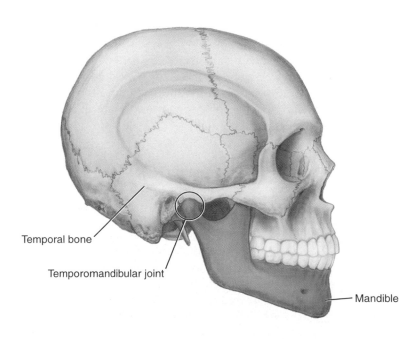

Temporal bone

Temporomandibular joint

Mandible

FIGURE 3-49 Lateral view of the skull showing the mandible and the temporomandibular joint.

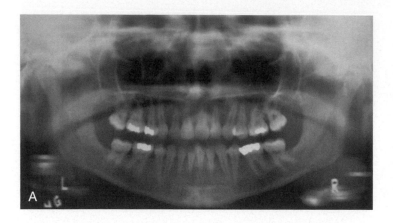

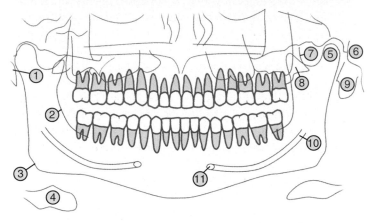

1. Styloid process
2. External oblique line
3. Angle of mandible
4. Hyoid bone
5. Mandibular condyle
6. Vertebra
7. Coronoid process
8. Pterygoid plates
9. Ear lobe
10. Mandibular canal
11. Mental foramen

B

FIGURE 3-50 A, Panoramic radiograph.
B, Panoramic anatomy of the lower face. (**A,** From Bath-Balogh M, Fehrenbach MJ: *Illustrated dental embryology, histology, and anatomy*, ed 6, St. Louis, 2006, Saunders. **B,** Modified from Olson SS: *Dental radiography laboratory manual*, Philadelphia, 1995, WB Saunders.)

articulation with the temporal bones at each temporomandibular joint (see Chapter 5). The mandible also articulates with each of the maxillae by way of their contained respective lower and upper dentition. The mandible is more effectively studied when it is temporarily removed from the skull model. The mandible can be studied from three views: the anterior, lateral, and medial views.

Anterior View of the Mandible.

On the anterior surface of the mandible are many important landmarks (Figures 3-51 to 3-53). The **mental protuberance** (**ment**-il pro-**too**-ber-ins), the bony prominence of the chin, is located deep to the roots of the mandibular incisors. The mental protuberance is more pronounced in males but can be visualized and palpated in females. In the midline on the surface of the mandible is a faint ridge, an indication of the mandibular **symphysis** (**sim**-fi-sis),

where the bone is formed by the fusion of right and left processes. Like other symphyses in the body, this is a midline articulation where the bones are joined by fibrocartilage, but this articulation fuses together in early childhood.

Farther posteriorly on the surface of the mandible, typically between the apices of the first and second mandibular premolars, is an opening called the **mental foramen** (see Figures 3-50 to 3-52 and Table 3-3). As mandibular growth proceeds in young children, the mental foramen alters in direction from anterior to posterosuperior. The mental foramen allows the entrance of the mental nerve and blood vessels into the mandibular canal (discussed later).

The mental foramen's posterosuperior opening in adults signifies the changed direction of the emerging mental nerve. This is an important landmark to note intraorally and on a radiograph before administration of a mental or incisive local anesthetic block. Not confusing the mental foramen on a radiograph with a

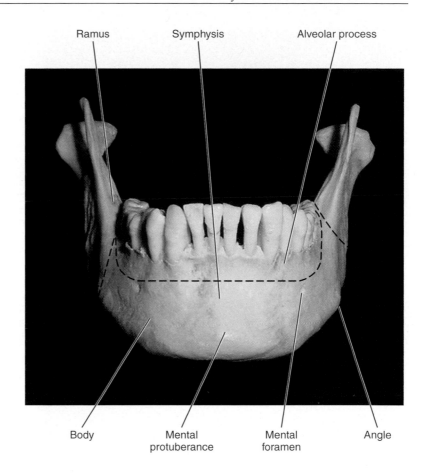

FIGURE 3-51 Anterior view of the mandible and its associated landmarks.

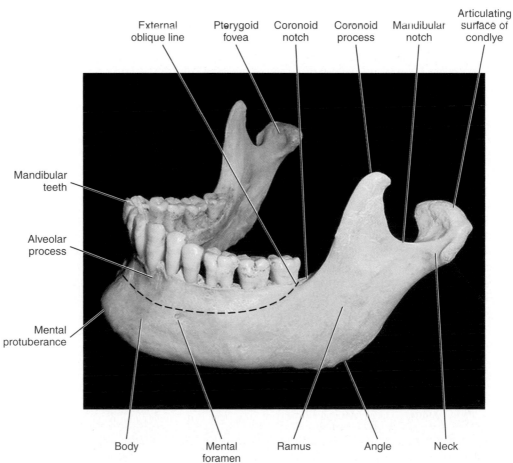

FIGURE 3-52 Slightly oblique lateral view of the mandible and its associated landmarks.

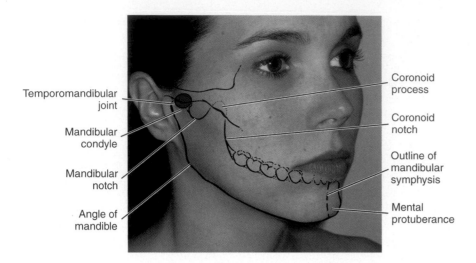

Temporomandibular joint

Mandibular condyle

Mandibular notch

Angle of mandible

Coronoid process

Coronoid notch

Outline of mandibular symphysis

Mental protuberance

FIGURE 3-53 Lateral view of the face showing the landmarks of the mandible.

periapical lesion related to the teeth or other oral radiolucent lesions is also important.

The heavy horizontal portion of the lower jaw inferior to the mental foramen is called the **body of the mandible** (see Figure 3-51). Superior to this, the portion of the lower jaw that usually contains the roots of the mandibular teeth is the alveolar process of the mandible (see Figure 3-52 and Table 3-4). The body of the mandible, along with the alveolar process, elongates to provide space for additional teeth as the child nears adulthood.

The mandibular alveolar process can become resorbed if a patient becomes completely edentulous in the mandibular arch (occasionally noted also in partially edentulous cases). This resorption can occur to such an extent that the mental foramen is virtually on the superior border of the mandible, instead of opening on the anterior surface, changing its relative position. The body of the mandible is not affected and remains thick and rounded.

The alveolar process of the mandibular incisors is less dense than the body of the mandible and even less dense than the alveolar process of the posterior teeth, allowing local infiltration of the mandibular incisors by a local anesthetic agent with varying degrees of success (see Chapter 9). The density of the mandibular bone in an area also determines the route that a dental infection takes with abscess and fistula formation (see Chapter 12). Finally, the differences in alveolar process density determine the easiest and most convenient areas of bony fracture used during tooth extraction. Thus the mandibular third molar is mechanically easier to remove by fracturing the thinner lingual surface (being careful of the nearby lingual nerve) rather than the thicker buccal surface.

Lateral View of the Mandible.
On the lateral aspect of the mandible, the stout, flat plate of the **ramus** (**ray**-mus) extends superiorly and

posteriorly from the body of the mandible on each side (see Figure 3-52). During growth of the body, the body of the mandible and alveolar process elongates posterior to the mental foramen, providing space for three additional permanent teeth. The ramus, which serves as the primary area for the attachment of the muscles of mastication, grows superiorly and posteriorly, displacing the mental protuberance of the chin inferiorly and anteriorly as one nears adulthood.

The anterior border of the ramus is a thin, sharp margin that terminates in the **coronoid process** (**kor**-ah-noid) (see Table 3-4). The main portion of the anterior border of the ramus forms a concave forward curve called the **coronoid notch.** The coronoid notch is a landmark for the administration of the inferior alveolar local anesthetic block. Inferior to the coronoid notch, the anterior border of the ramus becomes the **external oblique line** (ob-**leek**). The external oblique line or ridge is a crest where the ramus joins the body of the mandible. The line is noted as a radiopaque line on a radiograph superior to the mylohyoid line. Many clinicians use this line intraorally to help locate the coronoid notch.

The posterior border of the ramus is thickened and extends from the **angle of the mandible** to a projection, the **condyle of the mandible** with its neck (see Figures 3-50 to 3-53). The **articulating surface of the condyle** (ar-**tik**-you-late-ing) is an oval head involved in the temporomandibular joint. Between the coronoid process and the condyle is a depression, the **mandibular notch** (man-**dib**-you-lar).

Medial View of the Mandible.
Visible on the internal or medial view of the mandible are the body of the mandible, alveolar process of the mandible (see Table 3-4), and ramus (Figure 3-54). In addition, near the midline of the mandible is a cluster of small projections called the **genial tubercles** (ji-**ni**-il) or mental spines, which is another muscle attachment area.

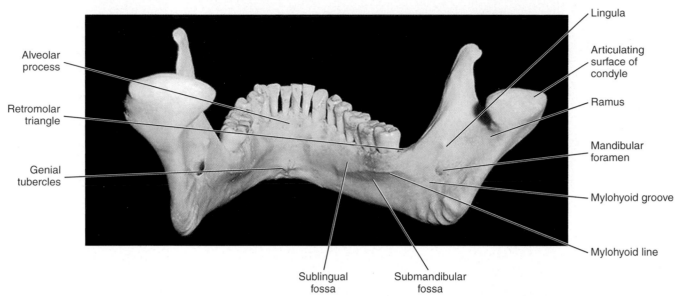

FIGURE 3-54 Internal or medial view of the mandible and its associated landmarks.

At the lateral edge of each mandibular alveolar process is a rounded, roughened area, the **retromolar triangle** (re-tro-**moh**-lar), just posterior to the most distal molar of the mandibular dentition. The retromolar triangle is a bony landmark that, when covered with soft tissue, is the retromolar pad.

Along each medial surface of the body of the mandible is the **mylohyoid line** (my-lo-**hi**-oid) or internal oblique ridge that extends posteriorly and superiorly, becoming more prominent as it ascends each body. The mylohyoid line is the point of attachment of the mylohyoid muscle that forms the floor of the mouth. The roots of the posterior mandibular teeth often extend internally inferior to the mylohyoid line. The line can be noted on a radiograph as the radiopaque line inferior to the external oblique line.

A shallow depression, the **sublingual fossa** (sub-**ling**-gwal), which contains the sublingual salivary gland, is located superior to the anterior portion of the mylohyoid line. Inferior to the posterior portion of the mylohyoid line and inferior to the posterior mandibular teeth is a deeper depression, the **submandibular fossa** (sub-man-**dib**-you-lar), which contains the submandibular salivary gland.

On the internal surface of the ramus is a central opening, the **mandibular foramen** (man-**dib**-you-lar), which is the opening of the **mandibular canal** (see Figure 3-54 and Table 3-3). The mandibular foramen is three-fourths the distance from the coronoid notch to the posterior border of the ramus. The inferior alveolar nerve and blood vessels exit the mandible through the mandibular foramen after traveling in the mandibular canal. With age and tooth loss, the alveolar process is absorbed so that the mandibular canal is nearer the

superior border. Sometimes with excessive alveolar process absorption, the mandibular canal disappears entirely and leaves the inferior alveolar nerve without its bony protection, although it is still covered by soft tissues.

Rarely, a patient may have a bifid inferior alveolar nerve, in which case a second mandibular foramen, more inferiorly placed, exists and can be detected by noting a doubled mandibular canal on a radiograph (see Chapter 8). Keeping this anatomical variant concerning the mandibular foramen, as well as its usual location, in mind is important when administering an inferior alveolar local anesthetic block.

Overhanging the mandibular foramen is a bony spine, the **lingula** (**lin**-gu-lah), which serves as an attachment for the sphenomandibular ligament associated with the temporomandibular joint (see Chapter 5). A small groove, the **mylohyoid groove**, passes forward and downward from the mandibular foramen. The mylohyoid nerve and blood vessels travel in the mylohyoid groove.

The **articulating surface of the condyle** (ar-**tik**-you-late-ing) can be seen in this view. This is where the mandible articulates with the temporal bone at the temporomandibular joint (see Chapter 5). Inferior to the articular surface of the condyle on the anterior surface is a triangular depression, the **pterygoid fovea** (**fo**-vee-ah) (see Figure 3-52).

Paranasal Sinuses

The **paranasal sinuses** (pare-ah-**na**-zil) are paired, air-filled cavities in bone (Figures 3-55 and 3-56). These sinuses are lined with mucous membranes. The para-

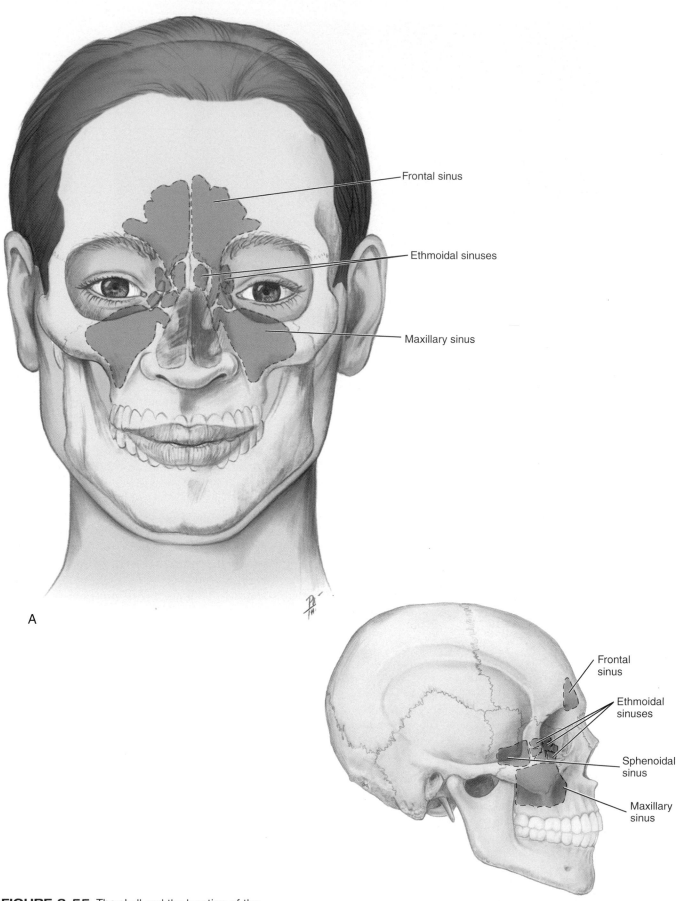

A

B

FIGURE 3-55 The skull and the location of the paranasal sinuses: anterior view **(A)** and lateral view **(B).**

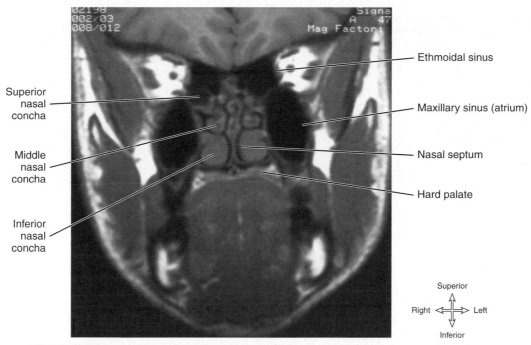

FIGURE 3-56 Coronal magnetic resonance imaging of the nasopharynx and oropharynx showing the ethmoid and maxillary sinuses. (From Reynolds PA, Abrahams PH: *McMinn's interactive clinical anatomy: head and neck*, ed 2, London, 2001, Mosby Ltd.)

nasal sinuses include the frontal, sphenoidal, ethmoidal, and maxillary sinuses. The sinuses communicate with the nasal cavity through small ostia or openings in the lateral nasal wall.

The sinuses serve to lighten the skull bones, act as sound resonators, and provide mucus for the nasal cavity. The mucous membranes of the sinuses can become inflamed and congested with mucus as in a **primary sinusitis** (sy-nu-**si**-tis). A primary sinusitis can involve allergies or an infection occurring in the sinus. The symptoms of sinusitis are headache, usually near the involved sinus, and foul-smelling nasal or pharyngeal discharge, possibly with some systemic signs of infection such as fever and weakness. The skin over the involved sinus can be tender, hot, and red due to the inflammatory process in the area.

Recent studies have found that the cause of chronic sinus infections lies in the nasal mucus, not in the nasal and sinus tissue targeted by standard treatment. This suggests a beneficial effect in treatments that target primarily the underlying and presumably damage-inflicting nasal and sinus membrane inflammation, instead of the secondary bacterial infection that has been the primary target of treatments for the disease. Also, some surgeons have already started to change the way they perform surgery for patients with chronic sinus infections: they now focus on removing the mucus, which is loaded with toxins from the inflammatory cells, rather than the tissue during surgery. Leaving the mucus behind might predispose patients for early recurrence of the chronic sinus infection. If any surgery

is performed, it is to enlarge the ostia in the lateral walls of the nasal cavity, creating adequate drainage.

An infection in one sinus can travel through the nasal cavity to other sinuses, leading to serious complications for the patient. Because the maxillary posterior teeth are in close proximity to the maxillary sinus, this can also create clinical problems if there are any disease processes are present, such as an infection in any of these teeth (discussed later and also in Chapter 12). These clinical problems can include a **secondary sinusitis,** inflammation of the sinuses from another source such as an infection of the adjacent teeth. A **perforation,** an abnormal hole in the wall of the sinus, also can occur with infection.

FRONTAL SINUSES

The paired frontal sinuses are located in the frontal bone just superior to the nasal cavity (see Figures 3-23 and 3-25). These two paranasal sinuses are asymmetrical (approximately 2 to 3 cm in diameter), but the left and right sinuses are always separated by a septum. Each frontal sinus communicates with and drains into the nasal cavity by a constricted canal to the middle nasal meatus, the **frontonasal duct** (frunt-o-**na**-zil). Standing near the patient during an extraoral examination, visually inspect and bilaterally palpate the frontal sinuses (Figure 3-57).

SPHENOIDAL SINUSES

The paired sphenoidal sinuses are located in the body of the sphenoid bone and cannot be palpated during

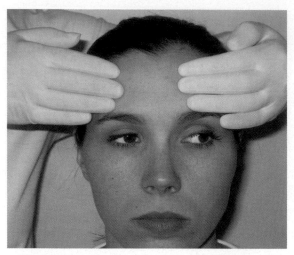

FIGURE 3-57 Palpation of the frontal sinuses.

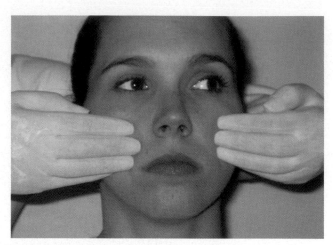

FIGURE 3-58 Palpation of the maxillary sinuses.

an extraoral examination (see Figure 3-33). These two paranasal sinuses are frequently asymmetrical (approximately 1.5 to 2.5 cm in diameter). The sphenoidal sinuses communicate with and drain into the nasal cavity through an opening superior to each superior nasal concha.

ETHMOIDAL SINUSES

The ethmoidal sinuses or ethmoid air cells are a variable number of small cavities in the lateral mass of each of the ethmoid bones and cannot be palpated during an extraoral examination (see Figure 3-37). These paranasal sinuses are roughly divided into the anterior, middle, and posterior ethmoid air cells. The posterior ethmoid air cells open into the superior meatus of the nasal cavity, and the middle and anterior ethmoid air cells open into the middle meatus.

MAXILLARY SINUSES

The maxillary sinuses are paired paranasal sinuses, each located in the body of the maxilla, just posterior to the maxillary canine and premolars (see Figures 3-45 and 3-46). The size varies according to individuals and their ages. These pyramid-shaped sinuses are the largest of the paranasal sinuses, and each one has an apex, three walls, a roof, and a floor. A portion of the sinuses can be seen on radiographs of the maxillary posterior teeth. During an extraoral examination, the maxillary sinuses (Figure 3-58) are visually inspected and bilaterally palpated.

The apex of the pyramid of the maxillary sinus points into the zygomatic arch, and the medial wall is formed by the lateral wall of the nasal cavity. The anterior wall corresponds with the anterior or facial wall of the maxilla, and the posterior wall is the infratemporal surface of the maxilla, the maxillary tuberosity. The roof of the maxillary sinus is the orbital floor, and the floor is the alveolar process of each maxilla.

Each maxillary sinus is divided into communicating compartments by bony walls or septa.

Due to the close proximity of the maxillary sinus to the alveolar process containing the roots of the maxillary posterior teeth, the periodontal tissues of these teeth may be in direct contact with the mucosa of the maxillary sinus. This close proximity can cause serious clinical problems such as secondary sinusitis and perforation during infection (see Chapter 12), extraction, or trauma related to the maxillary posterior teeth. The discomfort associated with a primary maxillary sinus infection can mimic the same discomfort with an endodontic or periodontal infection of the maxillary posterior teeth.

With age, the enlarging maxillary sinus may surround the roots of the maxillary posterior teeth and extend its margins into the body of the zygoma. If the maxillary posterior teeth are lost, the maxillary sinus may expand even more, thinning the bony floor of the alveolar process so that only a thin shell of bone is present.

The maxillary sinus drains into the middle meatus on each side. Drainage of the maxillary sinus is complicated and may promote a prolonged or chronic sinusitis because the ostium of each sinus is higher than the floor of the sinus cavity. Surgery may be required in the case of chronic maxillary sinusitis.

Fossae of the Skull

Three deeper depressions or fossae are present on the external surface of the skull. The bony boundaries for these paired fossae—the temporal, infratemporal, and pterygopalatine fossae—should be located on the skull model and skull diagrams (Table 3-6). These fossae are important landmarks of the skull for locating muscles, blood vessels, and nerves (Table 3-7).

TABLE 3-6

BOUNDARIES OF FOSSAE OF THE SKULL

Boundaries of Fossae	Temporal Fossa	Infratemporal Fossa	Pterygopalatine Fossa
Superior	Inferior temporal line	Greater wing of sphenoid bone	Inferior surface of sphenoid bone body
Anterior	Frontal process of zygomatic bone	Maxillary tuberosity	Maxillary tuberosity
Medial	Surface of temporal bone	Lateral pterygoid plate	
Lateral	Zygomatic arch	Mandibular ramus and zygomatic arch	Pterygomaxillary fissure
Inferior	Infratemporal crest of sphenoid bone	No bony border	Pterygopalatine canal
Posterior	Inferior temporal line	No bony border	Pterygoid process of sphenoid bone

TABLE 3-7

MUSCLES, BLOOD VESSELS, AND NERVES OF FOSSAE OF THE SKULL

	Temporal Fossa	Infratemporal Fossa	Pterygopalatine Fossa
Muscles	Temporalis muscle	Pterygoid muscles	
Blood vessels	Area blood vessels	Pterygoid plexus and maxillary artery (second portion) and branches including middle meningeal artery, inferior alveolar artery, and posterior superior alveolar artery	Maxillary artery (third portion) and branches including infraorbital and sphenopalatine arteries
Nerves	Area nerves	Mandibular nerve including inferior alveolar and lingual nerves	Pterygopalatine ganglion and maxillary nerve

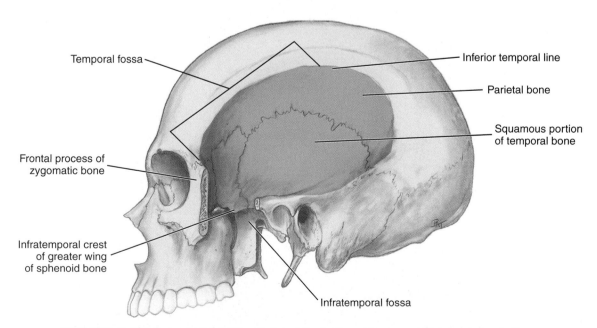

FIGURE 3-59 Lateral view of the skull and the temporal fossa and its boundaries *(with portions of the zygomatic and temporal bones removed).*

TEMPORAL FOSSA

The temporal fossa is a flat, fan-shaped paired depression on the lateral surface of the skull (Figure 3-59; see Figure 3-13). The temporal fossa is formed by portions of five bones: the zygomatic, frontal, greater wing of the sphenoid, temporal, and parietal bones.

The boundaries of the temporal fossa are: superiorly and posteriorly, the inferior temporal line; anteriorly, the frontal process of the zygomatic bone; medially, the surface of the temporal bone; and laterally, the zygomatic arch. Inferiorly, the boundary between the temporal fossa and the infratemporal fossa is the infratemporal crest on the greater wing of the sphenoid bone.

The temporal fossa includes a narrow strip of the parietal bone, the squamous portion of the temporal bone, the temporal surface of the frontal bone, and the temporal surface of the greater wing of the sphenoid bone. The temporal fossa contains the body of the temporalis muscle and area blood vessels and nerves.

INFRATEMPORAL FOSSA

The infratemporal fossa is a paired depression that is inferior to the anterior portion of the temporal fossa (see Figure 3-59). The temporal fossa and infratemporal fossa are divided by the infratemporal crest on the greater wing of the sphenoid bone. The infratemporal fossa can also be viewed from the inferior aspect of the skull model after temporarily removing the mandible (Figure 3-60).

The boundaries of the infratemporal fossa include: superiorly, the greater wing of the sphenoid bone; anteriorly, the maxillary tuberosity; medially, the lateral pterygoid plate; and laterally, the ramus of the mandible and zygomatic arch. No bony inferior or posterior boundary exists.

Many structures pass from the infratemporal fossa into the orbit through the inferior orbital fissure, which is located at the anterior and superior end of the fossa. Other structures pass into the infratemporal fossa from the cranial cavity.

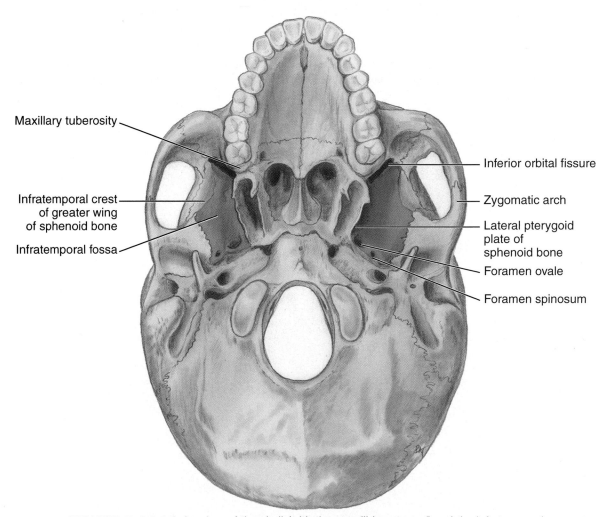

FIGURE 3-60 Inferior view of the skull *(with the mandible removed)* and the infratemporal fossae and boundaries.

The infratemporal fossa contains the mandibular division of the fifth cranial or trigeminal nerve (including the inferior alveolar and lingual nerves), which enters by way of the foramen ovale (see Table 3-3). The fossa also contains the pterygoid plexus and the pterygoid muscles.

The maxillary artery and its branches are also located here, including the middle meningeal artery, which goes into the cranial cavity through the foramen spinosum; the inferior alveolar artery, which enters the mandible through the mandibular foramen; and the posterior alveolar artery, which enters the maxilla through the posterior superior alveolar foramina (see Table 3-3).

PTERYGOPALATINE FOSSA

The pterygopalatine fossa is a cone-shaped paired depression deep to the infratemporal fossa (Figure 3-61). This small but important fossa is located between the pterygoid process and the maxillary tuberosity, close to the apex of the orbit.

The boundaries of the pterygopalatine fossa are: superiorly, the inferior surface of the body of the sphenoid bone; anteriorly, the maxillary tuberosity; medially, the vertical plate of the palatine bone; laterally, the pterygomaxillary fissure; inferiorly, the pterygopalatine canal; and posteriorly, the pterygoid process of the sphenoid bone.

The pterygopalatine fossa contains the maxillary artery and nerve and their branches arising here, including the infraorbital and sphenopalatine arteries, the maxillary division of the fifth cranial or trigeminal nerve and branches, and the pterygopalatine ganglion (see Table 3-3). The foramen rotundum is the entrance route for the maxillary nerve. A second foramen in the pterygoid process, the pterygoid canal, transmits autonomic fibers to the ganglion. The pterygopalatine canal connects with the greater and lesser palatine foramina of the palatine bones of the hard palate.

Bones of the Neck

CERVICAL VERTEBRAE

The **cervical vertebrae** (ver-teh-bray) are located in the vertebral column between the skull and the

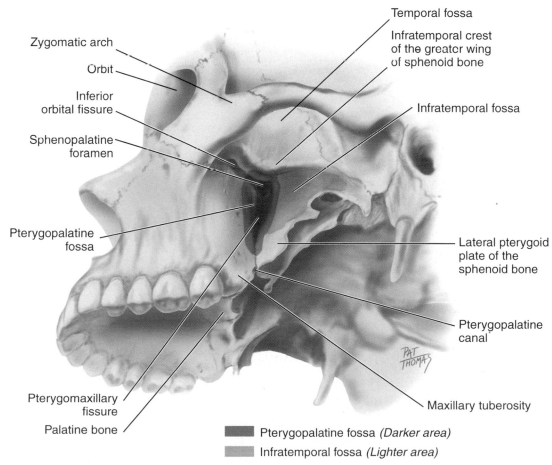

FIGURE 3-61 Oblique lateral view of the base of the skull and the roof of the pterygopalatine fossa and its boundaries.

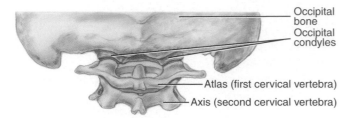

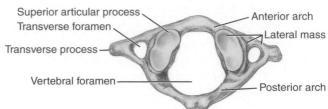

FIGURE 3-62 Posterior view of the skull and the first and second cervical vertebrae.

FIGURE 3-63 Superior view of the first cervical vertebra, the atlas.

thoracic vertebrae. All seven cervical vertebrae have a central **vertebral foramen** (**ver**-teh-brahl) for the spinal cord and associated tissues. In contrast to other vertebrae, the cervical vertebrae are characterized by the presence of a **transverse foramen** in the **transverse process** on each side of the vertebral foramen. The vertebral artery runs through these transverse foramina.

Damage to any of the vertebrae can affect dental treatment as the patient may experience a range of problems, from difficulty in movement to paralysis. Only the first two cervical vertebrae are described because their anatomy is unusual and they are located near the skull.

First Cervical Vertebra.
The first cervical vertebra or **atlas** (**at**-lis) articulates with the skull at the occipital condyles of the occipital bone (Figure 3-62). The atlas has the form of an irreg-

ular ring consisting of two **lateral masses** connected by a short **anterior arch** and a longer **posterior arch** (Figure 3-63). This cervical bone lacks a body and a spine.

The lateral masses can be effectively palpated by placing fingers between the two mastoid processes and the angles of the mandible. More medially, the lateral masses present large concave **superior articular processes** for the corresponding occipital condyles of the skull. The lateral masses also have circular **inferior articular processes** for articulation with the second cervical vertebra.

Second Cervical Vertebra.
The second cervical vertebra or **axis** (**ak**-sis) is characterized by the **dens** (denz) or odontoid process (Figure 3-64). The dens articulates anteriorly with the anterior arch of the first cervical vertebra (Figure 3-65). The body of the axis is inferior to the dens. The spine of the

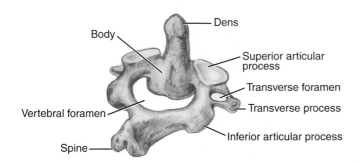

FIGURE 3-64 Posterosuperior view of the second cervical vertebra, the axis.

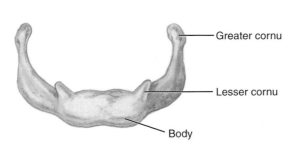

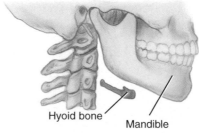

FIGURE 3-65 Anterior view of the hyoid bone with its location demonstrated on a lateral view of the lower skull and the upper vertebral bones.

axis is located posterior to the body. The body and the adjoining transverse process present superior articular processes for an additional articulation with the inferior articulating surfaces of the atlas. The inferior aspect of the axis presents inferior articular processes for articulating with the articular processes of the third cervical vertebra.

HYOID BONE

The **hyoid bone** (hi-oid) is suspended in the neck. It forms the base of the tongue and larynx. Many muscles attach to the hyoid bone (see Chapter 4). The hyoid bone is superior and anterior to the thyroid cartilage of the larynx. This bone is typically at the level of the third cervical vertebra but is raised during swallowing and other activities. The hyoid bone can be effectively palpated by feeling inferior to and medial to the angles of the mandible. Do not confuse the hyoid bone with the inferiorly placed thyroid cartilage (the "Adam's apple") (see Chapters 2 and 7).

The hyoid bone does not articulate with any other bones, giving it its characteristic mobility, which is necessary for mastication, swallowing, and speech. This bone is horizontally suspended from the end of the styloid process by the stylohyoid ligament and is connected by the broad thyrohyoid membrane with the thyroid cartilage.

The U-shaped hyoid bone consists of five portions as seen from an anterior view (see Figure 3-65). The anterior portion is the midline **body of the hyoid bone.** There is also a pair of projections on each side of the hyoid bone, the **greater cornu** and **lesser cornu.** These horns serve as attachments for muscles and ligaments.

Lateral Sagittal View of the Skull

Now that the external and internal portions of the skull have been viewed, as well as the individual bones of the skull, it is useful to consider an internal view of the skull on the lateral sagittal section in order to understand the overall placement of bony structures (Figure 3-66).

ABNORMALITIES OF BONE

Abnormalities of bone can include bony enlargements and fractures that may heal with abnormal contours. The dental professional needs to record any abnormal areas of bone and make any appropriate referrals. Because many facial bones are shared by two or more soft tissue components of the face, it is important to remember that an abnormality of one facial bone often involves many soft tissue components. A fracture

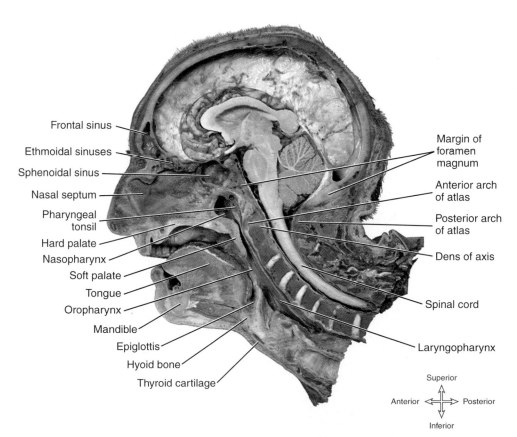

FIGURE 3-66 A lateral sagittal section skull and associated tissues. (From Reynolds PA, Abrahams PH: *McMinn's interactive clinical anatomy: head and neck*, ed 2, London, 2001, Mosby Ltd.)

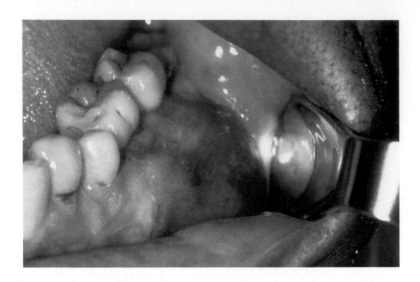

FIGURE 3-67 Nodular bony enlargements may occur in the oral cavity such as in this case of ameloblastoma, a tumor of dental tissues in the mandible. This may result in facial asymmetry.

of the frontal bone may clinically involve both the forehead and the eyes.

Bony enlargements can lead to facial asymmetry as well as nodular intraoral areas (Figures 3-67 and 68). Some, such as palatal or mandibular tori, are normal variations, but others can be due to endocrine diseases causing abnormal bone growth. Bone can also enlarge with tumorous growth of bone or other tissues such as dental tissues, as in the case of an ameloblastoma.

Bone may also fracture with severe blows to the face. Fractures of the facial skeleton tend to occur at its points of buttress with the cranium. These buttress points include the medial aspect of the orbit, articulation of the zygoma with the frontal and temporal bones, articulation of the pterygoid plates, and the palatine bones and maxillae. The fracture of the bone may be detected by gentle palpation. If the fracture is bilateral, the entire facial skeleton can be pushed posteriorly, resulting in upper respiratory tract obstruction. These fractures may heal poorly and result in abnormal bony contours.

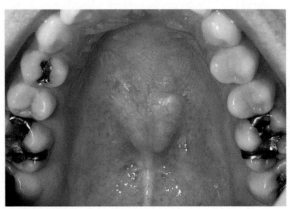

FIGURE 3-68 Nodular bony enlargements may occur in the oral cavity such as in this case of a palatal torus, a benign growth of bone.

Identification Exercises

Identify the structures on the following diagrams by filling in each blank with the correct anatomical term. You can check your answers by looking back at the figure indicated in parentheses for each identification diagram.

1. (Figure 3-4)

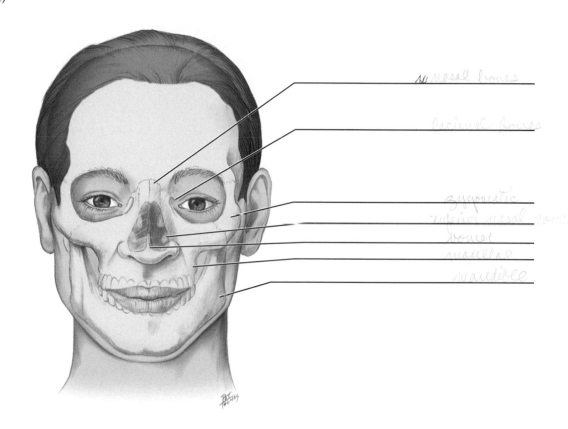

N nasal bones

lacrimal bones

zygomatic

inferior nasal concha

vomer

maxilla

mandible

2. (Figures 3-5, 3-6, and 3-7)

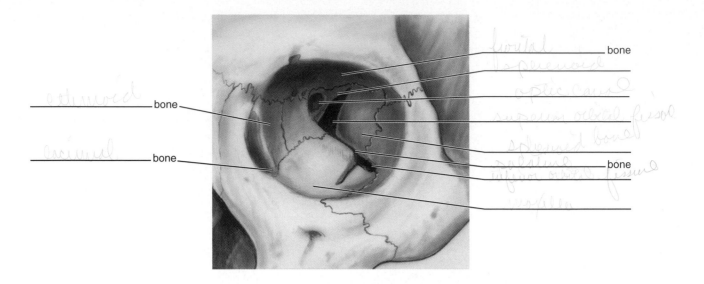

3. (Figures 3-20, 3-23, and 3-27)

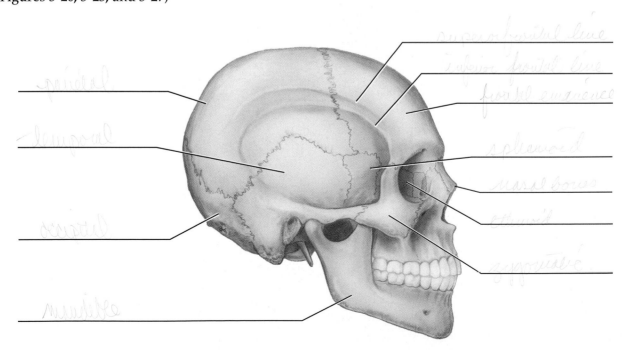

4. (Figure 3-22)

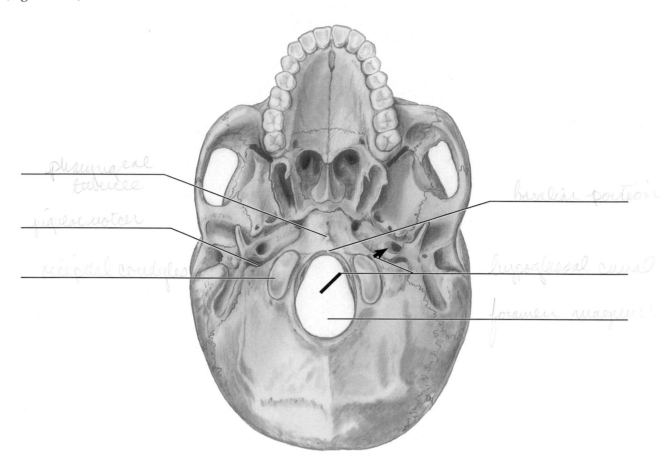

pharyngeal tubercle

jugular notch

occipital condyles

basilar portion

hypoglossal canal

foramen magnum

5. (Figures 3-28, 3-29, and 3-30)

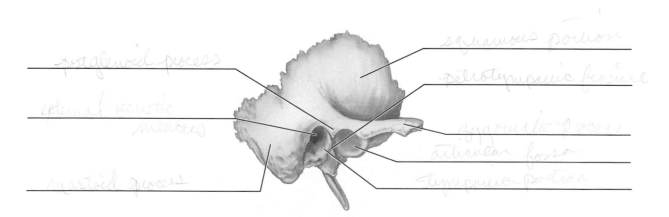

postglenoid process

external acoustic meatus

mastoid process

squamous portion

petrotympanic fissure

zygomatic process

articular fossa

tympanic portion

6. (Figures 3-31 and 3-32, *A*)

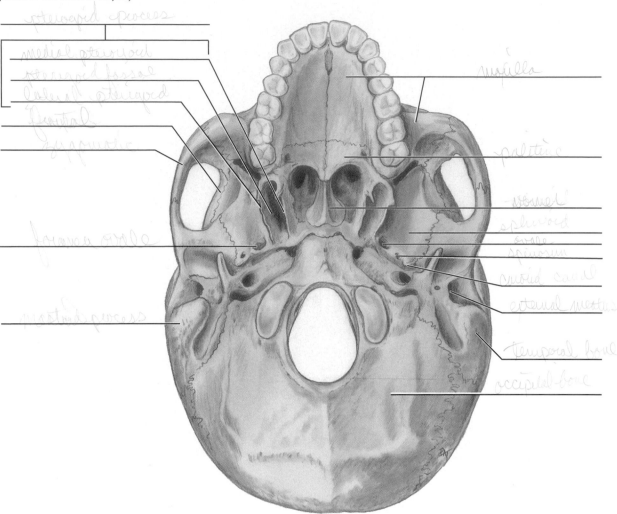

pterygoid process
medial pterygoid
pterygoid fossa
lateral pterygoid
frontal
zygomatic
foramen ovale
mastoid process

maxilla
palatine
vomer
sphenoid
ovale
spinosum
carotid canal
external meatus
temporal bone
occipital bone

7. (Figure 3-33, *A*)

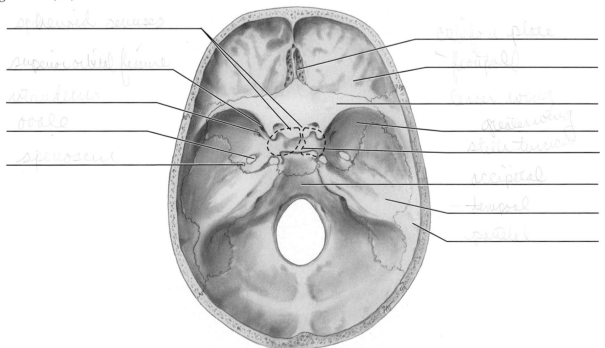

sphenoid sinuses
superior orbital fissure
rotundum
ovale
spinosum

cribriform plate
frontal
lesser wing
greater wing
sella turcica
occipital
temporal
parietal

8. (Figure 3-35)

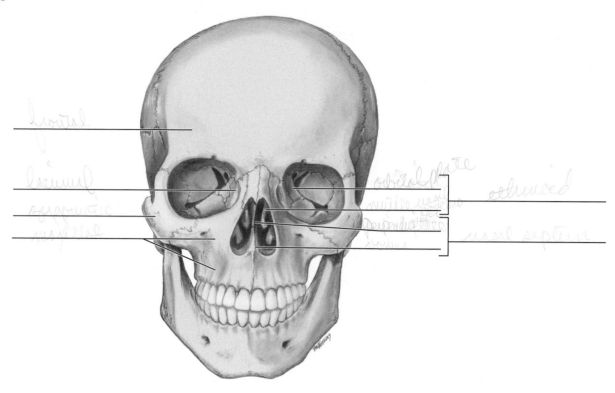

frontal

lacrimal

zygomatic

maxilla

orbital plate

middle nasal

perpendicular

ethmoid

nasal septum

9. (Figure 3-38)

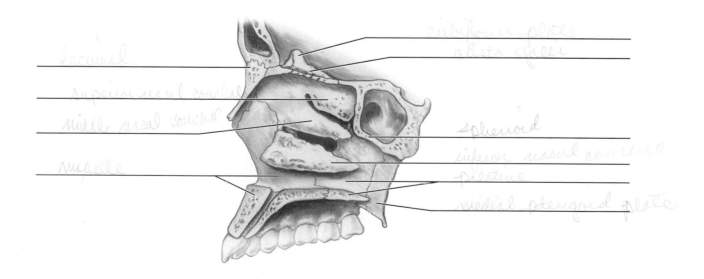

frontal

superior nasal concha

middle nasal concha

maxilla

cribriform plate

crista galli

sphenoid

inferior nasal concha

palatine

medial pterygoid plate

10. (Figures 3-40 and 3-41)

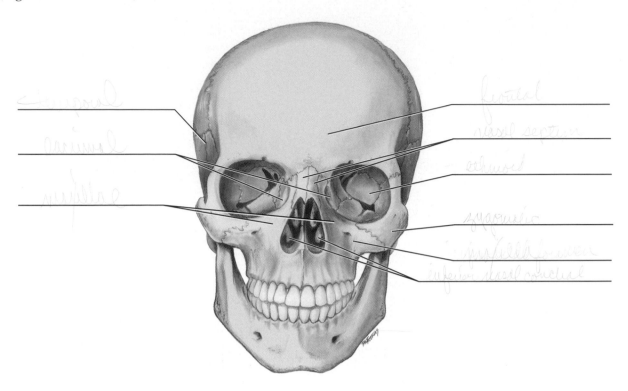

11. (Figure 3-42)

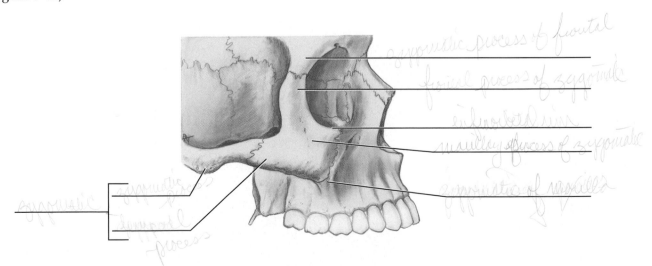

12. (Figure 3-44)

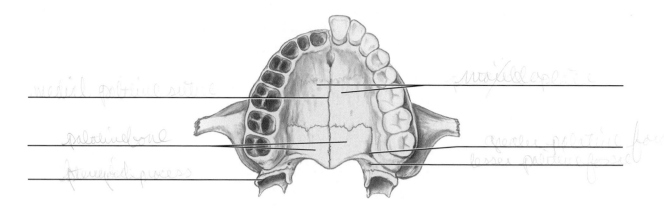

13. (Figure 3-45)

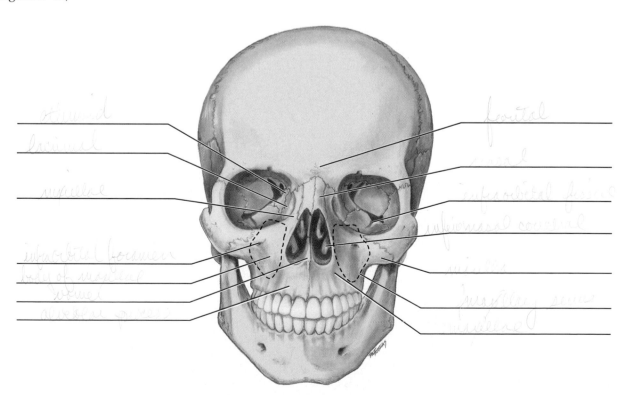

14. (Figure 3-47)

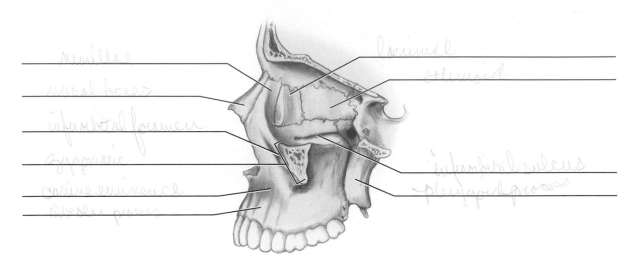

maxilla

nasal bones

infraorbital foramen

zygomatic

canine eminence

alveolar process

lacrimal

ethmoid

infraorbital sulcus

pterygoid process

15. (Figures 3-49 and 3-55, B)

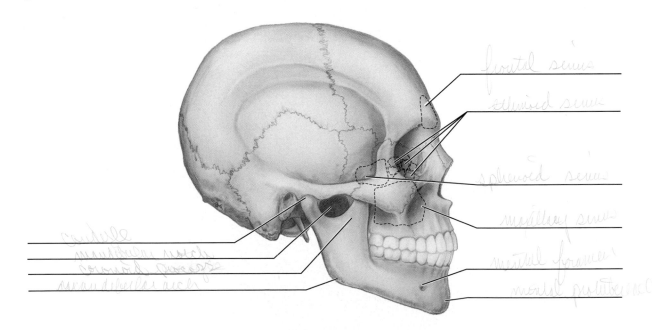

frontal sinus

ethmoid sinus

sphenoid sinus

maxillary sinus

mental foramen

mental protuberance

condyle

mandibular notch

coronoid process

mandibular arch

16. (Figure 3-60)

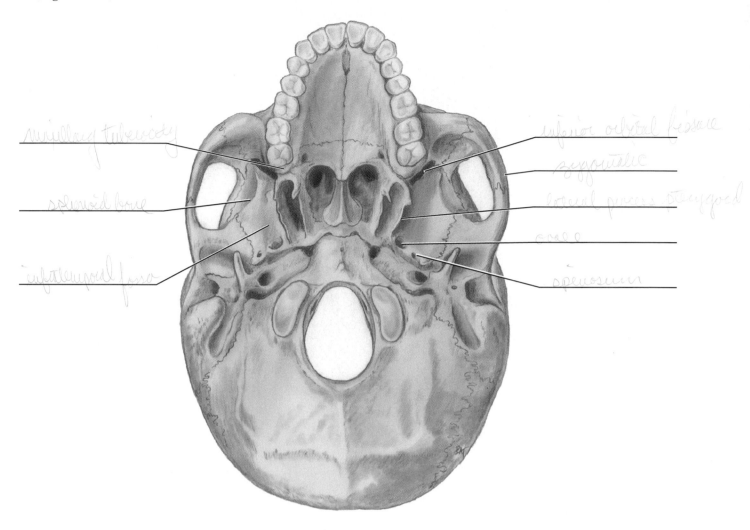

maxillary tuberosity

sphenoid bone

infratemporal fossa

inferior orbital fissure

zygomatic

lateral process pterygoid

ovale

spinosum

17. (Figure 3-61)

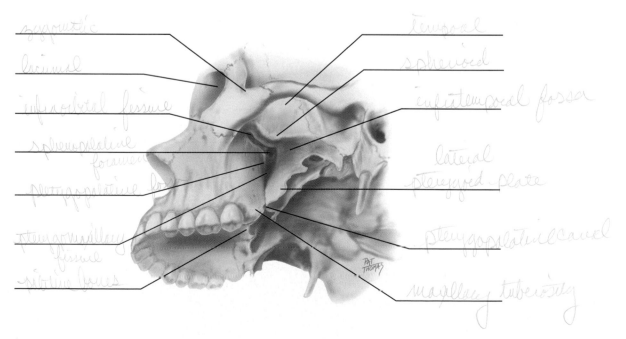

zygomatic

lacrimal

infraorbital fissure

sphenopalatine foramen

pterygopalatine fossa

pterygomaxillary fissure

palatine bones

temporal

sphenoid

infratemporal fossa

lateral pterygoid plate

pterygopalatine canal

maxillary tuberosity

18. (Figure 3-62)

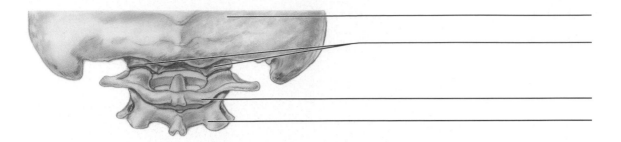

19. (Figure 3-65)

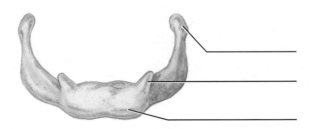

20. (Figure 3-65)

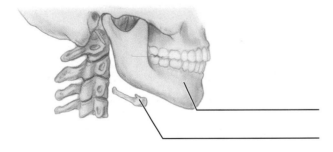

■ REVIEW QUESTIONS

1. Which of the following features is located on the temporal bone?
   A. Superior temporal line
   B. Foramen rotundum
   C. External acoustic meatus
   D. Cribriform plate
   E. Orbital plate

2. Which area is immediately posterior to the most distal tooth in the upper arch?
   A. Retromolar triangle
   B. Postglenoid process
   C. Cribriform plate
   D. Maxillary tuberosity
   E. Hamular process

3. In addition to the zygomatic bone, which of the following bones has a process that forms the zygomatic arch?
   A. Temporal bone
   B. Maxilla
   C. Sphenoid bone
   D. Palatine bone

4. Which of the following is the name of the articulation of the parietal bones and the occipital bone?
   A. Coronal suture
   B. Squamosal suture
   C. Sagittal suture
   D. Lambdoidal suture

5. Which of the following bony landmarks form an articulation?
   A. Occipital condyles with the atlas
   B. Occipital condyles with the axis
   C. Mandibular fossa with the coronoid notch
   D. Mandibular fossa with the coronoid process

6. Which of the following features is located on the lateral surface of the mandible?
   A. Lingula
   B. Submandibular fossa
   C. Genial tubercles
   D. External oblique line
   E. Mandibular foramen

7. The orbital apex is composed of the lesser wing of the sphenoid bone and the:
   A. Ethmoid bone
   B. Frontal bone
   C. Maxilla
   D. Palatine bone
   E. Lacrimal bone

8. Which of the following landmarks is formed by the maxillae?
   A. Mental spine
   B. Median palatine suture
   C. Retromolar triangle
   D. Hamulus
   E. Inferior orbital fissure

9. Which of the following structures is located in the infratemporal fossa?
   A. Masseter muscle
   B. Pterygopalatine ganglion
   C. Posterior superior alveolar artery
   D. Maxillary division of the fifth cranial nerve

10. The concavity on the anterior border of the coronoid process of the ramus is called the:
    A. Mandibular notch
    B. Coronoid notch
    C. Temporal fossa
    D. Infratemporal fossa

11. Which of the following landmarks serves to help locate the hyoid bone?
    A. Level of the first cervical vertebra
    B. Superior and anterior to the thyroid cartilage
    C. Articulation with the cartilage of the larynx
    D. Inferior and posterior to the Adam's apple

12. Which of the following structures forms the floor of each maxillary sinus?
    A. Alveolar process of the maxilla
    B. Facial wall of the maxilla
    C. Infratemporal surface of the maxilla
    D. Lateral wall of the nasal cavity

13. Which of the following processes is located just inferior and medial to the external acoustic meatus?
    A. Pterygoid process
    B. Styloid process
    C. Mastoid process
    D. Hamulus

14. The spaces under the three conchae of the lateral walls of the nasal cavity are called:
    A. Ostia
    B. Ducts
    C. Meatus
    D. Inferior nasal conchae
    E. Vestibules

15. Which of the following bones and their processes form the hard palate?
   A. Maxillary processes of the maxillae and the horizontal plates of the palatine bones
   B. Palatal processes of the maxillae and the maxillary plates of the palatine bones
   C. Horizontal plates of the palatine bones and the palatine processes of the maxillae
   D. Maxillary plates of the palatine bones and the horizontal processes of the maxillae

16. Which of the following nerves is associated with the stylomastoid foramen?
   A. Fifth cranial nerve
   B. Seventh cranial nerve
   C. Ninth cranial nerve
   D. Tenth cranial nerve
   E. Eleventh cranial nerve

17. Which of the following bones of the skull is paired?
   A. Sphenoid bone
   B. Ethmoid bone
   C. Occipital bone
   D. Vomer
   E. Parietal bone

18. Which of the following plates is perforated to allow the passage of the olfactory nerves for the sense of smell?
   A. Medial plate of the sphenoid bone
   B. Lateral plate of the sphenoid bone
   C. Perpendicular plate of the ethmoid bone
   D. Cribriform plate of the ethmoid bone

19. Which of the following bones of the skull is considered a cranial bone?
   A. Vomer
   B. Maxilla
   C. Sphenoid bone
   D. Zygomatic bone
   E. Mandible

20. In which portion of the temporal bone is the temporomandibular joint located?
   A. Squamous portion
   B. Tympanic portion
   C. Petrous portion
   D. Mastoid portion

21. Which is a single bone located at the midline of the skull?
   A. Temporal
   B. Zygomatic
   C. Sphenoid
   D. Inferior nasal conchae

22. Which of the following structures is a normal, short, windowlike opening in bone?
   A. Fossa
   B. Foramen
   C. Fissure
   D. Perforation

23. Which of the following bones helps form the jugular foramen along with the jugular notch of the temporal bone?
   A. Occipital
   B. Mandible
   C. Parietal
   D. Sphenoid

24. Which of the following is a faint ridge noted where the right and left mandibular processes fused together in early childhood?
   A. Mylohyoid line
   B. Mental protuberance
   C. Mandibular symphysis
   D. External oblique line

25. In which bone are the infraorbital foramen and canal located?
   A. Frontal
   B. Maxilla
   C. Sphenoid
   D. Zygomatic

26. Which of the following structures is a large, roughened projection on the petrous portion of the temporal bone?
   A. Notch
   B. Process
   C. Air cells
   D. Sinus

27. Which of the following landmarks is an anterior process on the sphenoid bone?
   A. Wing
   B. Notch
   C. Body
   D. Angle

28. The lacrimal gland is located just inside the lateral portion of the:
   A. Glabella
   B. Supraorbital ridge
   C. Supraorbital notch
   D. Nasion

29. The occipital condyles are located _____ and _____ to the foramen magnum.
   A. medial, anterior
   B. lateral, anterior
   C. medial, posterior
   D. lateral, posterior

30. Which bone forms both the superior and middle nasal conchae?
   A. Occipital bone
   B. Mandibular bone
   C. Maxillary bone
   D. Frontal bone
   E. Ethmoid bone

Muscular System

LEARNING OBJECTIVES

After studying this chapter, the reader should be able to do the following:

1. Define and pronounce all the key terms and anatomical terms in this chapter.
2. Locate and identify the muscles of the head and neck on a diagram, skull, and patient.
3. Describe the origin, insertion, and action of each muscle of the head and neck.
4. State the nerve(s) that innervate each muscle of the head and neck.
5. Discuss the processes of mastication, speech, and swallowing with regard to anatomical considerations.
6. Correctly complete the review questions and activities for this chapter.
7. Integrate the knowledge about the muscles of the head and neck into the clinical dental practice.

KEY TERMS

Action Movement accomplished by a muscle when the muscle fibers contract.

Facial Paralysis (pah-**ral**-i-sis) Loss of action of the facial muscles.

Insertion End of the muscle that is attached to the more movable structure.

Muscle Type of body tissue that shortens under neural control, causing soft tissue and bony structures to move.

Origin End of the muscle that is attached to the least movable structure.

OVERVIEW OF THE MUSCULAR SYSTEM

A **muscle** in the muscular system shortens under neural control, causing soft tissue and bony structures of the body to move. Each muscle has two ends attached to these structures, and they are categorized according to their role in movement. The **origin** is the end of the muscle that is attached to the least movable structure. The **insertion** is the other end of the muscle and is attached to the more movable structure.

Generally, the insertion of the muscle moves toward the origin when the muscle is contracted. The movement that is accomplished when the muscle fibers contract is the **action** of the muscle. The muscles have specific innervation that is discussed in this chapter, but a more thorough explanation of the nervous system can be found in Chapter 8. The blood supply to the muscular area is further discussed in Chapter 6. It is important to remember that unlike innervation to the muscles, which is a one-to-one relationship, arterial supply is regional. Arteries supply all structures in their vicinity, and muscles receive blood from all nearby arteries.

MUSCLES OF THE HEAD AND NECK

The dental professional needs to determine the location and action of many muscles of the head and neck in order to perform a thorough patient examination. This information is important because the placement of many other structures such as bones, blood vessels, nerves, and lymph nodes is related to the location of the muscles. The muscles may also malfunction and be involved in temporomandibular joint disorders (see Chapter 5), occlusal dysfunction, and certain nervous system diseases. Muscles of the head and neck and their attachments are also a consideration in the spread of dental infections (see Chapter 12).

The muscles of the head and neck can be divided into several groups by function. Thus the muscles of the head and neck are divided into seven main groups: the cervical muscles, muscles of facial expression, muscles of mastication, hyoid muscles, muscles of the tongue, muscles of the soft palate, and muscles of the pharynx. Muscle groups to the ears, eyes, and nose are not included in this chapter.

Cervical Muscles

The two **cervical muscles** considered in this text are both superficial and easily palpated on the neck. These cervical muscles are the sternocleidomastoid and trapezius muscles.

STERNOCLEIDOMASTOID MUSCLE

One of the largest and most superficial cervical muscles is the paired **sternocleidomastoid muscle (SCM)** (stir-no-klii-do-**mass**-toid). The SCM is thick and serves as a primary muscular landmark of the neck during an extraoral examination of a patient. The SCM is effectively palpated on each side of the neck when the patient moves the head to the opposite side (Figure 4-1). The SCM divides the neck region into anterior and posterior cervical triangles (see Chapter 2).

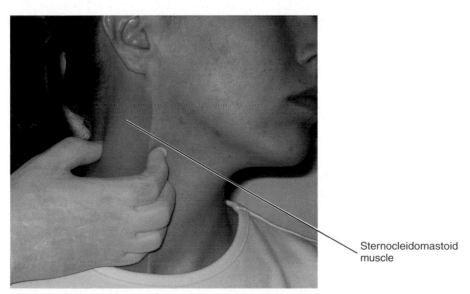

Sternocleidomastoid muscle

FIGURE 4-1 Palpation of the right sternocleidomastoid muscle of a patient by having the patient turn the head to the opposite side *(muscle highlighted)*.

Origin and Insertion. The SCM originates from the medial portion of the clavicle and the sternum's superior and lateral surfaces and passes posteriorly and superiorly to insert on the mastoid process of the temporal bone (Figure 4-2). This insertion is just posterior and inferior to the external acoustic meatus of each ear.

Action. If one muscle contracts, the head and neck bend to the same side, and the face and front of the neck rotate to the opposite side. If both muscles contract, the head will flex at the neck and extend at the junction between the neck and skull.

Innervation. The SCM is innervated by the eleventh cranial or accessory nerve.

TRAPEZIUS MUSCLE

The other important superficial cervical muscle is the paired **trapezius muscle** (trah-**pee**-zee-us), which covers the lateral and posterior surfaces of the neck. The trapezius muscle is a broad, flat, triangular muscle.

Origin and Insertion. The trapezius muscle originates from the external surface of the occipital bone and the posterior midline of the cervical and thoracic regions. This muscle inserts on the lateral third of the clavicle and portions of the scapula (Figure 4-3).

Action. The cervical fibers of the muscle act to lift the clavicle and scapula, as when the shoulders are shrugged.

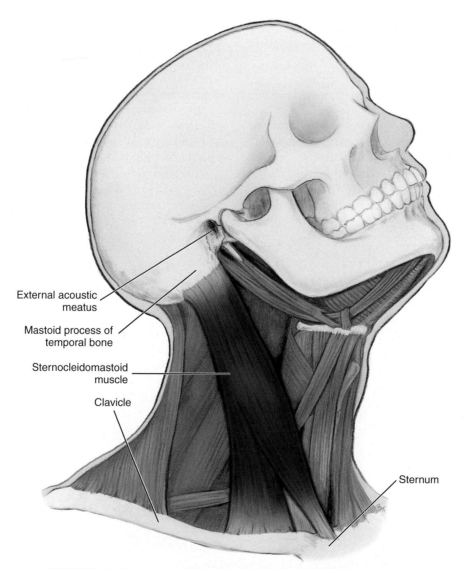

External acoustic meatus

Mastoid process of temporal bone

Sternocleidomastoid muscle

Clavicle

Sternum

FIGURE 4-2 Origin and insertion of the right sternocleidomastoid muscle.

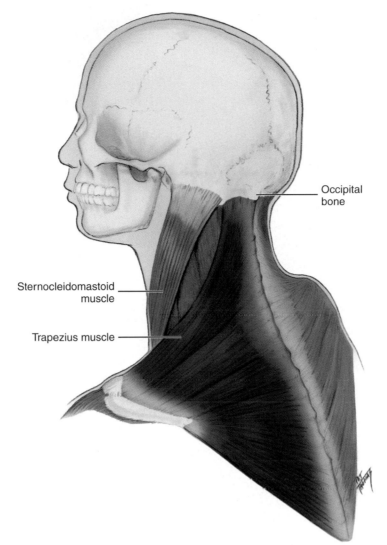

FIGURE 4-3 Origin and insertion of the left trapezius muscle.

Innervation. The trapezius muscle is innervated by the eleventh cranial or accessory nerve and the third and fourth cervical nerves.

Muscles of Facial Expression

The **muscles of facial expression** are paired muscles in the superficial fascia of the facial tissues (Figures 4-4 and 4-5). Use of these muscles is noted during an extraoral examination. All the muscles of facial expression originate from the surface of the skull bone (rarely the fascia) and insert on the dermis of skin tissue. When they contract, the skin moves. These muscles also cause wrinkles at right angles to the muscles' action line. Again, the use of your mirror image as various facial expressions are made is helpful in learning about these muscles. Smiling is easier than frowning, as our grandparents would say. It does take only 17 muscles to smile, but it takes a lot of extra effort by your facial muscles (43, to be exact) to frown.

Origin and Insertion. The locations of the muscles of facial expression vary. These muscles may be further grouped according to whether they are situated in the scalp, eye, or mouth region. The specific origin and insertion of each muscle of facial expression are listed in Table 4-1.

Action. During facial expression, the muscles of facial expression all act in various combinations, similar to the muscles of mastication, to vary the appearance of the face (Table 4-2). An inability to form facial expressions on one side of the face may be the first sign of damage to the nerve of these muscles.

Innervation. All muscles of facial expression are innervated by the seventh cranial or facial nerve, each nerve serving one side of the face. Damage to the

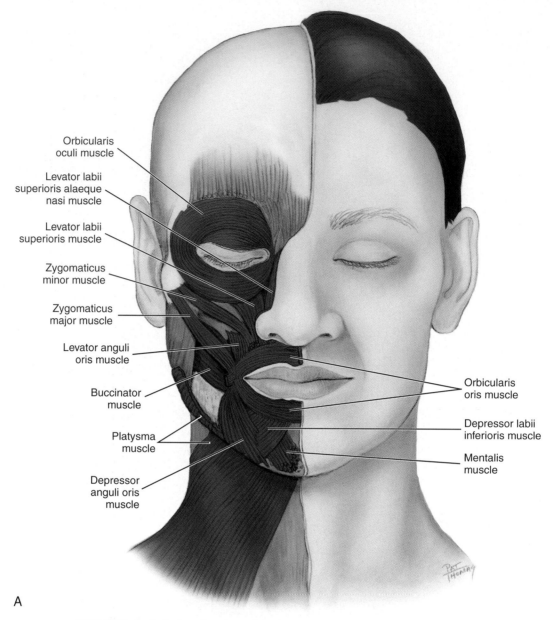

Orbicularis
oculi muscle

Levator labii
superioris alaeque
nasi muscle

Levator labii
superioris muscle

Zygomaticus
minor muscle

Zygomaticus
major muscle

Levator anguli
oris muscle

Buccinator
muscle

Platysma
muscle

Depressor
anguli oris
muscle

Orbicularis
oris muscle

Depressor labii
inferioris muscle

Mentalis
muscle

A

FIGURE 4-4 A, Anterior view of most of the muscles of facial expression.

facial nerve results in **facial paralysis** of facial expression on the involved side (Figure 4-6). Paralysis is the loss of voluntary muscle action. The facial nerve can become damaged permanently or temporarily (see Chapter 8). This damage can occur with a stroke (cerebrovascular accident), Bell's palsy (as in this case), and parotid salivary gland cancer (malignant neoplasm) because the facial nerve travels through the gland. The gland can also be damaged permanently by surgery or temporarily by trauma, as with an incorrectly given inferior alveolar local anesthetic block (see Chapter 9). These situations of paralysis not

only inhibit facial expression but also seriously impair the patient's ability to speak, either permanently or temporarily.

MUSCLES OF FACIAL EXPRESSION IN THE SCALP REGION

Epicranial Muscle.

The **epicranial muscle** (ep-ee-**kray**-nee-al) or epicranius is a muscle of facial expression located in the scalp region. This muscle has two bellies, the frontal and occipital bellies. The bellies are separated by a large,

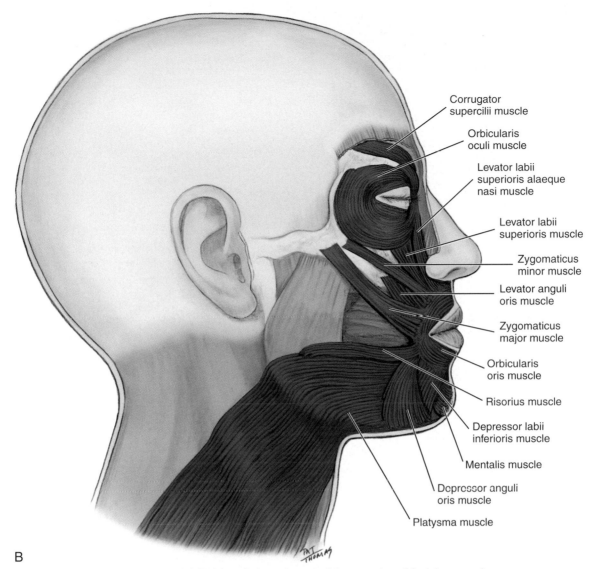

FIGURE 4-4, cont'd B, Lateral view of most of the muscles of facial expression.

Corrugator supercilii muscle

Orbicularis oculi muscle

Levator labii superioris alaeque nasi muscle

Levator labii superioris muscle

Zygomaticus minor muscle

Levator anguli oris muscle

Zygomaticus major muscle

Orbicularis oris muscle

Risorius muscle

Depressor labii inferioris muscle

Mentalis muscle

Depressor anguli oris muscle

Platysma muscle

B

spread-out scalpal tendon. This muscle and its tendon are one of the layers that form the scalp.

Origin and Insertion. The frontal belly arises from the **epicranial aponeurosis** (ap-o-new-**row**-sis) or galea aponeurotica, a scalpal tendon (Figure 4-7). The epicranial aponeurosis is located over the area where the parietal and occipital bones meet, the most superior portion of the skull. The frontal belly then inserts into the skin tissue of the eyebrow and root of the nose. The occipital belly originates from the occipital bone and mastoid process of the temporal bone and then inserts in the epicranial aponeurosis.

Action. The epicranial muscle raises the eyebrows and scalp, as when a person shows surprise (Figure 4-8). The two bellies can act independent of each other during facial expressions.

MUSCLES OF FACIAL EXPRESSION IN THE EYE REGION

The muscles of facial expression in the eye region include the orbicularis oculi and corrugator supercilii muscles (Figure 4-9).

Orbicularis Oculi Muscle.

The **orbicularis oculi muscle** (or-bik-you-**laa**-ris **oc**-yule-eye) is a muscle of facial expression that encircles the eye. This muscle has important functions in protecting and moistening the eye, as well as in facial expression.

Origin and Insertion. This muscle originates on the orbital rim, nasal process of the frontal bone, and frontal process of the maxilla. Most of the fibers insert

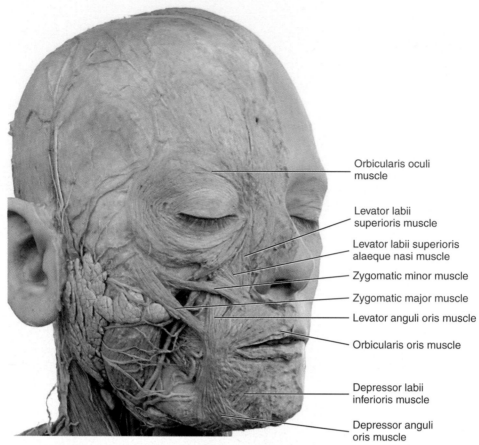

Orbicularis oculi
muscle

Levator labii
superioris muscle

Levator labii superioris
alaeque nasi muscle

Zygomatic minor muscle

Zygomatic major muscle

Levator anguli oris muscle

Orbicularis oris muscle

Depressor labii
inferioris muscle

Depressor anguli
oris muscle

FIGURE 4-5 Superficial dissection of the face showing many of the muscles of facial expression. (From Reynolds PA, Abrahams PH: *McMinn's interactive clinical anatomy: head and neck*, ed 2, London, 2001, Mosby Ltd.)

in the skin tissue at the lateral region of the eye, although some inner fibers completely encircle the eye.

   Action. This muscle closes the eyelid. If all fibers are active, the eye can be squinted, and wrinkles form in the lateral portions of the eye or "crow's feet."

Corrugator Supercilii Muscle.

The **corrugator supercilii muscle** (cor-rew-**gay**-tor soo-per-**sili**-eye) is a muscle of facial expression in the eye region, deep to the superior portion of the orbicularis oculi muscle.

   Origin and Insertion. This muscle originates on the frontal bone in the supraorbital region. It then passes superiorly and laterally to insert in the skin tissue of the eyebrow.

   Action. This muscle draws the skin tissue of the eyebrow medially and inferiorly toward the nose, which causes vertical wrinkles in the glabella area of the forehead and horizontal wrinkles at the bridge of the nose, as when a person frowns (see Figure 4-14, *B*). It works in concert with the muscles of the nasal region.

MUSCLES OF FACIAL EXPRESSION IN THE MOUTH REGION

The largest group of facial muscles is associated with the mouth. The muscles of facial expression in the mouth region include the orbicularis oris, buccinator, risorius, levator labii superioris, levator labii superioris alaeque nasi, zygomaticus major, zygomaticus minor, levator anguli oris, depressor anguli oris, depressor labii inferioris, mentalis, and platysma muscles.

Orbicularis Oris Muscle.

The **orbicularis oris muscle** (or-bik-you-**laa**-ris **or**-is) is an important muscle of facial expression in the mouth region. This muscle acts to shape and control the size of the mouth opening and is important for creating the lip positions and movements during speech.

   Origin and Insertion. This muscle encircles the mouth and inserts in the skin tissue at the angle of the

TABLE 4-1

ORIGIN AND INSERTION OF THE MUSCLES OF FACIAL EXPRESSION

Muscles	Origin	Insertion
Epicranial	Frontal belly: epicranial aponeurosis Occipital belly: occipital and temporal bone	Frontal belly: eyebrow and root of nose Occipital belly: epicranial aponeurosis
Orbicularis oculi	Orbital rim, frontal and maxillary bones	Lateral region of eye, some encircle eye
Corrugator supercilii	Frontal bone	Eyebrow
Orbicularis oris	Encircles mouth	Angle of mouth
Buccinator	Maxilla, mandible, and pterygomandibular raphe	Angle of mouth
Risorius	Fascia superficial to masseter muscle	Angle of mouth
Levator labii superioris	Maxilla	Upper lip
Levator labii superioris alaeque nasi	Maxilla	Ala of nose and upper lip
Zygomaticus major	Zygomatic bone	Angle of mouth
Zygomaticus minor	Zygomatic bone	Upper lip
Levator anguli oris	Maxilla	Angle of mouth
Depressor anguli oris	Mandible	Angle of mouth
Depressor labii inferioris	Mandible	Lower lip
Mentalis	Mandible	Chin
Platysma	Clavicle and shoulder	Mandible and muscles of mouth

mouth (Figure 4-10). In the upper lip, fibers also insert on the ridges of the philtrum.

Action. This muscle has four relatively distinct movements: a pressing together (closing the lips), a tightening and thinning (pursing the lips), a rolling inward between the teeth (grimacing), and a thrusting outward (pouting and kissing).

Buccinator Muscle.

The **buccinator muscle** (buck-**sin**-nay-tor) is a muscle of facial expression that forms the anterior portion of the cheek or the lateral wall of the oral cavity.

Origin and Insertion. This muscle originates from three areas: the alveolar processes of the maxilla and mandible and a fibrous structure, the **pterygomandibular raphe** (teh-ri-go-man-**dib** yule lar **ra** fe) (Figure 4-11). The pterygomandibular raphe extends

from the hamulus and passes inferiorly to attach to the posterior end of the mandible's mylohyoid line. The buccinator and superior pharyngeal constrictor muscles of the pharynx are attached to each other at the raphe. The pterygomandibular raphe is noted in the oral cavity as the **pterygomandibular fold.** The buccinator runs horizontally to insert into the skin tissue at the angle of the mouth. Thus the muscle has different fiber groups: the deep vertical fibers between the alveolar processes and the superficial horizontal fibers from the raphe to the corner of the mouth.

Action. This muscle pulls the angle of the mouth laterally and shortens the cheek both vertically and horizontally. This action causes the muscle to keep food pushed back on the occlusal surface of teeth, as when a person chews. By keeping the food in the correct position when chewing, the muscle assists the

TABLE 4-2

MUSCLES OF FACIAL EXPRESSION AND THEIR ASSOCIATED FACIAL EXPRESSIONS

Muscles	Facial Expression
Epicranial	Surprise
Orbicularis oculi	Closing eyelid
Corrugator supercilii	Frowning
Orbicularis oris	Closing and pursing lips, as well as pouting and grimacing
Buccinator	Chewing
Risorius	Stretching lips
Levator labii superioris	Raising upper lip
Levator labii superioris alaeque nasi	Raising upper lip and dilating nostrils in a sneer
Zygomaticus major	Smiling
Zygomaticus minor	Raising upper lip, assisting in smiling
Levator anguli oris	Smiling
Depressor anguli oris	Frowning
Depressor labii inferioris	Lowering lower lip
Mentalis	Raising chin and protruding lower lip
Platysma	Raising neck skin and grimacing

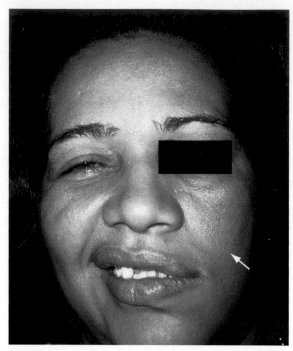

FIGURE 4-6 Patient trying to smile with unilateral paralysis of the facial muscles due to muscle damage from Bell's palsy. Patient is unable to show facial expression on that side *(arrow).*

muscles of mastication. In infants the muscle provides suction for suckling. In addition, because of its importance in expelling air through pursed lips, blowpipes, or wind instruments, it has been called the "trumpet muscle."

Risorius Muscle.
The **risorius muscle** (ri-**soh**-ree-us) is a thin muscle of facial expression in the mouth region.

Origin and Insertion. The risorius muscle originates from fascia superficial to the masseter muscle and passes anteriorly to insert in the skin tissue at the angle of the mouth (Figure 4-12).

Action. It acts to stretch the lips laterally, retracting the labial commissures and widening the oral cavity. The risorius muscle has been thought (erroneously) to produce "grinning" or "smiling" but really

produces more of a grimace. It has a connection with the platysma in that it often contracts with it.

Levator Labii Superioris Muscle.
A broad, flat muscle of facial expression in the mouth region is the **levator labii superioris muscle** (le-**vate**-er **lay**-be-eye soo-per-ee-**or**-is).

Origin and Insertion. This muscle originates from the infraorbital rim of the maxilla. It then passes inferiorly to insert in the skin tissue of the upper lip (Figure 4-13).

Action. This muscle elevates the upper lip (Figure 4-14, *A*).

Levator Labii Superioris Alaeque Nasi Muscle.
The **levator labii superioris alaeque nasi muscle** (le-**vate**-er **lay**-be-eye soo-per-ee-**or**-is a-lah-cue **naz**-eye) is also a muscle of facial expression in the mouth region.

Origin and Insertion. This muscle originates from the frontal process of the maxilla. It then passes inferiorly to insert into two areas: the skin tissue of the ala (or wing) of the nose and the upper lip (see Figure 4-13).

Action. This muscle elevates the upper lip and ala of the nose, thus also dilating the nostrils, as in a sneering expression (Figure 4-14, *B*).

Zygomaticus Major Muscle.
Another muscle of facial expression in the mouth region is the **zygomaticus major muscle** (zy-go-**mat**-i-kus).

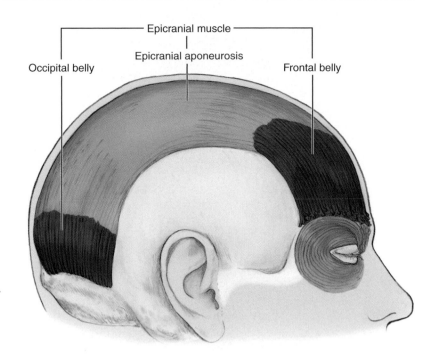

FIGURE 4-7 Origin and insertion of the frontal belly and occipital belly of the right epicranial muscle.

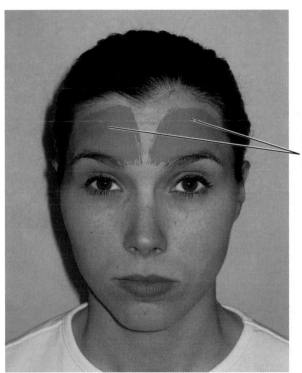

Epicranial muscles (frontal belly)

FIGURE 4-8 Facial expression of surprise on a patient using the epicranial muscle to raise the eyebrows and scalp *(muscle highlighted)*.

Origin and Insertion. This muscle originates from the zygomatic bone, lateral to the zygomaticus minor muscle. The muscle then passes anteriorly and inferiorly to insert in the skin tissue at the angle of the mouth (see Figure 4-13).

Action. This muscle elevates the angle of the upper lip and pulls it laterally, as when a person smiles (see Figure 4-14, *A*). Some research suggests that the difference between a genuine smile and a perfunctory (or lying) smile is that when a person truly feels happy,

Continued on p. 106

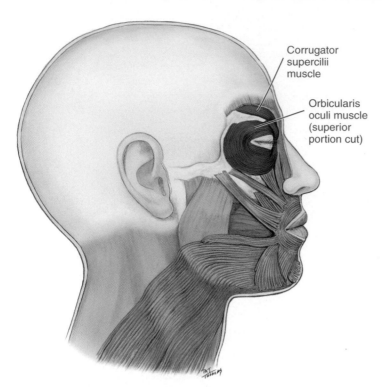

FIGURE 4-9 Orbicularis oculi muscle and corrugator supercilii muscle.

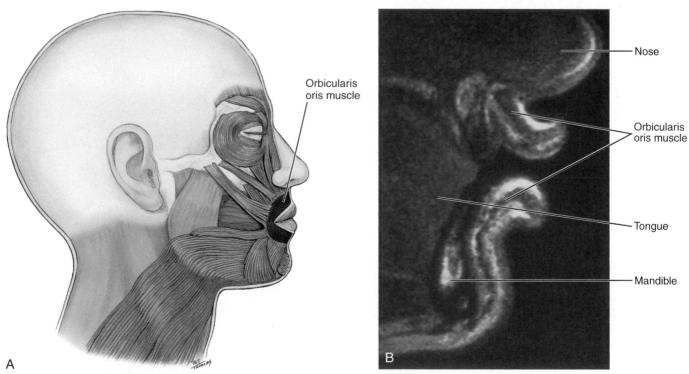

FIGURE 4-10 Orbicularis oris muscle: diagram (A) and (B) sagittal magnetic resonance imaging of a kiss. (B, From Reynolds PA, Abrahams PH: *McMinn's interactive clinical anatomy: head and neck*, ed 2, London, 2001, Mosby Ltd.)

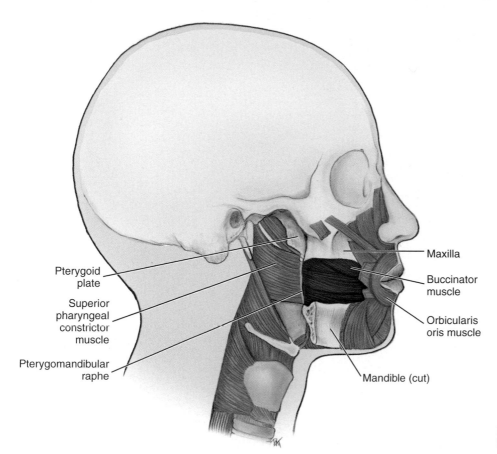

Pterygoid plate

Superior pharyngeal constrictor muscle

Pterygomandibular raphe

Maxilla

Buccinator muscle

Orbicularis oris muscle

Mandible (cut)

FIGURE 4-11 Origin and insertion of the buccinator muscle.

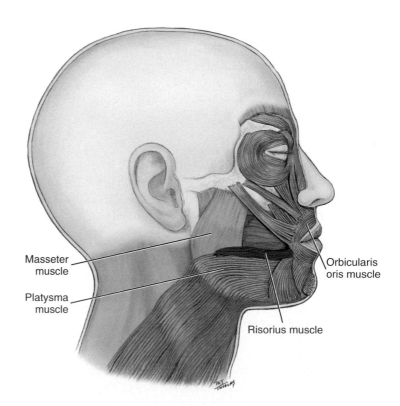

Masseter muscle

Platysma muscle

Orbicularis oris muscle

Risorius muscle

FIGURE 4-12 Origin and insertion of the risorius muscle.

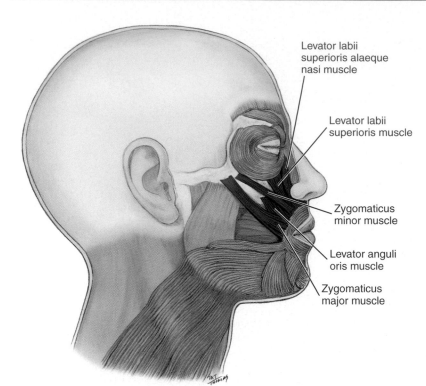

Levator labii
superioris alaeque
nasi muscle

Levator labii
superioris muscle

Zygomaticus
minor muscle

Levator anguli
oris muscle

Zygomaticus
major muscle

FIGURE 4-13 Levator labii superioris alaeque nasi muscle, levator labii superioris muscle, zygomaticus minor muscle, levator anguli oris muscle, and zygomaticus major muscle.

Text continued from p. 103

the zygomatic major muscle contracts together with the orbicularis oculi muscle.

Zygomaticus Minor Muscle.

The **zygomaticus minor muscle** (zy-go-**mat**-i-kus) is a small muscle of facial expression in the mouth region, medial to the zygomaticus major muscle.

Origin and Insertion. This muscle originates on the body of the zygomatic bone. It then inserts in the skin tissue of the upper lip adjacent to the insertion of the levator labii superioris muscle (see Figure 4-13).

Action. This muscle elevates the upper lip (see Figure 4-14, *A*), assisting in smiling.

Levator Anguli Oris Muscle.

Deep to both the zygomaticus major and zygomaticus minor muscles is the **levator anguli oris muscle** (le-**vate**-er **an**-gu-lie), another muscle of facial expression in the mouth region.

Origin and Insertion. This muscle originates on the canine fossa of the maxilla, usually superior to the root of the maxillary canine. The muscle then passes inferiorly to insert in skin tissues at the angle of the mouth (see Figure 4-13).

Action. This muscle elevates the angle of the mouth, as when a person smiles (see Figure 4-14, *A*).

Depressor Anguli Oris Muscle.

The **depressor anguli oris muscle** (de-**pres**-er **an**-gu-lie) is a triangular muscle of facial expression in the lower mouth region.

Origin and Insertion. This muscle originates on the lower border of the mandible and passes superiorly to insert in the skin tissue at the angle of the mouth (Figure 4-15).

Action. This muscle depresses the angle of the mouth, as when a person frowns (see Figure 4-14, *B*).

Depressor Labii Inferioris Muscle.

Deep to the depressor anguli oris muscle is the **depressor labii inferioris muscle** (de-**pres**-er **lay**-be-eye in-**fere**-ee-o-ris), another muscle of facial expression in the mouth region.

Origin and Insertion. This muscle also originates from the lower border of the mandible and passes superiorly to insert in the skin tissue of the lower lip (see Figure 4-15).

Action. This muscle depresses the lower lip, exposing the mandibular incisor teeth. Some experts have suggested that it expresses irony.

Mentalis Muscle.

The **mentalis muscle** (men-**ta**-lis) is a short, thick muscle of facial expression superior and medial to the mental nerve in the mouth region.

Origin and Insertion. This muscle originates on the mandible near the midline and inserts in the skin tissue of the chin (Figure 4-16).

Action. This muscle raises the chin, causing the displaced lower lip to protrude and narrowing the oral vestibule. When active, these fibers may dislodge a complete denture in an edentulous patient who has

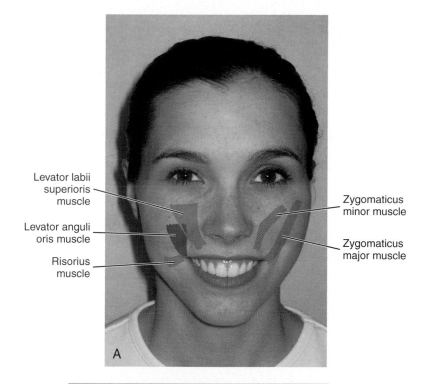

Levator labii superioris muscle

Levator anguli oris muscle

Risorius muscle

Zygomaticus minor muscle

Zygomaticus major muscle

A

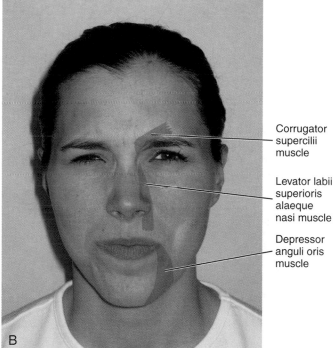

Corrugator supercilii muscle

Levator labii superioris alaeque nasi muscle

Depressor anguli oris muscle

B

FIGURE 4-14 A, Patient using some of the muscles of facial expression when smiling *(muscles highlighted and labeled)*. **B,** Patient using some of the muscles of facial expression while looking disgusted *(muscles highlighted and labeled).*

lost alveolar ridge height. The mentalis is so named because it is associated with thinking or concentration; it also has been said to express doubt.

Platysma Muscle.

The **platysma muscle** (plah-**tiz**-mah) is a muscle of facial expression that runs from the neck all the way to the mouth, covering the anterior cervical triangle.

Origin and Insertion. This muscle originates in the skin tissue superficial to the clavicle and shoulder. It then passes anteriorly to insert on the lower border of the mandible and the muscles surrounding the mouth (Figure 4-17).

Action. This muscle raises the skin of the neck to form noticeable vertical and horizontal ridges and depressions. It can also pull the corner of the mouth down, as when a person grimaces (Figure 4-18).

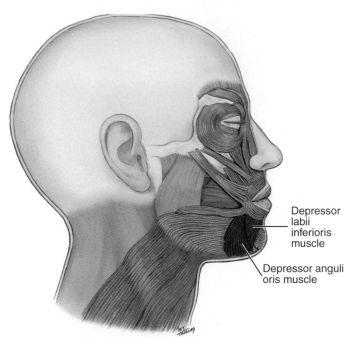

FIGURE 4-15 Depressor labii inferioris muscle and depressor anguli oris muscle.

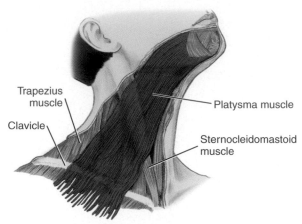

FIGURE 4-17 Origin and insertion of the right platysma muscle.

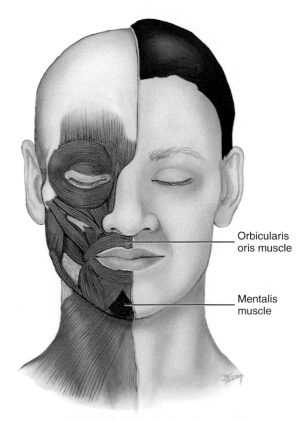

FIGURE 4-16 Mentalis muscle.

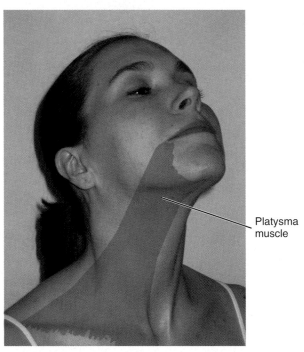

FIGURE 4-18 Patient using the right platysma muscle to raise the skin of the neck *(muscle highlighted)*.

Muscles of Mastication

The **muscles of mastication** (mass-ti-**kay**-shun) are four pairs of muscles attached to the mandible: the masseter, temporalis, medial pterygoid, and lateral pterygoid muscles.

Origin and Insertion. The origin and insertion of each muscle are discussed (Table 4-3).

Action. The muscles of mastication are responsible for closing the jaws, moving the lower jaw forward or backward, and shifting the lower jaw to one side. These jaw movements involve the movement

TABLE 4-3

ORIGIN AND INSERTION OF THE MUSCLES OF MASTICATION

Muscles	Origin	Insertion
Masseter	Superficial head: anterior two thirds of lower border of zygomatic arch Deep head: posterior third and medial surface of zygomatic arch	Superficial head: angle of mandible Deep head: ramus of mandible
Temporalis	Temporal fossa	Coronoid process of mandible
Medial pterygoid	Pterygoid fossa of sphenoid bone	Angle of mandible
Lateral pterygoid	Superior head: greater wing of sphenoid bone Inferior head: lateral pterygoid plate from sphenoid bone	Both heads: pterygoid fovea of mandible

of the mandible, while the rest of the skull remains relatively stable. These muscles of mastication work with the temporomandibular joint to accomplish these movements of the mandible (see Chapter 5). The dental professional needs to understand the association of the muscles of mastication with the movements of the mandible: depression, elevation, protrusion, retraction, and lateral deviation (Table 4-4).

TABLE 4-4

MUSCLES OF MASTICATION WITH ASSOCIATED MOVEMENTS OF MANDIBLE

Muscles	Mandibular Movements
Masseter	Elevation of mandible (during jaw closing)
Temporalis	Elevation of mandible (during jaw closing) Retraction of mandible (lower jaw backward)
Medial pterygoid	Elevation of mandible (during jaw closing)
Lateral pterygoid	Inferior heads: slight depression of mandible (during jaw opening) One muscle: lateral deviation of mandible (shift lower jaw to opposite side) Both muscles: protrusion of mandible (lower jaw forward)

Innervation. All muscles of mastication are innervated by the mandibular division of the fifth cranial or trigeminal nerve.

MASSETER MUSCLE

The most obvious muscle of mastication is the **masseter muscle (mass**-et-er) (see Figure 2-6) since it is the most superficially located and one of the strongest. The masseter muscle is a broad, thick, rectangular muscle on each side of the face, anterior to the parotid salivary gland.

This muscle can become enlarged in patients who habitually clench or grind their teeth and even in those who constantly chew gum. This masseteric hypertrophy is asymptomatic and soft and is usually bilateral but can be unilateral. If the hypertrophy is bilateral, there still may be asymmetry of the face due to unequal enlargement of the muscles (Figure 4-19). This enlargement may be confused with parotid gland disease, dental infections, and maxillofacial neoplasms. However, no other signs are present except those involved in changes in occlusion intraorally, and the enlargement corresponds with the outline of the muscle. Most patients seek medical attention because of comments about facial appearance.

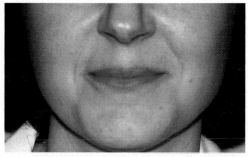

FIGURE 4-19 Bilateral enlargement of the masseter muscle.

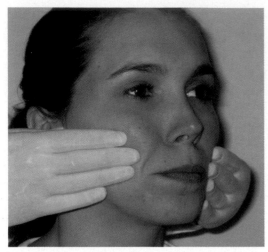

FIGURE 4-20 Palpation of the masseter muscle by having patient clench the teeth.

During an extraoral examination, stand near the patient and visually inspect and bilaterally palpate the masseter muscle. Place the fingers of each hand over the muscle and ask the patient to clench the teeth together several times (Figure 4-20). This muscle has two heads, a superficial head and a deep head.

Origin and Insertion. The superficial head of the muscle originates from the anterior two thirds of the lower border of the zygomatic arch. The deep head originates from the posterior third and the entire medial surface of the zygomatic arch. Both these heads pass inferiorly to insert on the mandible. The superficial head inserts on the lateral surface of the angle, and the deep head inserts on the ramus superior to the angle (Figure 4-21).

Action. The action of the muscle during bilateral contraction of the entire muscle is to elevate the mandible, raising the lower jaw. Elevation of the mandible occurs during the closing of the jaws.

TEMPORALIS MUSCLE

The **temporalis muscle** (tem-poh-**ral**-is) is a broad, fan-shaped muscle of mastication on each side of the head that fills the temporal fossa, superior to the zygomatic arch.

Origin and Insertion. This muscle originates from the entire temporal fossa that is bound at the top by the inferior temporal line and at the bottom by the infratemporal crest. It then passes inferiorly to insert on the coronoid process of the mandible (Figure 4-22).

Action. If the entire muscle contracts, the main action is to elevate the mandible, raising the lower jaw. Elevation of the mandible occurs during the closing of the jaws. If only the posterior portion contracts, the muscle moves the lower jaw backward. Moving the lower jaw backward causes retraction of the mandible. Retraction of the jaw often accompanies the closing of the jaws.

MEDIAL PTERYGOID MUSCLE

Deeper, yet similar in form to the superficial masseter muscle, is another muscle of mastication, the **medial pterygoid muscle** (**teh**-ri-goid) or internal pterygoid muscle.

Origin and Insertion. The muscle originates from the pterygoid fossa on the medial surface of the

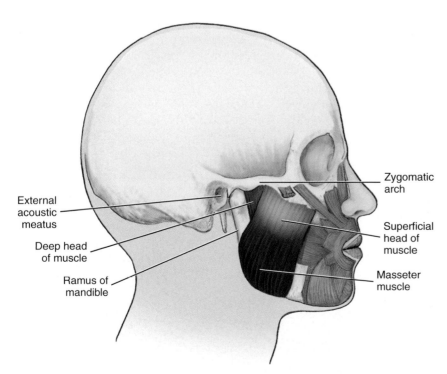

External acoustic meatus

Deep head of muscle

Ramus of mandible

Zygomatic arch

Superficial head of muscle

Masseter muscle

FIGURE 4-21 Masseter muscle with its superficial head and its deep head.

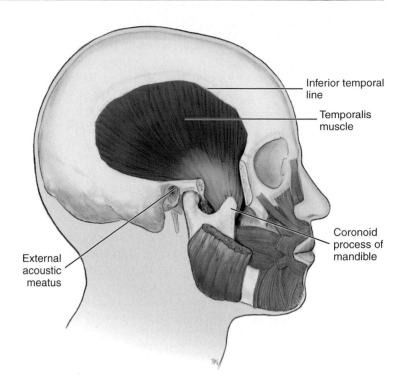

FIGURE 4-22 Origin and insertion of the temporalis muscle (*zygomatic arch and superior portion of the masseter muscle have been removed*).

lateral pterygoid plate of the sphenoid bone. It then passes inferiorly, posteriorly, and laterally to insert on the medial surface of the angle of the mandible (Figure 4-23).

Action. The muscle elevates the mandible, raising the lower jaw. Elevation of the mandible occurs during the closing of the jaws. This muscle is weaker than the masseter muscle in this action.

LATERAL PTERYGOID MUSCLE

The **lateral pterygoid muscle** or external pterygoid muscle is a muscle of mastication. This muscle has two separate heads of origin, the superior head and inferior head. The two heads of the muscle are separated by a slight interval anteriorly but fuse posteriorly. The entire muscle lies within the infratemporal fossa, deep to the temporalis muscle (see Chapter 3).

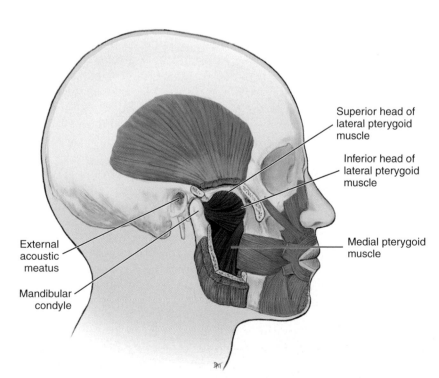

FIGURE 4-23 Medial pterygoid muscle and lateral pterygoid muscle with its superior head and its inferior head (*lower portion of the temporalis muscle, zygomatic arch, and most of the mandibular ramus have been removed*).

Origin and Insertion. The superior head originates from the inferior surface of the greater wing of the sphenoid bone (the roof of the infratemporal fossa). The inferior head originates from the lateral surface of the lateral pterygoid plate of the sphenoid bone. Both heads then unite, passing posteriorly to insert on the anterior surface of the neck of the mandibular condyle at the pterygoid fovea (see Figure 4-23). A few of the most superior fibers insert on the capsule of the temporomandibular joint.

Action. The inferior head has a slight tendency to depress the mandible, lowering the lower jaw. Depression of the mandible occurs during the opening of the jaws. The main action when both muscles contract is to bring the lower jaw forward, thus causing the protrusion of the mandible. Protrusion of the mandible often occurs during opening of the jaws. If only one muscle is contracted, the lower jaw shifts to the opposite side, causing lateral deviation of the mandible.

Hyoid Muscles

The **hyoid muscles** (hi-oid) assist in the actions of mastication and swallowing. Most of these muscles are in a superficial position in the neck tissues. These can be grouped according to whether they are suprahyoid or infrahyoid muscles (Box 4-1).

Origin and Insertion. Both groups of the hyoid muscles are attached in some way to the **hyoid bone** (Figure 4-24). The hyoid bone is a horseshoe-shaped bone suspended inferior to the mandible (see Chapter 3). The hyoid bone does not articulate with any other bone and has only muscular and ligamentary attachments. The designation for each muscle group, suprahyoid or infrahyoid, is based on its vertical position in relationship to the hyoid bone. The specific origin and insertion of each muscle are discussed in Table 4-5.

BOX 4-1

Hyoid Muscles and Their Group, Suprahyoid or Infrahyoid, Based on Their Relationship to the Hyoid Bone

Suprahyoid
Digastric
Mylohyoid
Stylohyoid
Geniohyoid

Infrahyoid
Sternothyroid
Sternohyoid
Omohyoid
Thyrohyoid

SUPRAHYOID MUSCLES

The **suprahyoid muscles** (soo-prah-**hi**-oid) are located superior to the hyoid bone (Figures 4-25 and 4-26; see Figure 4-24). These muscles may be further divided according to their anterior or posterior position to the hyoid bone. The **anterior suprahyoid muscle group** includes the anterior belly of the digastric, mylohyoid, and geniohyoid muscles. The **posterior suprahyoid muscle group** includes the posterior belly of the digastric and stylohyoid muscles.

Action. Two actions associated with mastication result from muscle contraction. One action of both the anterior and posterior suprahyoid muscles is to cause the elevation of the hyoid bone and larynx if the mandible is stabilized by contraction of the muscles of mastication. This action occurs during swallowing.

The other action associated with mastication results from only the contraction of the anterior suprahyoid muscles, which causes the mandible to depress and the jaws to open when the hyoid bone is stabilized by the contraction of the posterior suprahyoid muscles and infrahyoid muscles, the other hyoid muscle group. Thus normal jaw opening involves the lateral pterygoid muscles, which protrude the mandible, and the anterior suprahyoid muscles, which lower the mandible. Some of the suprahyoid muscles have additional specific actions that are also discussed.

Digastric Muscle.

The **digastric muscle** (di-**gas**-trik) is a suprahyoid muscle that has two separate bellies, the anterior and posterior bellies. The anterior belly is a portion of the anterior suprahyoid muscle group, and the posterior belly is a portion of the posterior suprahyoid muscle group. Each digastric muscle demarcates the superior portion of the anterior cervical triangle, forming (with the mandible) a submandibular triangle on each side of the neck. The right and left anterior bellies of the muscle form a midline submental triangle.

Origin and Insertion. The anterior belly originates on a tendon loosely attached to the body and greater cornu of the hyoid bone called the **intermediate tendon** and passes superiorly and anteriorly to insert close to the symphysis on the inner surface of the mandible. The posterior belly arises from the mastoid notch, medial to the mastoid process of the temporal bone, and passes anteriorly and inferiorly to insert on the intermediate tendon.

Innervation. The anterior belly is innervated by the mylohyoid nerve, a branch of the mandibular division of the fifth cranial or trigeminal nerve. The posterior belly is innervated by the posterior digastric nerve, a branch of the seventh cranial or facial nerve.

Mylohyoid Muscle.

The **mylohyoid muscle** (my-lo-**hi**-oid) is an anterior suprahyoid muscle that is deep to the digastric

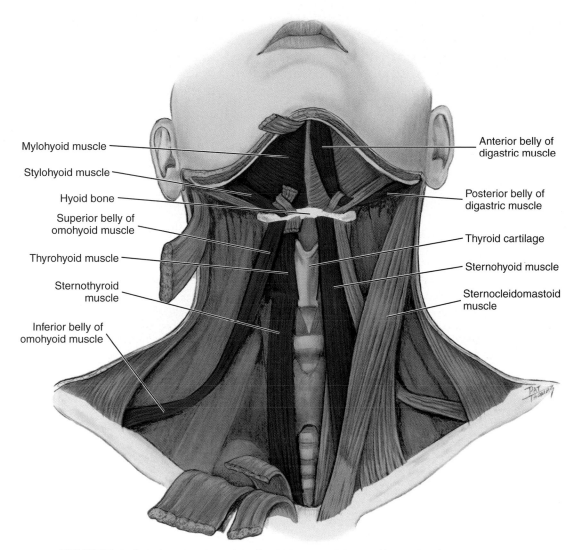

FIGURE 4-24 Anterior view of the hyoid bone and the hyoid muscles (*except the geniohyoid muscle*).

muscle, with fibers running transversely between the two sides of the mandible.

Origin and Insertion. This muscle originates from the mylohyoid line on the inner surface of the mandible. The right and left muscles pass inferiorly to unite medially, forming the floor of the mouth. The most posterior fibers of the muscle insert on the body of the hyoid bone.

Action. In addition to either elevating the hyoid bone or depressing the mandible, the muscle also forms the floor of the mouth and helps elevate the tongue.

Innervation. This muscle is innervated by the mylohyoid nerve, a branch of the mandibular division of the fifth cranial or trigeminal nerve.

Stylohyoid Muscle.

The **stylohyoid muscle** (sty-lo-**hi**-oid) is a thin posterior suprahyoid muscle, anterior and superficial to the posterior belly of the digastric muscle.

Origin and Insertion. This muscle originates from the styloid process of the temporal bone and passes anteriorly and inferiorly to insert on the body of the hyoid bone.

Innervation. This muscle is innervated by the stylohyoid nerve, a branch of the seventh cranial or facial nerve.

Geniohyoid Muscle.

The **geniohyoid muscle** (ji-nee-o-**hi**-oid) is an anterior suprahyoid muscle that is deep to the mylohyoid muscle.

Origin and Insertion. This muscle originates from the medial surface of the mandible. On this surface of the mandible, the muscle is attached near the symphysis at the genial tubercles (see Figure 4-24). The muscle then passes posteriorly and inferiorly to insert on the body of the hyoid bone.

Innervation. This muscle is innervated by the first cervical nerve, conducted by way of the twelfth cranial or hypoglossal nerve.

TABLE 4-5

ORIGIN AND INSERTION OF THE HYOID MUSCLES

Muscles	Origin	Insertion
Suprahyoid		
Digastric	Anterior belly: intermediate tendon Posterior belly: mastoid notch of temporal bone	Anterior belly: medial surface of mandible Posterior belly: intermediate tendon
Mylohyoid	Mylohyoid line of mandible	Body of hyoid bone
Stylohyoid	Styloid process of temporal bone	Body of hyoid bone
Geniohyoid	Genial tubercles of mandible	Body of hyoid bone
Infrahyoid		
Sternothyroid	Posterior surface of sternum	Thyroid cartilage
Sternohyoid	Posterior and superior surfaces of sternum	Body of hyoid bone
Omohyoid	Inferior belly: scapula Superior belly: inferior belly	Inferior belly: superior belly Superior belly: body of hyoid bone
Thyrohyoid	Thyroid cartilage	Body and greater cornu of hyoid bone

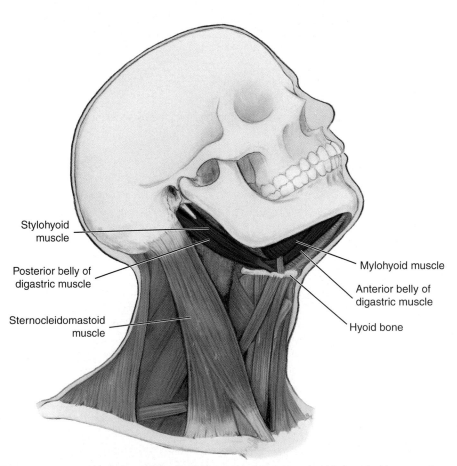

FIGURE 4-25 Lateral view of the hyoid bone and the suprahyoid muscles (*except the geniohyoid muscle*).

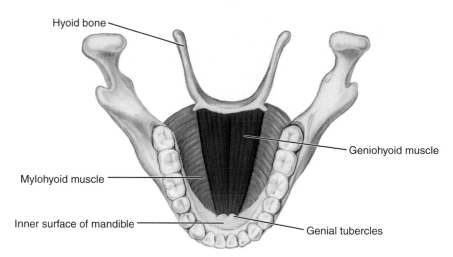

Hyoid bone

Geniohyoid muscle

Mylohyoid muscle

Inner surface of mandible

Genial tubercles

FIGURE 4-26 View from above the floor of the oral cavity showing the origin and insertion of the geniohyoid muscle.

INFRAHYOID MUSCLES

The **infrahyoid muscles** (in-frah-**hi**-oid) are four pairs of hyoid muscles inferior to the hyoid bone (Figure 4-27; see Figure 4-24). The muscles include the sternohyoid, sternothyroid, thyrohyoid, and omohyoid muscles.

Action. Most of the infrahyoid muscles depress the hyoid bone. Some of the muscles have additional specific actions that are also discussed.

Innervation. All the infrahyoid muscles are innervated by the second and third cervical nerves.

Sternothyroid Muscle.

The **sternothyroid muscle** (ster-no-**thy**-roid) is an infrahyoid muscle located superficial to the thyroid gland.

Origin and Insertion. This muscle originates from the posterior surface of the sternum, deep and medial to the sternohyoid muscle, at the level of the first rib. The muscle then passes superiorly to insert on the thyroid cartilage.

Action. This muscle depresses the thyroid cartilage and larynx, yet does not directly depress the hyoid bone.

Sternohyoid Muscle.

The **sternohyoid muscle** (ster-no-**hi**-oid) is an infrahyoid muscle superficial to the sternothyroid muscle as well as the thyroid gland and cartilage.

Origin and Insertion. This muscle originates from the posterior and superior surfaces of the sternum, close to where the sternum joins each clavicle. The muscle then passes superiorly to insert on the body of the hyoid bone.

Omohyoid Muscle.

The **omohyoid muscle** (o-mo-**hi**-oid) is an infrahyoid muscle lateral to both the sternothyroid and thyrohyoid muscles. This muscle has a superior belly and an inferior belly. The superior belly divides the inferior

portion of the anterior cervical triangle into the carotid and muscular triangles. In the posterior cervical triangle, the inferior belly serves to demarcate the subclavian triangle (inferiorly) from the occipital triangle (superiorly).

Origin and Insertion. The inferior belly originates from the scapula. The inferior belly then passes anteriorly and superiorly, crossing the internal jugular vein deep to the SCM, where it attaches by a short tendon to the superior belly. The superior belly originates from the short tendon attached to the inferior belly and then inserts on the lateral border of the body of the hyoid bone.

Thyrohyoid Muscle.

The **thyrohyoid muscle** (thy-ro-**hi**-oid) is covered by the omohyoid and sternohyoid muscles.

Origin and Insertion. This muscle originates on the thyroid cartilage and inserts on the body and greater cornu of the hyoid bone. It appears as a continuation of the sternothyroid muscle.

Action. In addition to depressing the hyoid bone, the muscle raises the thyroid cartilage and larynx.

Muscles of the Tongue

The **muscles of the tongue** can be grouped accord-ing to whether they are intrinsic or extrinsic tongue muscles (Figure 4-28). The tongue consists of symmetrical halves divided from each other by the **median septum** (**sep**-tum), a deep fibrous structure in the midline of the tongue. The median septum corresponds with the midline depression on the tongue's dorsal surface called the **median lingual sulcus** (see Chapter 2). Each half of the tongue has muscular groups arranged in various directions, with the intrinsic and extrinsic tongue muscles intertwining. The tongue is further divided into a base and body with an apex.

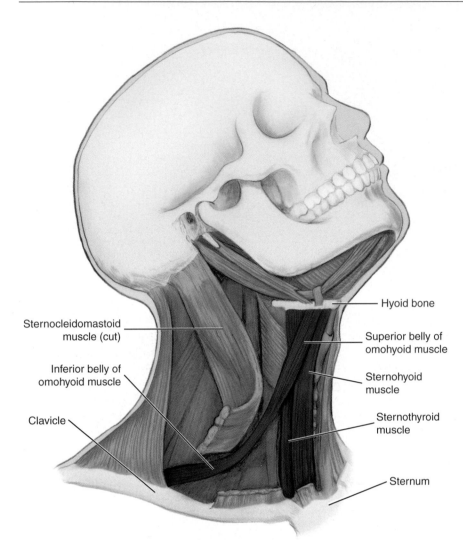

Sternocleidomastoid muscle (cut)

Inferior belly of omohyoid muscle

Clavicle

Hyoid bone

Superior belly of omohyoid muscle

Sternohyoid muscle

Sternothyroid muscle

Sternum

FIGURE 4-27 Lateral view of the hyoid bone and the infrahyoid muscles.

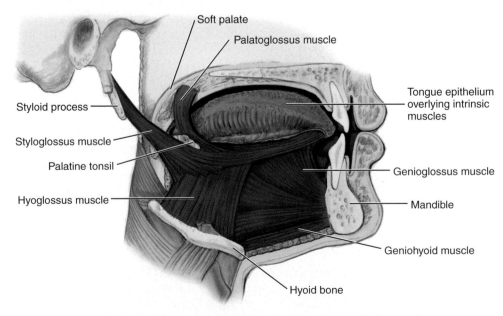

Soft palate

Palatoglossus muscle

Styloid process

Styloglossus muscle

Palatine tonsil

Hyoglossus muscle

Tongue epithelium overlying intrinsic muscles

Genioglossus muscle

Mandible

Geniohyoid muscle

Hyoid bone

FIGURE 4-28 The tongue with its intrinsic and extrinsic muscles.

Origin and Insertion. The intrinsic tongue muscles are all located inside the tongue. The muscles all have their origin outside the tongue yet have their insertion inside the tongue.

Action. The tongue has complex movements during mastication, speaking, and swallowing. These movements are a result of the combined action of muscles of the tongue. The intrinsic tongue muscles change the shape of the tongue. The muscles also move the tongue while suspending and anchoring the tongue to the mandible, styloid process, and hyoid bone. When studying the muscles of the tongue, try to visualize the movements produced by these muscles. The specific actions of each muscle of the tongue will be given.

INTRINSIC TONGUE MUSCLES

Four sets of **intrinsic tongue muscles** (in-**trin**-sik) exist, all located entirely inside the tongue (see Figure 4-28). These tongue muscles are named by their orientation. The intrinsic tongue muscles include the superior longitudinal, transverse, vertical, and inferior longitudinal muscles. Anatomists consider the intrinsic tongue muscles to be inseparable, so they are not usually treated as separate muscles.

Origin and Insertion. The **superior longitudinal muscle** is the most superficial of the intrinsic tongue muscles. This muscle runs in an oblique and longitudinal direction in the dorsal surface from the base to the apex. Deep to the superior longitudinal muscle is the **transverse muscle.** The transverse muscle runs in a transverse direction from the median septum to pass outward toward the lateral surface of the tongue. The **vertical muscle** runs in a vertical direction from the dorsal surface inward to the ventral surface in the body of the tongue. The **inferior longitudinal muscle** is located in the ventral surface of the tongue. This muscle runs in a longitudinal direction from the base to the apex of the tongue.

Action. The superior and inferior longitudinal muscles act together to change the shape of the tongue by shortening and thickening it and act singly to help it curl in various directions. The transverse and vertical muscles act together to make the tongue long and narrow.

Innervation. All the intrinsic tongue muscles are innervated by the twelfth cranial or hypoglossal nerve.

EXTRINSIC TONGUE MUSCLES

Three pairs of **extrinsic tongue muscles** (eks-**trin**-sik) have different origins outside the tongue and all their insertions inside the tongue (Table 4-6; see Figure 4-28). These muscles of the tongue have names ending in "glossus," the Greek word for tongue. The extrinsic tongue muscles include the genioglossus, styloglossus, and hyoglossus muscles. Some anatomists also include the palatoglossus muscle in this category because it is involved in tongue movement; the palatoglossus muscle is discussed with the muscles of the soft palate in this chapter.

Innervation. All the extrinsic tongue muscles are innervated by the twelfth cranial or hypoglossal nerve, a nerve with a name indicating its function and location.

Genioglossus Muscle.
The **genioglossus muscle** (ji-nee-o-**gloss**-us) is a fan-shaped extrinsic tongue muscle superior to the geniohyoid muscle.

Origin and Insertion. The muscle arises from the genial tubercles (or mental spines) on the internal surface of the mandible. A few of the most inferior fibers insert on the hyoid bone, but most of the fibers insert in the tongue from its base almost to the apex. The right and left muscles are separated by the tongue's median septum.

Action. Different portions of the muscle can protrude the tongue out of the oral cavity or depress portions of the tongue surface. The protrusive activity of the muscle helps to prevent the tongue from sinking back and obstructing respiration; therefore during general anesthesia, the mandible is sometimes pulled forward to achieve the same effect.

Styloglossus Muscle.
The **styloglossus muscle** (sty-lo-**gloss**-us) is another extrinsic tongue muscle.

Origin and Insertion. This muscle originates from the styloid process of the temporal bone. It then passes inferiorly and anteriorly to insert into two

TABLE 4-6

EXTRINSIC TONGUE MUSCLES WITH THEIR ORIGINS, INSERTIONS, AND ACTIONS*

Muscles	Origin	Insertion	Action
Genioglossus	Genial tubercles on mandible	Hyoid bone and tongue	Protrudes tongue and depresses portions
Styloglossus	Styloid process of temporal bone	Tongue	Retracts tongue
Hyoglossus	Greater cornu and body of hyoid bone	Tongue	Depresses tongue

*The palatoglossus muscle is noted under the muscles of the soft palate.

portions of the lateral surface of the tongue, its apex and at the border of the body and base.

Action. This muscle retracts the tongue, moving it superiorly and posteriorly.

Hyoglossus Muscle

The **hyoglossus muscle** (hi-o-**gloss**-us) is an extrinsic tongue muscle.

Origin and Insertion. This muscle originates on the greater cornu and a portion of the body of the hyoid bone. It then inserts into the lateral surface of the body of the tongue.

Action. This muscle depresses the tongue.

Muscles of the Pharynx

The **pharynx** (**far**-inks) is part of both the respiratory and digestive tracts and is connected to both the nasal and oral cavities. The pharynx consists of three portions: the nasopharynx, oropharynx, and laryngo-pharynx (see Chapter 2). The **muscles of the pharynx** are involved in speaking, swallowing, and middle ear function. These muscles are responsible for initiating the swallowing process. The muscles of the pharynx include the stylopharyngeus, pharyngeal constrictor, and soft palate muscles.

STYLOPHARYNGEUS MUSCLE

The **stylopharyngeus muscle** (sty-lo-fah-**rin**-je-us) is a paired longitudinal muscle of the pharynx.

Origin and Insertion. This muscle originates from the styloid process of the temporal bone. The muscle then inserts into the lateral and posterior pharyngeal walls (Figure 4-29).

Action. The muscle elevates the pharynx, and simultaneously widens the pharynx.

Innervation. This muscle is innervated by the ninth cranial or glossopharyngeal nerve.

PHARYNGEAL CONSTRICTOR MUSCLES

The **pharyngeal constrictor muscles** (fah-**rin**-je-il kon-**strik**-tor) consist of three paired muscles—the

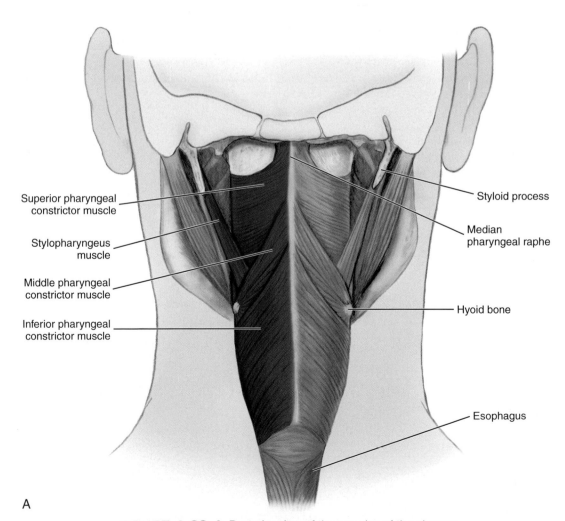

A

FIGURE 4-29 A, Posterior view of the muscles of the pharynx.

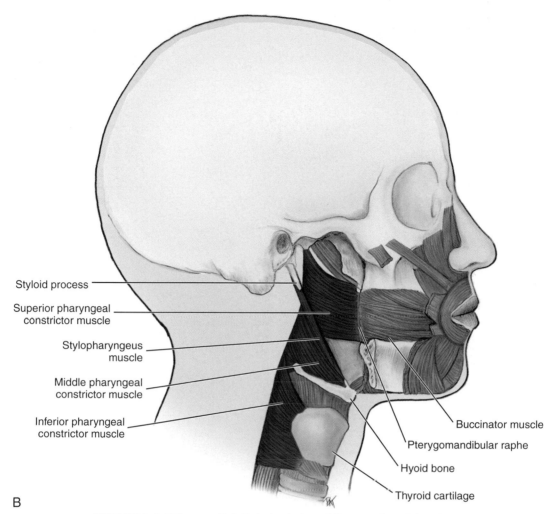

Styloid process

Superior pharyngeal
constrictor muscle

Stylopharyngeus
muscle

Middle pharyngeal
constrictor muscle

Inferior pharyngeal
constrictor muscle

Buccinator muscle

Pterygomandibular raphe

Hyoid bone

Thyroid cartilage

B

FIGURE 4-29, cont'd B, Lateral view of the muscles of the pharynx.

superior, middle, and inferior pharyngeal constrictor muscles—that form the lateral and posterior walls of the pharynx.

Origin and Insertion. The origin of each muscle is different, although the muscles overlap each other and have similar insertions (see Figure 4-29). The superior pharyngeal constrictor muscle originates from the pterygoid hamulus, mandible, and pterygomandibular raphe. The middle pharyngeal constrictor muscle originates on the hyoid bone and stylohyoid ligament. The inferior pharyngeal constrictor muscle originates from the thyroid and cricoid cartilages of the larynx. All three muscles overlap each other, the inferior being most superficial. These muscles then insert into the **median pharyngeal raphe,** a midline fibrous band of the posterior wall of the pharynx that is itself attached to the base of the skull.

Action. All three muscles raise the pharynx and larynx and help drive food inferiorly into the esophagus during swallowing.

Innervation. All three muscles are innervated by the pharyngeal plexus.

MUSCLES OF THE SOFT PALATE

The **soft palate** (**pal**-it) forms the nonbony posterior portion of the roof of the mouth or the oropharynx and connects laterally with the tongue (see Chapter 2). The muscles of the soft palate are involved in speaking and swallowing. The **muscles of the soft palate** include the palatoglossus, palatopharyngeus, levator veli palatini, and tensor veli palatini muscles and the muscle of the uvula (Figures 4-30 and 4-31, Table 4-7). Some anatomists consider the palatoglossus muscle to be an extrinsic muscle of the tongue because it is involved in tongue movement, but it will be considered only a muscle of the soft palate in this chapter.

Action. When the muscles of the soft palate are relaxed, the soft palate extends posteriorly over the anterior oropharynx. The combined actions of several muscles of the soft palate move the soft palate

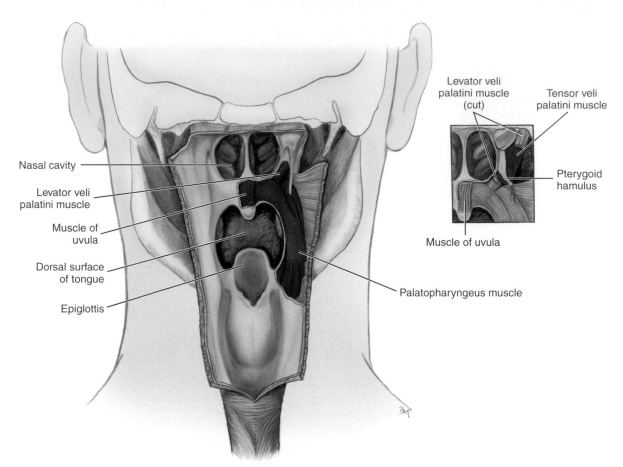

FIGURE 4-30 Posterior view of the muscles of the soft palate (pharyngeal constrictor muscles have been cut and mucous membranes partially removed).

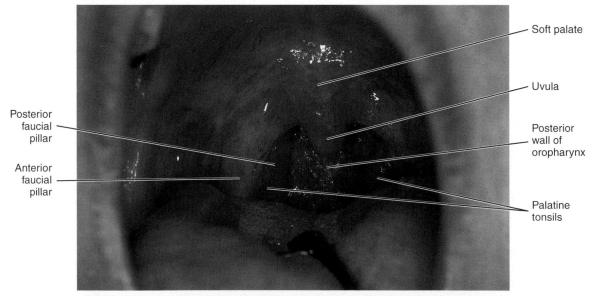

FIGURE 4-31 Intraoral view of the soft palate, uvula, and anterior and posterior faucial pillars with palatine tonsils. These oral landmarks are related to muscular tissue.

TABLE 4-7

MUSCLES OF THE SOFT PALATE WITH THEIR ORIGINS, INSERTIONS, AND ACTIONS

Muscles	Origin	Insertion	Action
Palatoglossus (anterior faucial pillar)	Median palatine raphe	Tongue	Elevates and arches tongue, depressing soft palate toward tongue
Palatopharyngeus (posterior faucial pillar)	Soft palate	Laryngopharynx and thyroid cartilage	Moves palate posteroinferiorly and posterior pharyngeal wall anterosuperiorly
Levator veli palatini	Temporal bone	Median palatine raphe	Raises soft palate to contact the posterior pharyngeal wall
Tensor veli palatini	Auditory tube and sphenoid	Median palatine raphe bone	Tenses and slightly lowers soft palate
Muscle of the uvula	Tissue projection that hangs inferiorly from posterior soft palate		Soft palate closely adapts to posterior pharyngeal wall

superiorly and posteriorly to contact the posterior pharyngeal wall that is being moved anteriorly. This movement of both the soft palate and pharyngeal wall brings a separation between the nasopharynx and oral cavity during swallowing to prevent food from entering the nasal cavity while eating. Specific actions of each muscle of the soft palate will also be discussed.

Innervation. All of the muscles except the tensor veli palatini muscle are innervated by the pharyngeal plexus. This muscle is supplied by the mandibular division of the fifth cranial or trigeminal nerve.

Palatoglossus Muscle.

The **palatoglossus muscle** (pal-ah-to-**gloss**-us) forms the **anterior faucial pillar** (**faw**-shawl) in the oral cavity, a vertical fold anterior to each palatine tonsil (see Figures 4-28 and 4-31 and Chapter 10).

Origin and Insertion. This muscle originates from the **median palatine raphe** (**pal**-ah-tine), a midline fibrous band of the palate. It then inserts into the lateral surface of the tongue.

Action. This muscle elevates the base of the tongue, arching the tongue against the soft palate, and depresses the soft palate toward the tongue. The muscles on both sides form a sphincter, separating the oral cavity from the pharynx.

Palatopharyngeus Muscle.

The **palatopharyngeus muscle** (pal-ah-to-fah-**rin**-je-us) forms the **posterior faucial pillar** in the oral cavity, a

vertical fold posterior to each palatine tonsil (see Figures 4-30 and 4-31 and Chapter 10).

Origin and Insertion. This muscle originates in the soft palate and inserts in the walls of the laryngopharynx and on the thyroid cartilage.

Action. It moves the palate posteroinferiorly and the posterior pharyngeal wall anterosuperiorly to help close off the nasopharynx during swallowing.

Levator Veli Palatini Muscle.

The **levator veli palatini muscle** (le-**vate**-er **vee**-lie pal-ah-**teen**-ee) is a muscle mainly situated superior to the soft palate (see Figure 4-30).

Origin and Insertion. This muscle originates from the inferior surface of the temporal bone. It then inserts into the median palatine raphe, a midline fibrous band of the palate (see Chapter 2).

Action. It raises the soft palate and helps bring it into contact with the posterior pharyngeal wall to close off the nasopharynx during speech and swallowing.

Tensor Veli Palatini Muscle.

The **tensor veli palatini muscle** (**ten**-ser **vee**-lie pal-ah-**teen**-ee) is a special muscle that stiffens the soft palate (see Figure 4-30). This muscle is probably active during all palatal movements. Some of its fibers are also responsible for opening the auditory tube to allow air to flow between the pharynx and middle ear cavity.

Origin and Insertion. This muscle originates from the auditory tube area and the inferior surface of the sphenoid bone. The muscle then passes inferiorly between the medial pterygoid muscle and medial pterygoid plate, forming a tendon near the pterygoid hamulus. The tendon winds around the hamulus, using it as a pulley, and then spreads out to insert in the median palatine raphe.

Action. This muscle tenses and slightly lowers the soft palate.

Muscle of the Uvula.
The **muscle of the uvula** (u-vu-lah) is a muscle of the soft palate.

Origin and Insertion. This muscle lies within the **uvula of the palate** (see Chapter 2). The uvula is a midline tissue structure that hangs inferiorly from the posterior margin of the soft palate (see Figures 4-30 and 4-31).

Action. This muscle shortens and broadens the uvula, changing the contour of the posterior portion of the soft palate. This change in contour allows the soft palate to adapt closely to the posterior pharyngeal wall to help close off the nasopharynx during swallowing.

Identification Exercises

Identify the structures on the following diagrams by filling in each blank with the correct anatomical term. You can check your answers by looking back at the figure indicated in parentheses for each identification diagram.

1. (Figure 4-4, *A*)

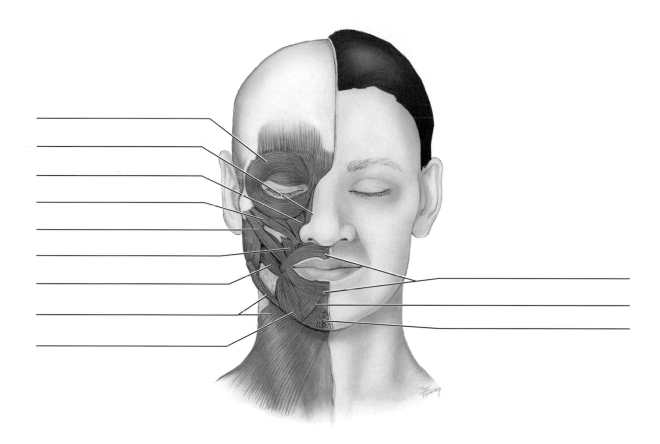

2. (Figure 4-4, *B*)

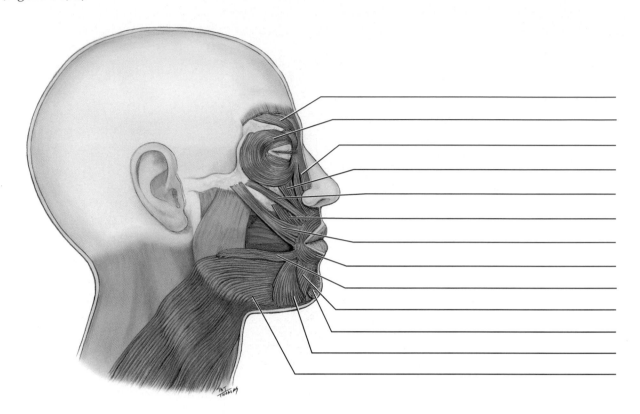

3. (Figures 4-22 and 4-23)

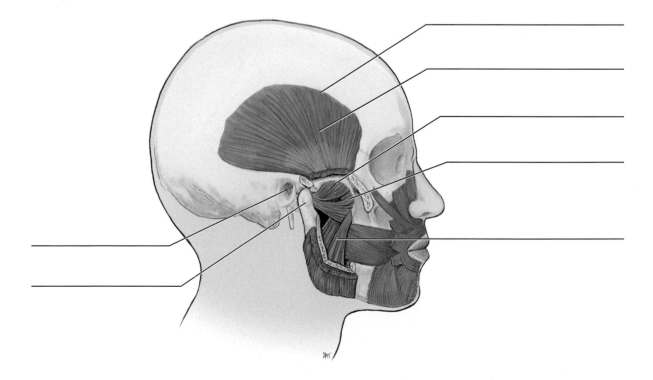

8. (Figure 4-30)

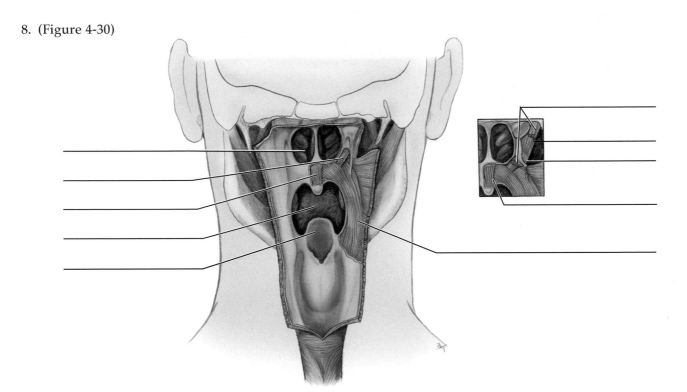

■ REVIEW QUESTIONS

1. Both the origin of the frontal belly of the epicranial muscle and the insertion of its occipital belly are at the:
   A. Clavicle and sternum
   B. Mastoid process
   C. Epicranial aponeurosis
   D. Pterygomandibular raphe

2. Which of the following muscles is considered a muscle of mastication?
   A. Buccinator muscle
   B. Risorius muscle
   C. Mentalis muscle
   D. Masseter muscle
   E. Corrugator supercilii muscle

3. The origin of a muscle is:
   A. The starting point of a muscle
   B. Where the muscle fibers join the bone tendon
   C. The muscle end attached to the least movable structure
   D. The muscle end attached to the most movable structure

4. Which of the following muscle pairs is divided by a median septum?
   A. Geniohyoid muscle
   B. Masseter muscle
   C. Digastric muscle
   D. Transverse muscle of the tongue
   E. Vertical muscle of the tongue

5. Which of the following paired muscles unites medially, forming the floor of the mouth?
   A. Geniohyoid muscle
   B. Omohyoid muscle
   C. Digastric muscle
   D. Mylohyoid muscle
   E. Transverse muscle of the tongue

6. Which of the following muscle groups depress the hyoid bone?
   A. Muscles of mastication
   B. Suprahyoid muscles
   C. Infrahyoid muscles
   D. Intrinsic tongue muscles
   E. Extrinsic tongue muscles

7. Which of the following muscles has two bellies, giving the muscle two different origins?
   A. Lateral pterygoid muscle
   B. Geniohyoid muscle
   C. Thyrohyoid muscle
   D. Stylohyoid muscle

8. Which of the following is the most important muscle used when the patient's lips close around the saliva ejector?
   A. Risorius muscle
   B. Mentalis muscle
   C. Mylohyoid muscle
   D. Buccinator muscle
   E. Orbicularis oris muscle

9. Which of the following muscle groups is involved in elevating the hyoid bone and depressing the mandible?
   A. Muscles of mastication
   B. Suprahyoid muscles
   C. Infrahyoid muscles
   D. Intrinsic tongue muscles
   E. Extrinsic tongue muscles

10. Which of the following muscle groups is innervated by the cervical nerves?
    A. Muscles of mastication
    B. Muscles of facial expression
    C. Suprahyoid muscles
    D. Infrahyoid muscles
    E. Intrinsic tongue muscles

11. Which muscle can make the patient's oral vestibule shallow, thereby making dental work difficult?
    A. Mentalis muscle
    B. Zygomaticus major muscle
    C. Depressor anguli oris muscle
    D. Levator anguli oris muscle

12. Which of the following muscle groups is innervated by the facial nerve?
    A. Intrinsic tongue muscles
    B. Extrinsic tongue muscles
    C. Muscles of facial expression
    D. Muscles of mastication

13. Which of the following muscle groups inserts directly on the hyoid bone?
    A. Geniohyoid, stylohyoid, and omohyoid muscles
    B. Masseter, stylohyoid, and digastric muscles
    C. Masseter, buccinator, and omohyoid muscles
    D. Palatopharyngeus and palatoglossus muscles and muscle of the uvula

14. Which of the following muscles is used when a patient grimaces?
    A. Epicranial muscle
    B. Corrugator supercilii muscle
    C. Risorius muscle
    D. Mentalis muscle

15. Which of the following muscles is an extrinsic muscle of the tongue?
    A. Geniohyoid muscle
    B. Hyoglossus muscle
    C. Mylohyoid muscle
    D. Transverse muscle
    E. Vertical muscle

16. Which of the following muscles compresses the cheeks during chewing, assisting the muscles of mastication?
    A. Risorius muscle
    B. Buccinator muscle
    C. Mentalis muscle
    D. Orbicularis oris muscle

17. The superior pharyngeal constrictor muscle:
    A. Originates from the larynx
    B. Inserts on the median pharyngeal raphe
    C. Overlaps the stylopharyngeus muscle
    D. Is a longitudinal muscle of the pharynx

18. Which of the following statements concerning the masseter muscle is correct?
    A. It is the most superficial muscle of facial expression.
    B. It originates from the zygomatic arch.
    C. It inserts on the medial surface of the mandible's angle.
    D. It depresses the mandible during jaw movement.

19. Which of the following muscles creates the anterior faucial pillar in the oral cavity?
    A. Palatoglossus muscle
    B. Palatopharyngeus muscle
    C. Stylopharyngeus muscle
    D. Tensor veli palatini muscle

20. Which of the following situations occurs when both sternocleidomastoid muscles are used by the patient?
    A. Neck is drawn laterally
    B. Head flexes at the neck
    C. Chin moves superiorly to the opposite side
    D. Head rotates and is drawn to the shoulders

21. Which muscle does *not* aid in smiling with the lips when it contracts?
    A. Zygomatic major muscle
    B. Levator anguli oris muscle
    C. Zygomaticus minor muscle
    D. Epicranial muscle

22. Which muscle lies just deep to the skin of the neck?
    A. Platysma muscle
    B. Buccinator muscle

    C. Risorius muscle
    D. Mentalis muscle

23. Which muscle is most superior?
    A. Corrugator supercilii muscle
    B. Zygomatic major muscle
    C. Superior pharyngeal constrictor muscle
    D. Superior belly of the omohyoid muscle

24. Which muscle, when contracted, causes a frown?
    A. Zygomaticus minor muscle
    B. Levator anguli oris muscle
    C. Depressor anguli oris muscle
    D. Risorius muscle

25. Which muscle is most superficial?
    A. Masseter muscle
    B. Medial pterygoid muscle
    C. Lateral pterygoid muscle
    D. Superior pharyngeal constrictor muscle

26. Which of the following are considered intrinsic tongue muscles?
    A. Superior longitudinal muscle
    B. Genioglossus muscle
    C. Styloglossus muscle
    D. Hyoglossus muscle

27. The muscles of the pharynx are involved in:
    A. Closing the jaws
    B. Facial expression
    C. Middle ear function
    D. Stabilization of the mandible

28. The posterior belly of the digastric muscle is also a(n):
    A. Muscle of facial expression
    B. Posterior suprahyoid muscle
    C. Intrinsic muscle of the tongue
    D. Extrinsic muscle of the tongue

29. Which of the following innervates the temporalis muscle?
    A. First cervical nerve by way of the hypoglossal nerve
    B. Ninth cranial nerve or glossopharyngeal nerve
    C. Maxillary branch of the trigeminal nerve
    D. Mandibular branch of the trigeminal nerve
    E. Seventh cranial nerve or facial nerve

30. Which muscle's activity helps to prevent the tongue from sinking back and obstructing respiration?
    A. Genioglossus muscle
    B. Stylopharyngeus muscle
    C. Inferior longitudinal muscle
    D. Palatoglossus muscle

Temporomandibular Joint

OUTLINE

- Overview of the Temporomandibular Joint
  - Bones of the Joint
  - Joint Capsule
  - Disc of the Joint
  - Ligaments Associated with the Joint
- Jaw Movements with Muscle Relationships
- Palpation of the Joint
- Disorders of the Joint

LEARNING OBJECTIVES

After studying this chapter, the reader should be able to do the following:

1. Define and pronounce all the key terms and anatomical terms in this chapter.
2. Locate and identify the specific anatomical landmarks of the temporomandibular joint on a diagram, skull, and patient.
3. Describe the movements of the temporomandibular joint and their relationship with the muscles in the head and neck region.
4. Discuss the disorders of the temporomandibular joint.
5. Correctly complete the review questions and activities for this chapter.
6. Integrate the knowledge about the anatomy of the temporomandibular joint into clinical dental practice.

KEY TERMS

Depression of the Mandible (de-**presh**-in) Lowering of the lower jaw.

Elevation of the Mandible (el-eh-**vay**-shun) Raising of the lower jaw.

Joint Site of a junction or union between two or more bones.

Lateral Deviation of the Mandible (de-vee-**ay**-shun) Shifting of the lower jaw to one side.

Ligament (**lig**-ah-mint) Band of fibrous tissue connecting bones.

Protrusion of the Mandible (pro-**troo**-shun) Bringing forward of the lower jaw.

Retraction of the Mandible (re-**trak**-shun) Bringing backward of the lower jaw.

Subluxation (sub-luk-**say**-shun) Acute episode of temporomandibular joint disorder in which both joints become dislocated, often due to excessive mandibular protrusion and depression.

Temporomandibular Disorder (TMD) (tem-poh-ro-man-**dib**-you-lar) Disorder involving one or both temporomandibular joints.

OVERVIEW OF THE TEMPOROMANDIBULAR JOINT

A **joint** is a site of a junction or union between two or more bones. The **temporomandibular joint (TMJ)** is a joint on each side of the head that allows for movement of the mandible for speech and mastication. A patient may have a disease process associated with one or both of the TMJs. Thus the dental professional needs to understand the anatomy of the TMJ, the normal movements involved with the joint, and any possible disorders associated with the joint.

The TMJ is innervated by the mandibular division of the fifth cranial or trigeminal nerve. The blood supply to the joint is from branches of the external carotid artery.

Bones of the Joint

The TMJ has two sets of articulations, one on each side of the head: the two temporal bones and the two condyles of the mandible (Figure 5-1). Both articulating bony surfaces of the joint are covered by fibrocartilage. Chapter 3 has more information on both of these bones of the joint.

TEMPORAL BONE

The **temporal bone (tem**-poh-ral) is a cranial bone that articulates with the mandible at the TMJ (Figure 5-2). The articulating area on the temporal bone of the joint is located on the bone's inferior aspect. This articulating area includes the bone's articular eminence and articular fossa. The **articular eminence** (ar-**tik**-you-ler) is positioned anterior to the articular fossa and consists of a smooth, rounded ridge.

The **articular fossa** or mandibular fossa is posterior to the articular eminence and consists of a depression on the temporal bone, posterior and medial to the **zygomatic process of the temporal bone** (zy-go-**mat**-ik). Posterior to the articular fossa is a sharper ridge, the **postglenoid process** (post-**gle**-noid).

MANDIBLE

The **mandible (man**-di-bl) is a facial bone that articulates with the temporal bone at the head of the **condyle of the mandible** with its **articulating surface of the condyle** (ar-**tik**-you-late-ing) (Figure 5-3). Posterior to the condyle is the **coronoid process (kor**-ah-noid). The depression of the **mandibular notch** (man-**dib**-you-lar) is located between the condyle and coronoid process.

Joint Capsule

A fibrous **joint capsule** completely encloses the TMJ (Figure 5-4). Superiorly, the capsule wraps around the margin of the temporal bone's articular eminence and articular fossa. Inferiorly, the capsule wraps around the circumference of the mandibular condyle including the condyle's neck.

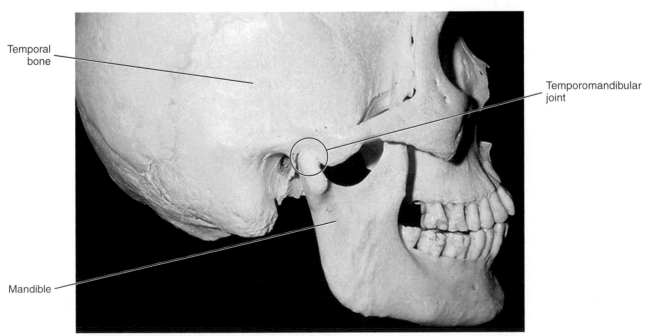

Temporal bone

Temporomandibular joint

Mandible

FIGURE 5-1 Lateral view of the skull showing the temporomandibular joint with the temporal bone and mandible.

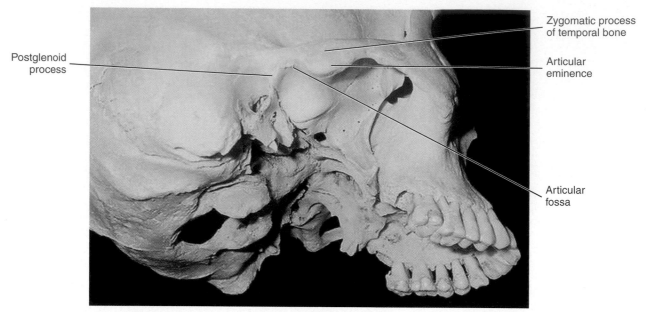

Postglenoid process

Zygomatic process of temporal bone

Articular eminence

Articular fossa

FIGURE 5-2 Inferolateral view of the skull with the temporal bone.

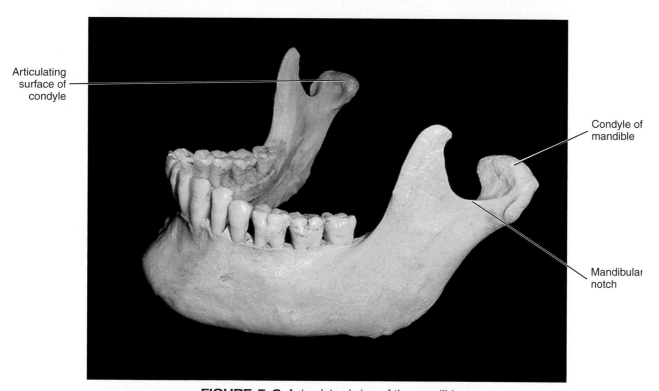

Articulating surface of condyle

Condyle of mandible

Mandibular notch

FIGURE 5-3 Anterolateral view of the mandible.

Disc of the Joint

The fibrous **disc of the joint** or meniscus of the joint is located between the temporal bone and condyle of the mandible on each side (see Figure 5-4). On parasagittal section, the disc appears caplike on the mandibular condyle, with its superior aspect concavoconvex from anterior to posterior and its inferior aspect concave.

This shape of the disc conforms with the shape of the adjacent articulating bones of the TMJ and is related to normal joint movements.

The disc completely divides the TMJ into two compartments or spaces. These two compartments are **synovial cavities** (sy-**no**-vee-al), an upper synovial cavity and a lower synovial cavity. The membranes

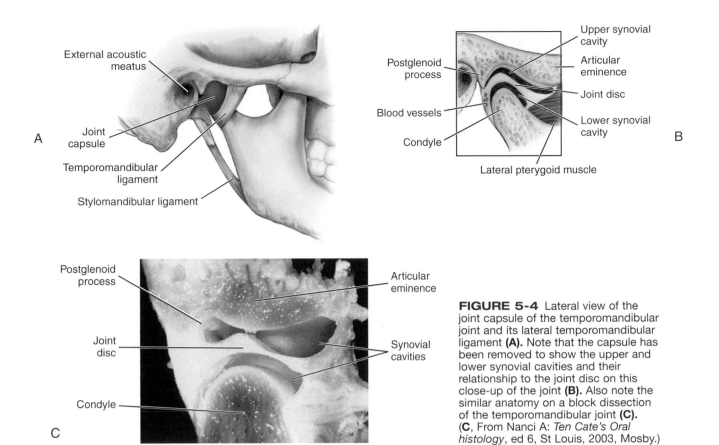

FIGURE 5-4 Lateral view of the joint capsule of the temporomandibular joint and its lateral temporomandibular ligament **(A).** Note that the capsule has been removed to show the upper and lower synovial cavities and their relationship to the joint disc on this close-up of the joint **(B).** Also note the similar anatomy on a block dissection of the temporomandibular joint **(C).** (**C,** From Nanci A: *Ten Cate's Oral histology*, ed 6, St Louis, 2003, Mosby.)

lining the inside of the joint capsule secrete **synovial fluid** that helps lubricate the joint and fills the synovial cavities. Synovial fluid is a clear, viscous liquid, rather like the white of an egg.

The disc is attached to the lateral and medial poles of the mandibular condyle. The disc is not attached to the temporal bone anteriorly, except indirectly through the capsule. Posteriorly, the disc is divided into two areas. The upper division of the posterior portion of the disc is attached to the temporal bone's postglenoid process, and the lower division attaches to the neck of the condyle. The disc blends with the capsule at these points. This posterior area of attachment of the disc to the capsule is one of the places where nerves and blood vessels enter the joint.

As a person ages or undergoes trauma to the area, the disc can become thinner or even perforated. Recent studies suggest that disc degeneration, which may occur as a result of aging or mechanical stress, causes calcifications within the disc. At any age, the disc may become dislocated forward by injury to the posterior attachment. Both perforation and displacement can lead to clinical problems (discussed later).

Ligaments Associated with the Joint

A **ligament** is a band of fibrous tissue that connects bones. Three paired ligaments are associated with the TMJ. These ligaments are the TMJ ligament, sphenomandibular ligament, and stylomandibular ligament (Figure 5-5).

TEMPOROMANDIBULAR JOINT LIGAMENT

The **TMJ ligament** is located on the lateral side of each joint and forms a reinforcement of the capsule of the TMJ. This ligament prevents the excessive retraction or moving backward of the mandible, a situation that might lead to problems with the TMJ.

SPHENOMANDIBULAR LIGAMENT

The **sphenomandibular ligament** (sfe-no-man-**dib**-you-lar) is not a portion of the TMJ but is located on the medial side of the mandible, some distance from the joint. This ligament runs from the angular spine of the sphenoid bone to the lingula of the mandibular foramen. The inferior alveolar nerve descends between the sphenomandibular ligament and the ramus of the mandible to gain access to the mandibular foramen. The sphenomandibular ligament, because of its attachment to the lingula, overlaps the opening of the foramen. It is a vestige of the embryonic lower jaw, Meckel's cartilage.

Although it is not a portion of the TMJ, the ligament becomes accentuated and taut when the mandible is

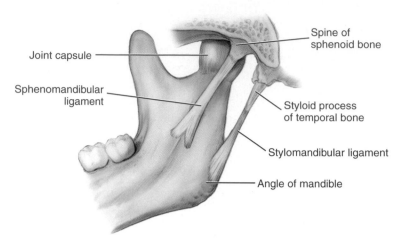

Joint capsule

Sphenomandibular
ligament

Spine of
sphenoid bone

Styloid process
of temporal bone

Stylomandibular ligament

Angle of mandible

FIGURE 5-5 Internal view of the temporomandibular joint with associated ligaments.

protruded. This ligament is a landmark for the administration of inferior alveolar local anesthetic block (see Chapter 9).

STYLOMANDIBULAR LIGAMENT

The **stylomandibular ligament** (sty-lo-man-**dib**-you-lar) is a variable ligament that is formed from a thickened cervical fascia in the area. This ligament runs from the styloid process of the temporal bone to the angle of the mandible. This ligament also becomes taut when the mandible is protruded.

JAW MOVEMENTS WITH MUSCLE RELATIONSHIPS

The TMJ allows for the movement of the mandible during speech and mastication. There are two basic types of movement performed by the joint and its associated muscles: a gliding movement and a rotational movement.

The gliding movement of the TMJ occurs mainly between the disc and the articular eminence of the temporal bone in the upper synovial cavity, with the disc plus the condyle moving forward or backward, down and up the articular eminence. The gliding movement allows the lower jaw to move forward or backward. Bringing the lower jaw forward involves **protrusion of the mandible.** Bringing the lower jaw backward involves **retraction of the mandible.** Protrusion involves the bilateral contraction of the lateral pterygoid muscles. The posterior portions of both temporalis muscles are involved during retraction of the mandible.

The rotational movement of the TMJ occurs mainly between the disc and the condyle of the mandible in the lower synovial cavity. The axis of rotation of the disc plus the condyle is transverse, and the movements accomplished are depression or elevation of the mandible. **Depression of the mandible** is the

lowering of the lower jaw. **Elevation of the mandible** is the raising of the lower jaw.

With these two types of movement, gliding and rotation, and with the right and left TMJs working together, the finer movements of the jaw can be accomplished. These include opening and closing the jaws and shifting the lower jaw to one side (Figure 5-6).

Opening the jaws during speech and mastication involves both depression and protrusion of the mandible. Closing the jaws involves both elevation and retraction of the mandible. Thus opening and closing the jaws involve a combination of gliding and rotational movements of the TMJs in their respective joint cavities. The disc plus the condyle glide on the articular fossa in the upper synovial cavity, moving forward or backward on the articular eminence. Roughly at the same time, the condyle of the mandible rotates on the disc in the lower synovial cavity.

Muscles are involved in lower jaw movements (see Chapter 4). The muscle of mastication involved in elevating the mandible during closing of the jaws are the bilateral masseter, temporalis, and medial pterygoid muscles. The anterior suprahyoid muscles are involved in depressing the mandible during opening of the jaws, when they bilaterally contract as the hyoid bone is stabilized by the other hyoid muscles. The inferior heads of the lateral pterygoid muscles may also be involved in depressing the mandible during opening of the jaws.

Lateral deviation, or lateral excursion of the mandible or shifting the lower jaw to one side, occurs during mastication. Lateral deviation involves both the gliding and rotational movements of the opposite TMJs in their respective joint cavities. During lateral deviation, one disc plus the condyle glide forward and medially on the articular eminence in the upper synovial cavity while the other condyle and disc remain relatively stable in position in the articular

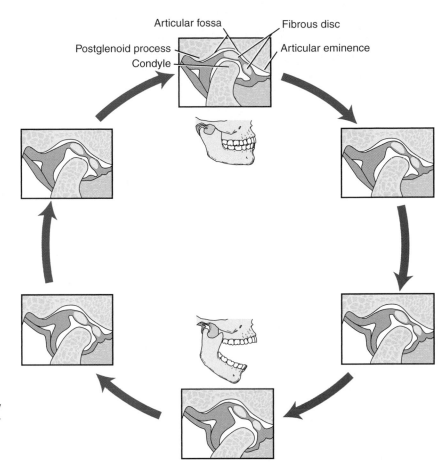

Articular fossa
Postglenoid process
Condyle
Fibrous disc
Articular eminence

FIGURE 5-6 Movements of the mandible related to the temporomandibular joint to show opening and closing of the mouth. (From Bath-Balogh M, Fehrenbach MJ: *Illustrated dental embryology, histology, and anatomy,* ed 6, St. Louis, 2006, WB Saunders.)

fossa. This produces a rotation around the more stable condyle.

Contraction of one of the lateral pterygoid muscles (the one on the protruding side) is involved during lateral deviation. When the mandible laterally deviates to the left, the right lateral pterygoid muscle contracts, moving the right condyle forward while the left condyle stays in position, thus causing the mandible to move to the left. The reverse situation occurs when the mandible laterally deviates to the right.

During mastication, the power stroke (when the teeth crunch the food) involves a movement from a laterally deviated position back to the midline. If the food is on the right, the mandible will be deviated to the right by the left lateral pterygoid muscle. The power stroke will return the mandible to the center, so the movement is to the left and involves a retraction of the left side. This is accomplished by the left posterior portion of the temporalis muscle. At the same time, all the closing jaw muscles on the right side contract to crush the food. The reverse situation occurs if the food is on the left.

The resting position of the TMJ is not with the teeth biting together. The muscular balance and proprioceptive feedback allow a freeway space of 2 to 4 mm to exist between the teeth at rest. When the teeth are lost, the jaw may overclose, which is often uncomfortable for the patient. Likewise, dentures that "jack" the jaw open are intolerable for a patient.

Palpation of the Joint

To palpate the joint and its associated muscles effectively, have the patient go through all the movements of the mandible (Table 5-1). The TMJ can be palpated just anterior to the external acoustic meatus of each ear (Figure 5-7). To assess the entire joint and its associated muscles effectively, use bilateral palpation and ask the patient to open and close the mouth several times. Then ask the patient to move the opened jaw left, then right, and then forward. Using digital palpation of the mandible moving at the TMJ, gently place a finger into the outer portion of the external acoustic meatus (Figure 5-8). Auscultation of the joint can also be done.

DISORDERS OF THE JOINT

A patient may have a disease process associated with one or both of the TMJs or a **temporomandibular disorder (TMD)**. The patient may experience chronic joint tenderness, swelling, and painful muscle spasms.

TABLE 5-1

MOVEMENT OF MANDIBLE AND TEMPOROMANDIBULAR JOINT WITH ASSOCIATED MUSCLES

Mandibular Movements	Temporomandibular Joint Movements	Associated Muscles
Protrusion of mandible, moving lower jaw forward	Gliding in both upper synovial cavities	Lateral pterygoid, bilateral contraction
Retraction of mandible, moving lower jaw backward	Gliding in both upper synovial cavities	Posterior portion of temporalis, bilateral contraction
Depression and protrusion of mandible, opening jaws	Gliding in both upper synovial cavities and rotation in both lower synovial cavities	Suprahyoids and inferior heads of lateral pterygoid, bilateral contraction
Lateral deviation of mandible, to shift lower jaw to opposite side	Gliding in one upper synovial cavity and rotation in opposite upper synovial cavity	Lateral pterygoid, unilateral contraction

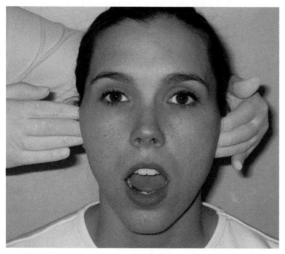

FIGURE 5-7 Palpation of the patient during movements of both temporomandibular joints.

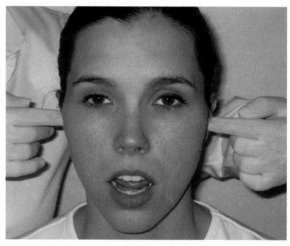

FIGURE 5-8 Palpation of the joint by gently placing a finger into the outer portion of the external acoustic meatus.

Also present may be difficulties of joint movement such as a limited or deviated mandibular opening. The dental professional plays an important role in the recognition, treatment, and maintenance of patients with this disorder.

Recognition of TMD includes palpation of the joint as the patient performs all the movements of the joint as well as palpation of the related muscles of mastication. All signs and symptoms related to TMD, such as the amount of mandibular opening and facial pain, as well as any parafunctional habits and related systemic diseases need to be recorded by the dental professional. The traditional skull radiograph of the joint area may be used, or magnetic resonance imaging (MRI) may be performed to aid in the diagnosis of

TMD. MRI is a noninvasive nuclear procedure for imaging soft tissue with high fat and water content. Thus MRI can make it possible to distinguish normal tissue from diseased tissue (Figure 5-9).

Not all patients with TMD have abnormalities in the joint disc or the joint itself. Most symptoms seem to come from the muscles. Most recent studies do not support the role of TMD in directly causing headaches, neck or back pain, or instability. Headaches are usually caused by muscle tension or vascular changes. Cyclic episodes of TMD and other incidents of chronic body pain are commonly encountered in the TMD population.

Joint sounds occur because of disc derangement. The posterior portion of the disc gets caught between

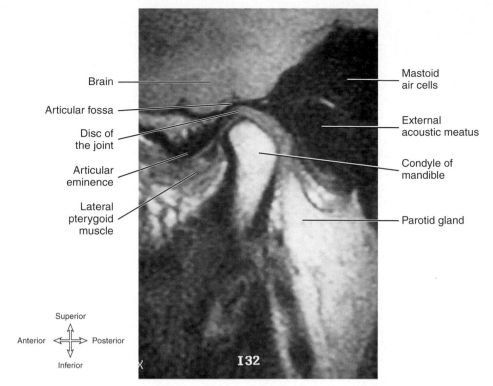

Brain

Articular fossa

Disc of
the joint

Articular
eminence

Lateral
pterygoid
muscle

Mastoid
air cells

External
acoustic meatus

Condyle of
mandible

Parotid gland

Superior

Anterior ⟵ ⟶ Posterior

Inferior

I 32

FIGURE 5-9 Coronal magnetic resonance imaging of a closed temporomandibular joint in an asymptomatic individual (MRI). (From Quinn PD: *Color atlas of temporomandibular joint surgery*, St Louis, 1998, Mosby.)

the condyle head and the articular eminence. Joint sounds are not a reliable indicator of TMD because they can change over time in a patient. Thus the clicking, grinding, and popping of the joint during movement that is commonly present with TMD is also found in 40% to 60% of persons without TMD.

An acute episode of TMD can occur when a patient opens the mouth too wide, causing maximal depression and protrusion of the mandible, as when yawning or receiving prolonged dental care. This causes **subluxation** or dislocation of both joints. Subluxation happens when the head of each condyle moves too far

anteriorly on the articular eminence. When the patient tries to close and elevate the mandible, the condylar heads cannot move posteriorly because the muscles have become spastic.

Treatment of subluxation consists of relaxing these muscles and carefully moving the mandible downward and back. The condylar heads will then be able to assume the normal posterior position in relationship to the articular eminence by the muscular action of the elevating muscles of mastication. Future care of these patients involves avoidance of extreme depression of the mandible.

Identification Exercises

Identify the structures on the following diagrams by filling in each blank with the correct anatomical term. You can check your answers by looking back at the figure indicated in parentheses for each identification diagram.

1. (Figures 5-1, 5-2. and 5-4, *A* and *B*)

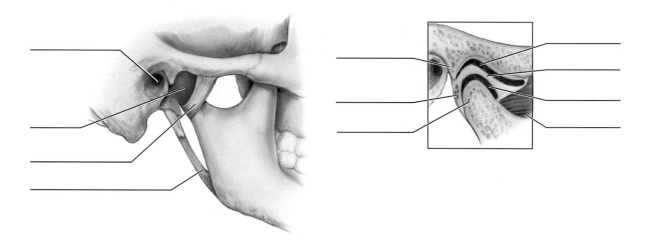

2. (Figures 5-3 and 5-5)

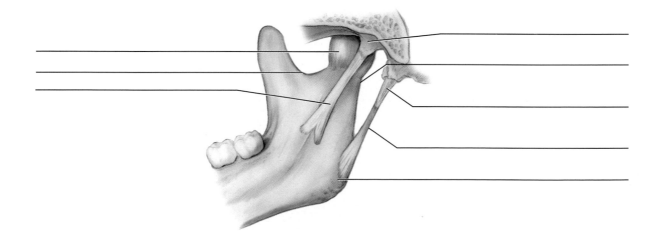

■ REVIEW QUESTIONS

1. Which of the following ligaments associated with the temporomandibular joint reinforces the joint capsule?
   A. Styloid ligament
   B. Stylomandibular ligament
   C. Temporomandibular ligament
   D. Sphenomandibular ligament

2. Which of the following landmarks is located on the mandible?
   A. Articular eminence
   B. Coronoid process
   C. Articular fossa
   D. Postglenoid process

3. Which of the following is a basic movement performed by the temporomandibular joint?
   A. Gliding movement only
   B. Rotational movement only
   C. Gliding and rotational movement
   D. No movement is performed

4. Which of the following muscles is involved in the lateral deviation of the mandible?
   A. Masseter muscle
   B. Medial pterygoid muscle
   C. Lateral pterygoid muscle
   D. Temporalis muscle
   E. Digastric muscle

5. Protrusion of the mandible primarily involves:
   A. Opening the jaws
   B. Closing the jaws
   C. Bringing the lower jaw forward
   D. Bringing the lower jaw backward
   E. Shifting the lower jaw to one side

6. Which of the following movements is assisted by the temporalis muscle?
   A. Mandibular depression only
   B. Mandibular elevation only
   C. Mandibular retraction only
   D. Mandibular depression and elevation
   E. Mandibular elevation and retraction

7. Which of the following ligaments associated with the temporomandibular joint has the inferior alveolar nerve descend nearby to gain access to the mandibular foramen?
   A. Sphenomandibular ligament only
   B. Stylomandibular ligament only
   C. Temporomandibular ligament only
   D. Sphenomandibular and stylomandibular ligaments
   E. Stylomandibular and temporomandibular ligaments

8. Which of the following statements about the temporomandibular disc is false?
   A. The disc separates the TMJ into synovial cavities.
   B. The disc is attached anteriorly and posteriorly to the condyle.
   C. Gliding movements take place between the disc and the temporal bone.
   D. The inferior surface of the disc is concave.

9. Which area of the mandible articulates with the temporal bone at the temporomandibular joint?
   A. Lingula
   B. Mandibular notch
   C. Coronoid process
   D. Condyle

10. During both mandibular protrusion and retraction, the rotation of the articulating surface of the mandible against the disc in the lower synovial cavity is prevented by:
    A. Facial muscles
    B. Infrahyoid muscles
    C. Muscles of mastication
    D. Ligaments of the temporomandibular joint

11. Which structure secretes synovial fluid?
    A. Mandibular condyle
    B. Disc of the joint
    C. Inner membranes lining the capsule
    D. Lateral pterygoid muscle

12. Which list is in order, from the most anterior structure to the most posterior structure?
    A. Articular fossa, postglenoid process, articular eminence
    B. Condyle, coronoid process, mandibular notch
    C. Articular eminence, articular fossa, postglenoid process
    D. Coronoid process, condyle, mandibular notch

13. At what position does a displaced disc usually lie?
    A. Anterior to its usual position
    B. Posterior to its usual position
    C. In the articular fossa
    D. In the mandibular notch

14. The joint capsule wraps around which structure?
A. Coronoid process
B. Mandibular notch
C. Condyle
D. Zygomatic arch

15. Which situation occurs with subluxation of the joint?
A. The head of condyle moves too far anteriorly on the articular eminence
B. The neck of condyle moves too far posteriorly on the articular eminence
C. The coronoid process moves too far anteriorly on the articular eminence
D. The coronoid process moves too far posteriorly on the articular eminence

16. Which of the following landmarks is located on the temporal bone?
A. Condyle
B. Articular fossa
C. Coronoid notch
D. External oblique line

17. Which of the following provides branches for the most *direct* blood supply to the temporomandibular joint?
A. Internal carotid artery
B. External carotid artery
C. Common carotid artery
D. Aorta

18. Which of the following is located posterior to the articular fossa in the region of the temporomandibular joint?
A. Postglenoid process
B. Articular eminence
C. Bony separation of the nasal septum
D. Zygomatic process of the temporal bone

19. Which of the following nerves innervates the temporomandibular joint?
A. Facial nerve
B. Hypoglossal nerve
C. Vagus nerve
D. Trigeminal nerve
E. Glossopharyngeal nerve

20. Which of the following can generally happen to the temporomandibular disc as a person ages?
A. Increased blood supply
B. Fewer calcifications
C. Perforations
D. Thickening

Vascular System

OUTLINE

LEARNING OBJECTIVES

After studying this chapter, the reader should be able to do the following:

1. Define and pronounce all the key terms and anatomical terms in this chapter.
2. Identify and trace the routes of the blood vessels of the head and neck on a diagram, skull, and patient.
3. Discuss the types of vascular lesions that can occur in the head and neck region.
4. Correctly complete the review questions and activities for this chapter.
5. Integrate the knowledge about the head and neck blood supply into clinical dental practice.

KEY TERMS

Anastomosis/Anastomoses (ah-nas-tah-**moe**-sis, ah-nas-tah-**moe**-sees) Communication of a blood vessel with another blood vessel by a connecting channel.

Arteriole (ar-**ter**-ee-ole) Smaller artery that branches off an artery and connects with a capillary.

Artery Type of blood vessel that carries blood away from the heart.

Atherosclerosis (ath-uh-roh-skluh-**roh**-sis) The narrowing and blockage of the arteries by a buildup of plaque.

(Continued)

141

KEY TERMS (continued)

Bacteremia (bak-ter-**ee**-me-ah) Bacteria traveling within the vascular system.

Capillary (**kap**-i-lare-ee) Smaller blood vessel that branches off an arteriole to supply blood directly to tissue.

Carotid Pulse (kah-**rot**-id) Reliable pulse palpated from the common carotid artery.

Embolus/Emboli (**em**-bol-us, **em**-bol-eye) Foreign material or thrombus traveling in the blood that can block the vessel.

Hematoma (hee-mah-**toe**-mah) Bruise that results when a blood vessel is injured and a small amount of blood escapes into the surrounding tissue and clots.

Hemorrhage (**hem**-ah-rij) Large amounts of blood that escape into the surrounding tissue without clotting when a blood vessel is seriously injured.

Plaque Substance which consists of cholesterol (mainly), calcium, clotting proteins, and other substances that can be found lining arteries.

Plexus (**plek**-sis) Network of blood vessels, usually veins.

Thrombus/Thrombi (**throm**-bus, **throm**-by) Clot that forms on the inner blood vessel wall.

Vein Type of blood vessel that travels to the heart, carrying blood.

Venous Sinuses (**vee**-nus) Blood-filled space between two layers of tissue.

Venule (**ven**-yule) Smaller vein that drains the capillaries of the tissue area and then joins larger veins.

OVERVIEW OF THE VASCULAR SYSTEM

The vascular system of the head and neck, as is the case in the rest of the body, consists of an arterial blood supply, a capillary network, and venous drainage. The dental professional must be able to locate the larger blood vessels of the head and neck because these vessels may become compromised due to a disease process or during a dental procedure such as a local anesthetic injection. Blood vessels may also spread infection in the head and neck area (see Chapter 12). The blood vessels may also spread cancerous cells from a tumor to distant sites and at a faster rate than lymphatic vessels.

Blood vessels are less numerous than lymphatic vessels, yet the venous portion mainly parallels the lymphatic vessels in location (see Chapter 10). A large network of blood vessels is called a **plexus.** The head and neck area contains certain important venous plexuses. Blood vessels also may communicate with each other by an **anastomosis** (plural, **anastomoses**), a connecting channel among the vessels.

An **artery** is a component of the vascular system that arises from the heart, carrying blood away from it. Each artery starts as a large vessel and branches into smaller vessels, each one a smaller artery or an **arteriole.** Each arteriole branches into even smaller vessels until it becomes a network of capillaries. Each **capillary** is smaller than an arteriole and can supply blood to a large tissue area only because there are so many of them.

A **vein** is another component of the vascular system. A vein, unlike an artery, travels to the heart and carries blood. Valves in the veins are mostly absent in the head and neck area, unlike in the rest of the body. This leads to two-way flow dictated by local pressure changes, which is the reason that facial or dental infections can lead to serious complications (see Chapter 12). After each smaller vein or **venule** drains the capillaries of the tissue area, the venules coalesce to become larger veins. Veins are much larger and more numerous than arteries. Veins anastomose freely and have a greater variability in location in comparison with arteries.

There are also different kinds of venous networks found in the body. Superficial veins are found immediately deep to the skin. Deeper veins usually accompany larger arteries in a more protected location within the tissue. **Venous sinuses** are blood-filled spaces between the two layers of tissue. All these networks are connected by anastomoses.

Reviewing the pathways of the arteries and veins as they exit and then enter the heart is important so as to understand the origins of the blood vessels of the head and neck. After the basic origins of the blood supply to the head and neck are understood, diagrams of the blood vessels overlying the skull figure are helpful in studying this system. Relating the tissues supplied and the area's blood vessels is an additional way of understanding the location of the various blood vessels. Remember that, unlike innervation supplied by the nerves to the muscles, which is a one-to-one relationship, blood supply is regional. Arteries supply all structures in their vicinity, and veins receive blood from all nearby structures.

ARTERIAL BLOOD SUPPLY TO THE HEAD AND NECK

The major arteries that supply the head and neck are the common carotid and subclavian arteries. The origins from the heart to the head and neck of these two arteries are different depending on the side of the body under consideration. The other arteries of the head and neck are symmetrically located on each side of the body.

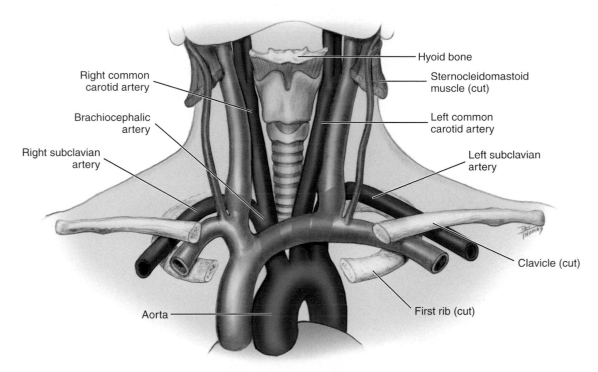

FIGURE 6-1 Origins from the heart of the arterial blood supply for the head and neck highlighting the pathways of the common carotid and subclavian arteries. Note that the pathways are different on the right and left sides of the body.

Origins to the Head and Neck

The origins from the heart of the common carotid and subclavian arteries that supply the head and neck are different for the right and left sides of the body (Figure 6-1). For the left side of the body, the common carotid and subclavian arteries arise directly from the **aorta** (**ay**-or-tah). For the right side of the body, the common carotid and subclavian arteries are both branches from the brachiocephalic artery. The **brachiocephalic artery** (bray-kee-o-sah-**fal**-ik) is a direct branch of the aorta.

The **common carotid artery** (kah-**rot**-id) is branchless and travels up the neck, lateral to the trachea and larynx, to the upper border of the thyroid cartilage (see Figure 6-1). The common carotid artery travels in a sheath deep to the sternocleidomastoid muscle. This sheath also contains the internal jugular vein and the tenth cranial or vagus nerve. The common carotid artery ends by dividing into the internal and external carotid arteries at about the level of the larynx (Figure 6-2).

Just before the common carotid artery bifurcates into the internal and external carotid arteries, it exhibits a swelling called the **carotid sinus** (see Figure 6-2). When the common carotid artery is palpated against the larynx, the most reliable arterial pulse of the body can be monitored. If the anterior border of the sternocleidomastoid muscle is rolled posteriorly at the level of the thyroid cartilage of the larynx or "Adam's apple," the **carotid pulse** can be felt in the groove of tissue produced. This pulse is most reliable because the common carotid is a major artery supplying the brain and therefore in an emergency situation (cardiopulmonary resuscitation) remains palpable by healthcare professionals when peripheral arteries such as the radial artery are not. The carotid pulse also is easily accessible during dental treatment.

The **subclavian artery** (sub-**klay**-vee-an) arises lateral to the common carotid artery (see Figure 6-1). The subclavian artery gives off branches to supply both intracranial and extracranial structures, but its major destination is the upper extremity (arm).

Internal Carotid Artery

The **internal carotid artery** is a division that travels upward in a slightly lateral position (in relationship to the external carotid artery) after leaving the common carotid artery (see Figure 6-2). This artery is hidden by the sternocleidomastoid muscle of the neck. The internal carotid artery has no branches in the neck but continues adjacent to the internal jugular vein within the carotid sheath to the skull base, where it enters the cranium. The internal carotid artery supplies intracranial structures and is the source of the **ophthalmic artery** (**of**-thal-mic), which supplies the eye, orbit, and lacrimal gland.

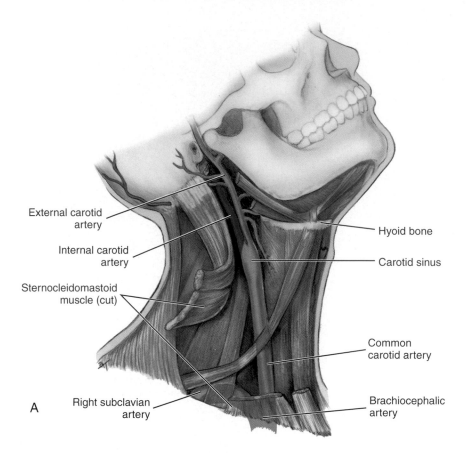

External carotid
artery

Internal carotid
artery

Sternocleidomastoid
muscle (cut)

Right subclavian
artery

A

Hyoid bone

Carotid sinus

Common
carotid artery

Brachiocephalic
artery

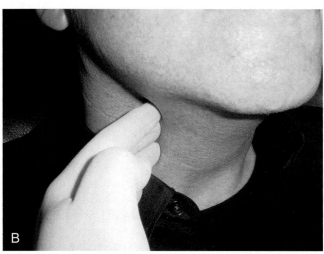

B

FIGURE 6-2 Pathway of the internal carotid artery after branching off the common carotid artery **(A).** Note where the carotid pulse can be palpated **(B).**

External Carotid Artery

As with the internal carotid artery, the **external carotid artery** begins at the superior border of the thyroid cartilage, at the termination of the common carotid artery and the carotid sheath. The external carotid artery travels upward in a more medial position (in relationship to the internal carotid artery) after arising from the common carotid artery (Figures 6-3 and 6-4). The external carotid artery supplies the extracranial tissues of the head and neck, including the oral cavity. The external carotid artery has four sets of branches

grouped according to their location to the main artery: the anterior, medial, posterior, and terminal branches (Table 6-1).

ANTERIOR BRANCHES OF THE EXTERNAL CAROTID ARTERY

Three anterior branches from the external carotid artery exist: the superior thyroid, lingual, and facial arteries (see Figure 6-4). The lingual and facial arteries continue to divide to serve areas of the head and neck that are of interest to dental professionals.

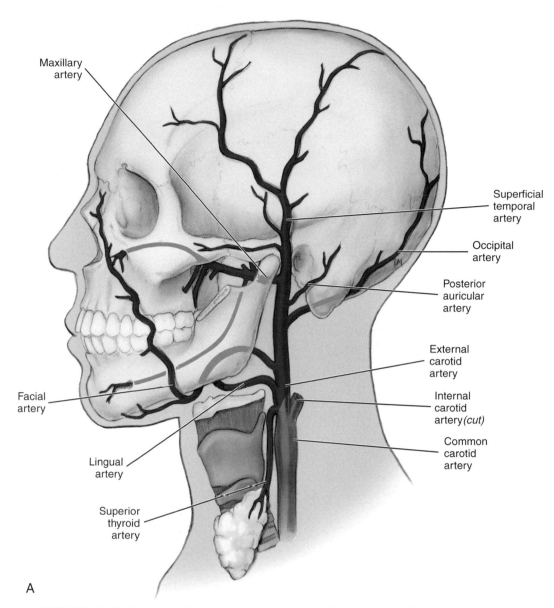

Maxillary
artery

Superficial
temporal
artery

Occipital
artery

Posterior
auricular
artery

External
carotid
artery

Internal
carotid
artery *(cut)*

Common
carotid
artery

Facial
artery

Lingual
artery

Superior
thyroid
artery

A

FIGURE 6-3 Pathway of the external carotid artery after branching off the common carotid artery. **A,** a diagram showing a lateral projection. Note that the medial branch of the external carotid artery, the ascending pharyngeal artery, cannot be seen. (From McMinn RMH, Hutchings RT, Logan BM. Color atlas of head and neck anatomy, 3 ed. St. Louis, Mosby, 2003.)   *Continued*

Superior Thyroid Artery.

The **superior thyroid artery** (**thy**-roid) is an anterior branch from the external carotid artery (see Figure 6-3). The superior thyroid artery has branches: the infrahyoid artery (in-frah-**hi**-oid), sternocleidomastoid branch (stir-no-klii-do-**mass**-toid), superior laryngeal artery (lah-**rin**-je-al), and cricothyroid branch. These branches supply the tissues inferior to the hyoid bone including the infrahyoid muscles, sternocleidomastoid muscle, muscles of the larynx, and thyroid gland.

Lingual Artery.

The **lingual artery** is an anterior branch from the external carotid artery and arises superior to the superior thyroid artery at the level of the hyoid bone (Figure 6-5; see Figure 6-3). The lingual artery travels anteriorly to the apex of the tongue by way of its inferior surface. The lingual artery supplies the tissues superior to the hyoid bone including the suprahyoid muscles and floor of the mouth by the dorsal lingual, deep lingual, sublingual, and suprahyoid branches.

The tongue is also supplied by branches of the lingual artery including several small dorsal lingual

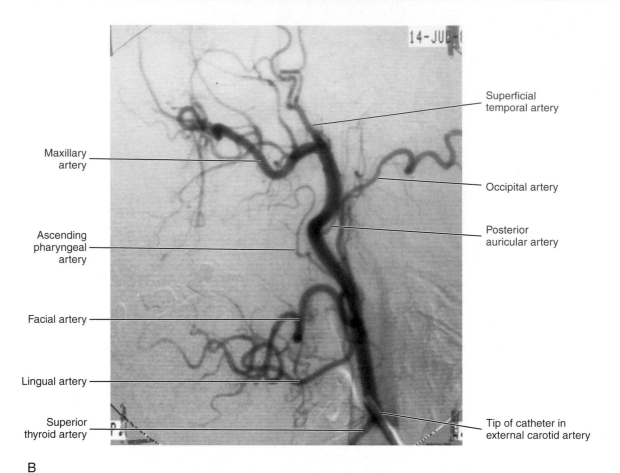

Maxillary artery

Ascending pharyngeal artery

Facial artery

Lingual artery

Superior thyroid artery

Superficial temporal artery

Occipital artery

Posterior auricular artery

Tip of catheter in external carotid artery

B

FIGURE 6-3, cont'd Pathway of the external carotid artery after branching off the common carotid artery. **B,** An arteriogram showing a lateral projection. (From McMinn RMH, Hutchings RT, Logan BM. Color atlas of head and neck anatomy, 3 ed. St. Louis, Mosby, 2003.)

TABLE 6-1

BRANCHES OF THE EXTERNAL CAROTID ARTERY

Branches of External Carotid Artery	Position of Branches	Further Branches
Superior thyroid	Anterior	Infrahyoid, sternocleidomastoid, superior laryngeal, and cricothyroid
Lingual	Anterior	Dorsal lingual, deep lingual, sublingual, and suprahyoid
Facial	Anterior	Ascending palatine, glandular, submental, inferior labial, superior labial, and angular
Ascending pharyngeal	Medial	Pharyngeal and meningeal
Occipital	Posterior	Muscular, sternocleidomastoid, auricular, and meningeal
Posterior auricular	Posterior	Auricular and stylomastoid
Superficial temporal	Terminal	Transverse facial, middle temporal, frontal, and parietal
Maxillary	Terminal	See Table 6-2

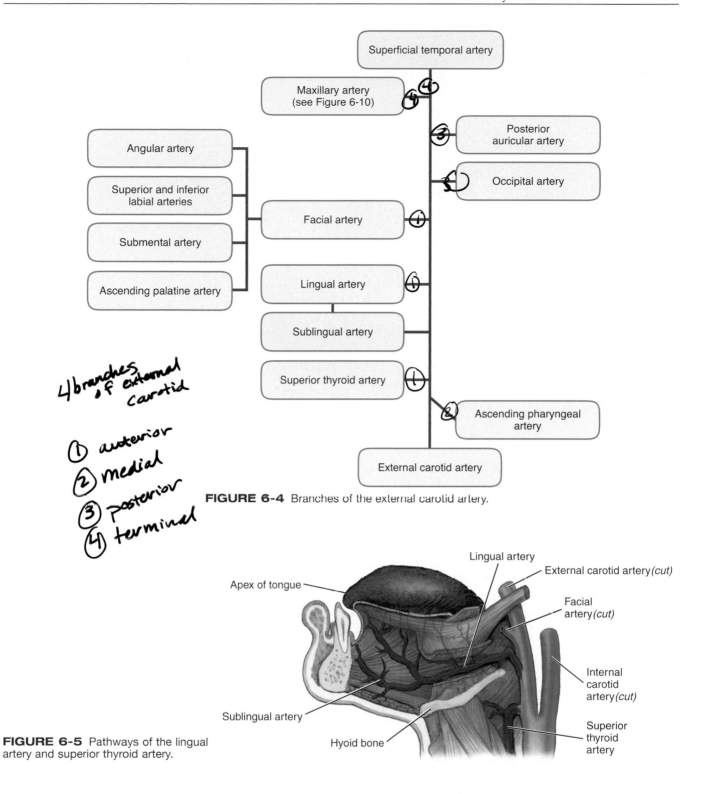

FIGURE 6-4 Branches of the external carotid artery.

(Handwritten notes)
4 branches of external carotid
① anterior
② medial
③ posterior
④ terminal

FIGURE 6-5 Pathways of the lingual artery and superior thyroid artery.

branches to the base and body and the deep lingual artery, the terminal portion of the lingual artery, to the apex.

The **sublingual artery** (sub-**ling**-gwal) supplies the mylohyoid muscle, sublingual salivary gland, and mucous membranes of the floor of the mouth. The small suprahyoid branch (soo-prah-**hi**-oid) supplies the suprahyoid muscles.

Facial Artery.

The **facial artery** is the final anterior branch from the external carotid artery (Figure 6-6; see Figure 6-5). The facial artery arises slightly superior to the lingual artery as it branches off anteriorly. Sometimes the facial and lingual arteries share a common trunk. The facial artery has a complicated path as it runs medial to the mandible, over the submandibular salivary

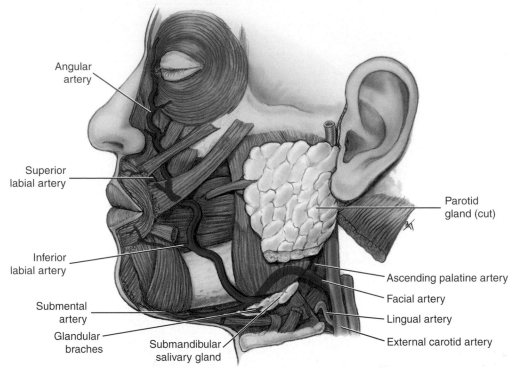

Angular
artery

Superior
labial artery

Inferior
labial artery

Submental
artery

Glandular
braches

Submandibular
salivary gland

Parotid
gland (cut)

Ascending palatine artery

Facial artery

Lingual artery

External carotid artery

FIGURE 6-6 Pathway of the facial artery.

gland, and then around the mandible's inferior border to its lateral side.

From the inferior border of the mandible, the facial artery runs anteriorly and superiorly near the angle of the mouth and along the side of the nose. The facial artery terminates at the medial canthus of the eye. Thus the facial artery supplies the face in the oral, buccal, zygomatic, nasal, infraorbital, and orbital regions.

The facial artery is paralleled by the facial vein in the head area, although they do not run together. In the neck the artery is separated from the vein by the posterior belly of the digastric muscle, stylohyoid muscle, and submandibular salivary gland. The facial artery's major branches include the ascending palatine, glandular branches, submental, inferior labial, superior labial, and angular arteries.

The **ascending palatine artery** (ah-**send**-ing **pal**-ah-tine) is the first branch from the facial artery (see Figure 6-6). The ascending palatine artery supplies the soft palate, palatine muscles, and palatine tonsils and can be the source of the serious blood loss or hemorrhage that may occur if it is injured during a tonsillectomy (blood vessel lesions are discussed later).

The glandular branches and **submental artery** (sub-**men**-tal) are branches from the facial artery that supply the submandibular lymph nodes, submandibular salivary gland, and mylohyoid and digastric muscles.

The **inferior labial artery** is another branch from the facial artery that supplies the lower lip tissues including the muscles of facial expression such as the depressor anguli oris muscle. The **superior labial artery** is also a branch from the facial artery that supplies the upper lip tissues.

The **angular artery** (**ang**-u-lar) is the termination of the facial artery and supplies the tissues along the side of the nose (see Figure 6-6).

MEDIAL BRANCH OF THE EXTERNAL CAROTID ARTERY

Only one medial branch comes from the external carotid artery, the small **ascending pharyngeal artery** (fah-**rin**-je-al) that arises close to the origin of the external carotid artery and cannot be seen in most lateral views of the head and neck. The ascending pharyngeal artery has many small branches such as the **pharyngeal branches** (fah-**rin**-je-al) and **meningeal branches** (me-**nin**-je-al) that supply the pharyngeal walls (where they anastomose with the ascending palatine artery), soft palate, and meninges of the brain.

POSTERIOR BRANCHES OF THE EXTERNAL CAROTID ARTERY

Two posterior branches of the external carotid artery exist: the occipital artery and posterior auricular artery (Figure 6-7).

Occipital Artery.

The **occipital artery** (ok-**sip**-it-al), a posterior branch of the external carotid artery, arises from the external carotid artery as it passes upward behind the ascending ramus of the mandible and travels to the posterior portion of the scalp (see Figure 6-7). The occipital artery supplies the suprahyoid and sternocleidomastoid muscles, as well as the scalp and meningeal tissues in the occipital region. The artery supplies these regions through the muscular branches, **sternocleidomastoid branches** (stir-no-klii-do-**mass**-toid), **auricular** (aw-**rik**-yule-lar), and **meningeal branches**. At its origin, the occipital artery is closely related to the twelfth cranial or hypoglossal nerve.

Posterior Auricular Artery.

The small **posterior auricular artery** is also a posterior branch of the external carotid artery (see Figure 6-7). The posterior auricular artery arises superior to the occipital artery and stylohyoid muscle at about the level of the tip of the styloid process. The posterior auricular artery supplies the internal ear by its auricular branch and the mastoid air cells by the **stylomastoid artery** (sty-lo-**mass**-toid).

TERMINAL BRANCHES OF THE EXTERNAL CAROTID ARTERY

The two terminal branches of the external carotid artery are the superficial temporal artery and the maxillary artery (Figures 6-8, 6-9, and 6-11). The external carotid artery splits into these terminal branches within the parotid salivary gland. In addition, both terminal branches give rise to many important arteries in the head and neck area.

Superficial Temporal Artery.

The **superficial temporal artery** (**tem**-poh-ral) is the smaller terminal branch of the external carotid artery (see Figure 6-8). The artery arises within the parotid salivary gland. This artery can sometimes be visible under the skin of the temporal region in the patient. The superficial temporal artery has several branches including the transverse facial artery, middle temporal artery, frontal branch, and parietal branch.

The small **transverse facial artery** supplies the parotid salivary gland duct and nearby facial tissues. The equally small **middle temporal artery** (**tem**-poh-ral) supplies the temporalis muscle. The **frontal branch**

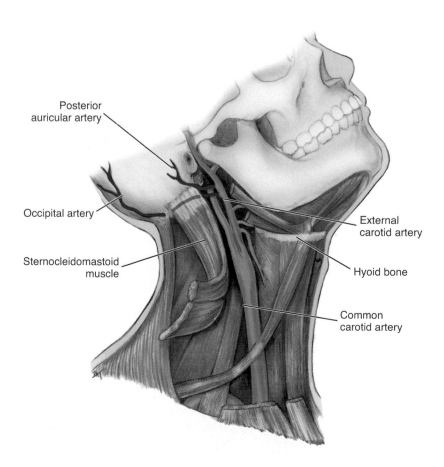

Posterior auricular artery

Occipital artery

Sternocleidomastoid muscle

External carotid artery

Hyoid bone

Common carotid artery

FIGURE 6-7 Pathways of the occipital artery and posterior auricular artery.

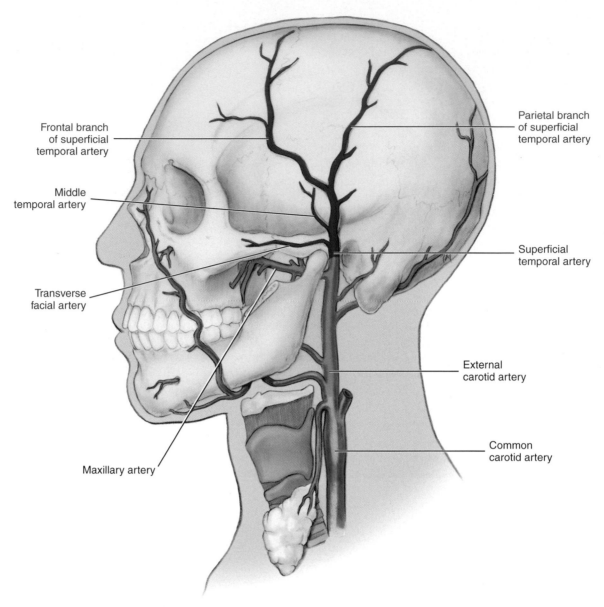

FIGURE 6-8 Pathway of the superficial temporal artery.

(**frunt**-il) and **parietal branch** (pah-**ry**-it-il) both supply portions of the scalp in the frontal and parietal regions.

Maxillary Artery

The **maxillary artery** (**mak**-sil-lare-ee) is the larger terminal branch of the external carotid artery (see Figures 6-9 and 6-11). The maxillary artery begins at the neck of the mandibular condyle within the parotid salivary gland. The maxillary artery runs between the mandible and the sphenomandibular ligament anteriorly and superiorly through the infratemporal fossa. The artery may run either superficial or deep to the lateral pterygoid muscle.

After traversing the infratemporal fossa, the maxillary artery enters the pterygopalatine fossa. The ptery-

gopalatine fossa is deep and inferior to the eye (see Chapter 3). Within the infratemporal and pterygopalatine fossae, the maxillary artery gives off many branches. The branches within the infratemporal fossa include the middle meningeal and inferior alveolar arteries and several arteries to muscles (Table 6-2).

The **middle meningeal artery** supplies the meninges of the brain by way of the foramen spinosum, located on the inferior surface of the skull, as well as the skull bones (see Figure 6-9).

The **inferior alveolar artery** (al-**ve**-o-lar) also arises from the maxillary artery in the infratemporal fossa (see Figure 6-9). The artery turns inferiorly to enter the mandibular foramen and then the mandibular canal, along with the inferior alveolar nerve. The mylohyoid

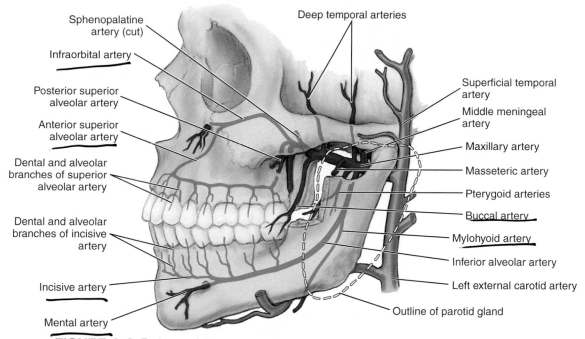

FIGURE 6-9 Pathway of the maxillary artery (*except those branches to the nasal cavity and palate*).

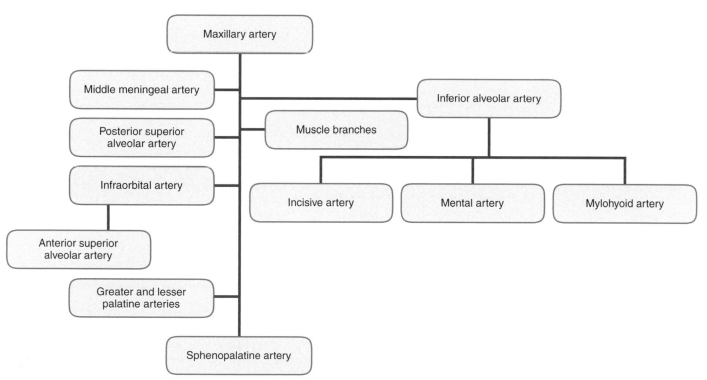

FIGURE 6-10 Branches of the maxillary artery.

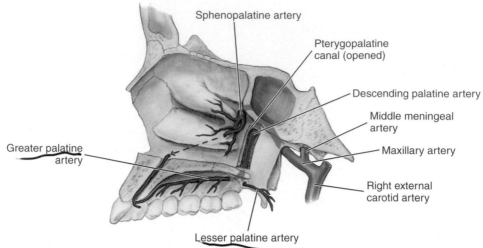

FIGURE 6-11 Pathways of the greater palatine artery, lesser palatine artery, and sphenopalatine artery.

TABLE 6-2

BRANCHES OF THE MAXILLARY ARTERY

Major Branches of Maxillary Artery	Further Branches	Tissues Supplied
Middle meningeal		Meninges of brain and bones of skull
Inferior alveolar	Mylohyoid, mental, and incisive	Mandibular teeth, mouth floor, and mental region
Deep temporal(s)		Temporalis muscle
Pterygoid(s)		Lateral and medial pterygoid muscles
Masseteric		Masseter muscle
Buccal		Buccinator muscle and buccal region
Posterior superior alveolar		Posterior maxillary teeth and maxillary sinus
Infraorbital	Orbital and anterior superior alveolar	Orbital region, face, and anterior maxillary teeth
Greater palatine	Lesser palatine(s)	Hard and soft palates
Sphenopalatine	Lateral nasal, septal, and nasopalatine	Nasal cavity and anterior hard palate

artery branches from the inferior alveolar artery before it enters the canal.

The **mylohyoid artery** (my-lo-**hi**-oid) arises from the inferior alveolar artery before the main artery enters the mandibular canal by way of the mandibular foramen (see Figure 6-9). The mylohyoid artery travels in the mylohyoid groove on the inner surface of the mandible and supplies the floor of the mouth and the mylohyoid muscle.

Within the mandibular canal, the inferior alveolar artery gives off the dental and alveolar branches

(see Figure 6-9). The dental branches of the inferior alveolar artery supply the pulp tissue of the mandibular posterior teeth by way of each tooth's apical foramen. The alveolar branches of the inferior alveolar artery supply the periodontium of the mandibular posterior teeth, including the gingiva. The inferior alveolar artery then branches into two arteries within the mandibular canal: the mental and incisive arteries.

The **mental artery** (**ment**-il) arises from the inferior alveolar artery and exits the mandibular canal by way of the mental foramen (see Figure 6-9). The mental foramen is located on the outer surface of the mandible, usually deep to the apices of the first and second mandibular premolar teeth. After the mental artery exits the canal, the artery supplies the tissues of the chin and anastomoses with the inferior labial artery.

The **incisive artery** (in-**sy**-ziv) branches off the inferior alveolar artery and remains in the mandibular canal to divide into dental and alveolar branches (see Figure 6-9). The dental branches of the incisive artery supply the pulp tissue of the mandibular anterior teeth by way of each tooth's apical foramen. The alveolar branches of the incisive artery supply the periodontium of the mandibular anterior teeth, including the gingiva, and anastomose with the alveolar branches of the incisive artery on the other side.

The maxillary artery also has branches that are located near the muscle they supply (see Figure 6-9). These arteries all accompany branches of the mandibular division of the fifth cranial or trigeminal nerve. The **deep temporal arteries** (**tem**-poh-ral) supply the anterior and posterior portions of the temporalis muscle. The **pterygoid arteries** (**the**-re-goid) supply the lateral and medial pterygoid muscles. The **masseteric artery** (mass-et-**tehr**-ik) supplies the masseter muscle. The **buccal artery** supplies the buccinator muscle and other soft tissues of the cheek.

Just as the maxillary artery leaves the infratemporal fossa and enters the pterygopalatine fossa, it gives off the **posterior superior alveolar artery** (see Figure 6-9). This artery enters the posterior superior alveolar foramina on the maxillary tuberosity and then gives off dental branches and alveolar branches. The posterior alveolar superior alveolar artery also anastomoses with the anterior superior alveolar artery.

The dental branches of the posterior superior alveolar artery supply the pulp tissue of the posterior maxillary teeth by way of each tooth's apical foramen. The alveolar branches of the posterior superior alveolar artery supply the periodontium of the posterior maxillary teeth, including the gingiva. Some branches also supply the maxillary sinus.

The **infraorbital artery** (in-frah-**or**-bit-al) branches from the maxillary artery in the pterygopalatine fossa and may share a common trunk with the posterior superior alveolar artery (see Figure 6-9). The infraorbital artery then enters the orbit through the inferior orbital fissure. While in the orbit, the artery travels in the infraorbital canal. Within the canal, the infraorbital artery provides orbital branches (**or**-bit-al) to the orbit and gives off the anterior superior alveolar artery.

The **anterior superior alveolar artery** arises from the infraorbital artery and gives off dental and alveolar branches (see Figure 6-9). The anterior superior alveolar artery also anastomoses with the posterior superior alveolar artery.

The dental branches of the anterior superior alveolar artery supply the pulp tissue of the anterior maxillary teeth by way of each tooth's apical foramen. The alveolar branches of the anterior superior alveolar artery supply the periodontium of the anterior maxillary teeth, including the gingiva.

After giving off these branches in the infraorbital canal, the infraorbital artery emerges onto the face from the infraorbital foramen (see Figure 6-9). The artery's terminal branches supply portions of the infraorbital region of the face and anastomose with the facial artery.

Also in the pterygopalatine fossa, the maxillary artery gives rise to the **descending palatine artery** (**pal**-ah-tine), which travels to the palate through the pterygopalatine canal which then terminates in both the **greater palatine artery** and **lesser palatine artery** by way of the greater and lesser palatine foramina to supply the hard and soft palates, respectively (see Figure 6-11). The maxillary artery ends by becoming the **sphenopalatine artery** (sfe-no-**pal**-ah-tine), which supplies the nasal cavity. The sphenopalatine artery gives rise to the posterior lateral nasal branches and septal branches, including a **nasopalatine branch** (nay-zo-**pal**-ah-tine) that accompanies the nasopalatine nerve through the incisive foramen on the maxilla (see Figure 6-11).

VENOUS DRAINAGE OF THE HEAD AND NECK

The veins of the head and neck start out as small venules and become larger as they near the base of the neck on their way to the heart. The veins of the head and upper neck are usually symmetrically located but have a greater variability in location than do the arteries, anastomosing freely. Veins are also generally larger and more numerous than arteries in the same tissue area.

The internal jugular vein drains the brain as well as most of the other tissues of the head and neck (Table 6-3), whereas the external jugular vein drains only a small portion of the extracranial tissues. However, the two veins have many anastomoses. The beginnings of both veins are discussed initially and, later, their route to the heart is discussed.

Facial Vein

The **facial vein** drains into the internal jugular vein, which is discussed later (Figure 6-12). The facial vein begins at the medial corner of the eye with the junction of two veins from the frontal region, the **supratrochlear vein** (soo-prah-**trok**-lere) and **supraorbital vein** (soo-prah-**or**-bit-al). The supraorbital vein also anastomoses with the ophthalmic veins. The **ophthalmic veins** (of-**thal**-mic) drain the tissues of the orbit. This anastomosis provides a communication

TABLE 6-3

VEINS OF THE HEAD

Region or Tributaries Drained	Drainage Veins	Major Veins
Meninges of brain	Middle meningeal	Pterygoid plexus
Lateral scalp area	Superficial temporal and posterior auricular	Retromandibular and external jugular
Frontal region	Supratrochlear and supraorbital	Facial and ophthalmic
Orbital region	Ophthalmic(s)	Cavernous sinus and pterygoid plexus
Superficial temporal and maxillary veins	Retromandibular	External jugular
Upper lip area	Superior labial	Facial
Maxillary teeth	Posterior superior alveolar	Pterygoid plexus
Lower lip area	Inferior labial	Facial
Mandibular teeth and submental region	Inferior alveolar	Pterygoid plexus
Submental region	Submental	Facial
Lingual and sublingual regions	Lingual	Facial or internal jugular
Deep facial areas and posterior superior alveolar and inferior alveolar veins	Pterygoid plexus	Maxillary
Pterygoid plexus of veins	Maxillary	Retromandibular

with the cavernous venous sinus, which may become fatally infected through the spread of dental infection (discussed later, see also Chapter 12). This is especially significant because the facial vein, like other veins of the head, has no valves to control the direction of blood flow.

The facial vein receives branches from the same areas of the face that are supplied by the facial artery. This vein anastomoses with the deep veins such as the pterygoid plexus in the infratemporal fossa and with the large retromandibular vein before joining the internal jugular vein at the level of the hyoid bone (discussed later).

The facial vein has some important tributaries in the oral region (see Figure 6-12). The **superior labial vein** drains the upper lip. The **inferior labial vein** drains the lower lip. The **submental vein** (sub-**men**-tal) drains the tissues of the chin as well as the submandibular region.

One excellent example of the venous variability concerns the **lingual veins.** These include the dorsal lingual veins that drain the dorsal surface of the tongue, the highly visible deep lingual veins that drain the ventral surface of the tongue, and the sublingual

veins that drain the floor of the mouth (see Chapter 2). These lingual veins may join to form a single vessel or may empty into larger vessels separately. They also may drain indirectly into the facial vein or directly into the internal jugular vein.

Retromandibular Vein

The **retromandibular vein** (reh-tro-man-**dib**-you-lar) will form the external jugular vein from a portion of its route. The retromandibular vein is formed by the merger of the superficial temporal vein and maxillary vein (Figure 6-13). The retromandibular vein emerges from the parotid salivary gland and courses inferiorly. This vein and its beginning venules drain areas similar to those supplied by the superficial temporal and maxillary arteries.

Inferior to the parotid gland, the retromandibular vein typically divides (see Figure 6-13). The anterior division joins the facial vein, and the posterior division continues its downward course on the surface of the sternocleidomastoid muscle. After being joined by the **posterior auricular vein** (aw-**rik**-you-lar), which drains the lateral scalp behind the ear, this posterior

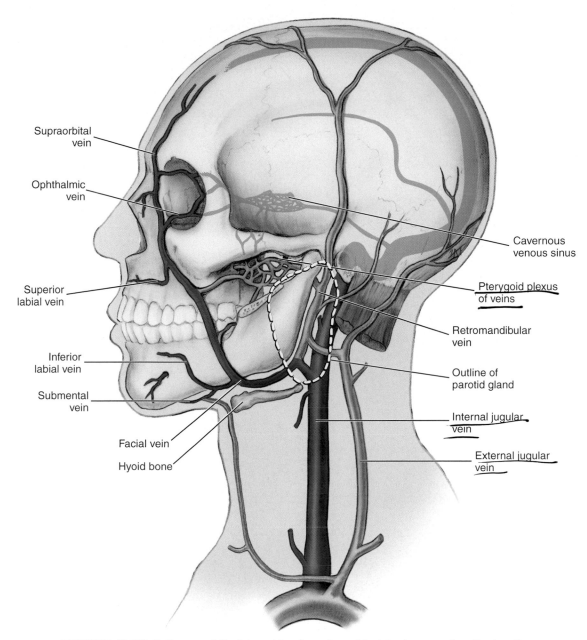

FIGURE 6-12 Pathways of the internal jugular vein and facial vein, as well as the location of the cavernous venous sinus.

division of the retromandibular veins becomes the external jugular vein. The external jugular vein is discussed later.

SUPERFICIAL TEMPORAL VEIN

The **superficial temporal vein** (**tem**-poh-ral) drains the lateral scalp and is superficially located (see Figure 6-13). The superficial temporal vein goes on to drain into and form the retromandibular vein, along with the deeper maxillary vein.

MAXILLARY VEIN

The **maxillary vein** (**mak**-sil-lare-ee) is deeper than the superficial temporal vein and begins in the infra-

temporal fossa by collecting blood from the pterygoid plexus, near the maxillary artery (see Figure 6-13). Through the pterygoid plexus, the maxillary vein receives the middle meningeal, posterior superior alveolar, inferior alveolar, and other veins such as those from the nose and palate (those areas served by the maxillary artery). After receiving these veins, the maxillary vein merges with the superficial temporal vein to drain into and form the retromandibular vein.

Pterygoid Plexus of Veins.

The **pterygoid plexus of veins** (**the**-ri-goid) is a collection of small anastomosing vessels located around the pterygoid muscles and surrounding the maxillary

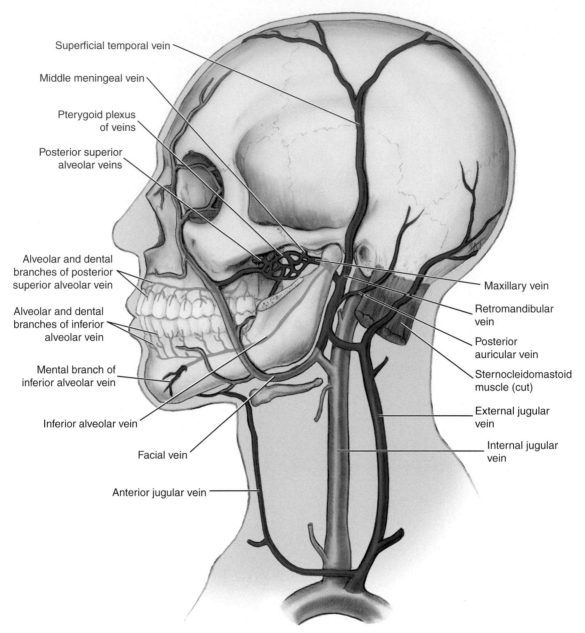

Superficial temporal vein

Middle meningeal vein

Pterygoid plexus
of veins

Posterior superior
alveolar veins

Alveolar and dental
branches of posterior
superior alveolar vein

Alveolar and dental
branches of inferior
alveolar vein

Mental branch of
inferior alveolar vein

Inferior alveolar vein

Facial vein

Anterior jugular vein

Maxillary vein

Retromandibular
vein

Posterior
auricular vein

Sternocleidomastoid
muscle (cut)

External jugular
vein

Internal jugular
vein

FIGURE 6-13 Pathways of the retromandibular vein and external jugular vein including the anterior jugular vein.

artery on each side of the face in the infratemporal fossa (see Figure 6-13). This plexus anastomoses with both the facial and retromandibular veins. The pterygoid plexus protects the maxillary artery from being compressed during mastication. By either filling or emptying, the pterygoid plexus can accommodate changes in volume of the infratemporal fossa that occur when the mandible moves.

The pterygoid plexus drains the veins from the deep portions of the face and then drains into the maxillary vein. The **middle meningeal vein** also drains the blood from the meninges of the brain into the pterygoid plexus of veins.

Some portions of the pterygoid plexus of veins are near the maxillary tuberosity, reflecting the drainage of dental tissues into the plexus. Thus there is a possibility of piercing the pterygoid plexus when a posterior superior alveolar local anesthetic block is performed if the needle is overinserted (see Chapter 9). When the pterygoid plexus of veins is pierced, a small amount of the blood escapes and enters the tissues, causing tissue tenderness, swelling, and the discoloration of a hematoma (discussed later).

A spread of infection along the needle tract deep into the tissues can also occur when the posterior superior alveolar local anesthetic block is incorrectly administered. This may involve a serious spread of infection to the cavernous venous sinus (discussed later; and see also Chapter 12).

Posterior Superior Alveolar Vein.

The pterygoid plexus of veins also drains the **posterior superior alveolar vein,** which is formed by the merging of its dental and alveolar branches (see Figure 6-13). The dental branches of the posterior superior alveolar vein drain the pulp tissue of the maxillary teeth by way of each tooth's apical foramen. The alveolar branches of the posterior alveolar vein drain the periodontium of the maxillary teeth, including the gingiva.

Inferior Alveolar Vein.

The **inferior alveolar vein** forms from the merging of its dental branches, alveolar branches, and mental branches in the mandible, where they also drain into the pterygoid plexus (see Figure 6-13). The dental branches of the inferior alveolar vein drain the pulp tissue of the mandibular teeth by way of each tooth's apical foramen. The alveolar branches of the inferior alveolar vein drain the periodontium of the mandibular teeth, including the gingiva.

The mental branches of the inferior alveolar vein enter the mental foramen after draining the chin area on the outer surface of the mandible, where they anastomose with branches of the facial vein. The mental foramen is on the surface of the mandible, usually between the apices of the mandibular first and second premolars.

Venous Sinuses

The **venous sinuses** in the brain are located in the meninges. Specifically, these sinuses are within the dura mater of the brain, a dense connective tissue that lines the inside of the cranium. These dural sinuses are channels by which blood is conveyed from the cerebral veins into the veins of the neck, particularly the internal jugular vein.

The venous sinus most important to dental professionals is the **cavernous venous sinus** (**kav**-er-nus) that is located on each side of the body of the sphenoid bone (see Figure 6-12). Each cavernous venous sinus communicates with the one on the opposite side and also with the pterygoid plexus of veins and superior ophthalmic vein, which anastomoses with the facial vein. The cavernous venous sinus may be involved with the spread of infection from the teeth or periodontium, which can lead to fatal results (see Chapter 12).

Internal Jugular Vein

The **internal jugular vein** (**jug**-you-lar) drains most of the tissues of the head and neck (Figure 6-14; see Figure 6-12). As mentioned earlier, the internal jugular vein, unlike many veins in other portions of the body, does not have any one-way valves, nor does any head

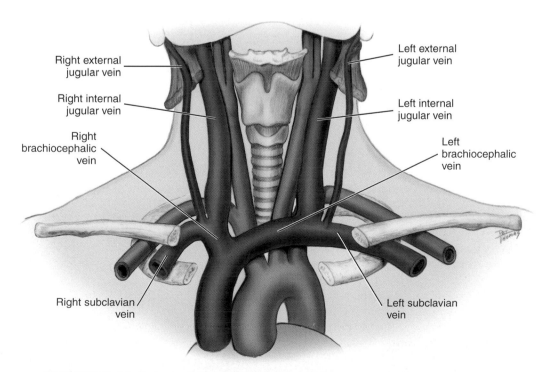

Right external jugular vein

Right internal jugular vein

Right brachiocephalic vein

Right subclavian vein

Left external jugular vein

Left internal jugular vein

Left brachiocephalic vein

Left subclavian vein

FIGURE 6-14 Pathways to the heart from the head and neck including the external and internal jugular veins, subclavian vein, brachiocephalic veins, and superior vena cava.

and neck vein (with the minor exception of the external jugular vein, discussed later). Not having any valves to prevent the backward flow of blood, this vein may become involved with the spread of infection (see Chapter 12).

The internal jugular vein originates in the cranial cavity and leaves the skull through the jugular foramen. It receives many tributaries including the veins from the lingual, sublingual, and pharyngeal areas as well as the facial vein. The internal jugular vein runs with the common carotid artery and its branches as well as the vagus nerve in the carotid sheath. Within the carotid sheath, the deep cervical group of lymph nodes form a chain along the internal jugular vein. The internal jugular vein descends in the neck to merge with the subclavian vein.

External Jugular Vein

As mentioned earlier, the posterior division of the retromandibular vein becomes the **external jugular vein.** The external jugular vein continues the descent inferiorly along the neck, terminating in the subclavian vein (see Figures 6-13 and 6-14). Alone among the veins of the head and neck, the external jugular vein has valves near its entry into the subclavian vein. Usually the external jugular vein is visible as it crosses the sternocleidomastoid muscle; to increase its visibility, it can be distended by gentle supraclavicular digital pressure to block outflow.

The **anterior jugular vein** drains into the external jugular vein (or directly into the subclavian vein) before it joins the subclavian vein (see Figure 6-13). The anterior jugular vein begins inferior to the chin, communicating with veins in the area, and descends near the midline within the superficial fascia, receiving branches from the superficial cervical structures. Only one anterior jugular vein may be present, but usually two veins are present, anastomosing with each other through a jugular venous arch.

Pathways to the Heart from the Head and Neck

On each side of the body, the external jugular vein joins the subclavian vein from the arm, and then the internal jugular vein merges with the **subclavian vein** (sub-**klay**-vee-an) to form the **brachiocephalic vein** (bray-kee-oo-sah-**fal**-ik) (see Figure 6-14). The brachiocephalic veins unite to form the **superior vena cava** (**vee**-na **kay**-va) and then travel to the heart. Because the superior vena cava is on the right side of the heart, the brachiocephalic veins are asymmetrical. The right brachiocephalic vein is short and vertical, and the left brachiocephalic vein is long and horizontal.

VASCULAR LESIONS

The narrowing and blockage of the arteries by a buildup of **plaque,** which consists of cholesterol (mainly), calcium, clotting proteins, and other substances, is called **atherosclerosis** (Figure 6-15). When this process occurs in the arteries leading to the heart, the result is cardiovascular disease (CVD). The process of **atherosclerosis** is now known to begin as early as in childhood. However, even late in adulthood, lifestyle changes can reduce the onset or severity of coronary artery disease.

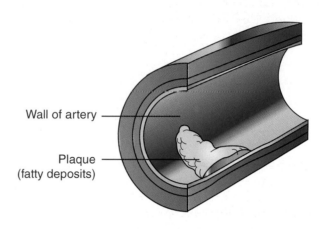

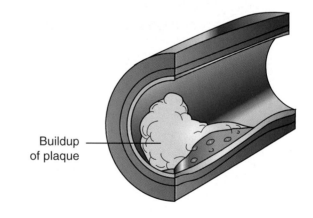

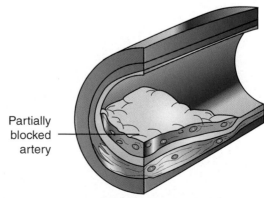

FIGURE 6-15 Plaque buildup in arteries with atherosclerosis during cardiovascular disease.

Blood vessels may become compromised in certain disease processes such as high blood pressure, infection, trauma, or endocrine pathology. These disease processes may lead to vascular lesions. One of these lesions is a clot or **thrombus** (plural, **thrombi**) that forms on the inner vessel wall (Figure 6-16).

A thrombus may dislodge from the inner vessel wall and travel as an **embolus** (plural, **emboli**) (Figure 6-17). Both of these vascular lesions can cause occlusion of the vessel in which the blood flow is blocked either partially or fully. Bacteria traveling in the blood can also cause a **bacteremia.** A transient bacteremia can occur with dental treatment and is serious in certain medically compromised patients (see Chapter 12).

This occlusion of the blood vessel can hamper blood circulation and cause further complications such as a stroke (cerebrovascular accident), a heart attack (myocardial infarction), or tissue destruction (gangrene), depending on the lesion's location. These thrombi may also be infected and spread infection by way of embolus formation to such areas as the cavernous venous sinus (see Chapter 12). A dental professional needs to keep in mind the possibility of vascular vessel lesions when treating a patient with vascular disease or dental-related infections.

When a blood vessel is seriously traumatized, large amounts of the blood can escape into the surrounding tissue without clotting, causing a **hemorrhage.** This is a serious, life-threatening vascular lesion. Other vascular lesions can involve tumorous or abnormal developmental growth of blood vessel tissues. A dental professional needs to be aware of the patient's

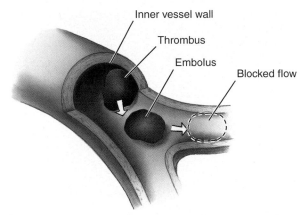

FIGURE 6-17 A dislodged thrombus forming an embolus and then traveling in a blood vessel and creating a blocked flow of blood.

health history with regard to these serious vascular diseases.

Blood vessels may also undergo localized trauma that results temporarily in a bruise. A bruise or **hematoma** results when a blood vessel is injured and a small amount of the blood escapes into the surrounding tissue and then clots (Figure 6-18). This escaped blood causes tissue tenderness, swelling, and discoloration that will last until the blood is broken down by the body.

An extraoral hematoma may result during a local anesthetic injection, especially when a posterior superior alveolar block near the pterygoid plexus of veins has been incorrectly administered (see Chapter

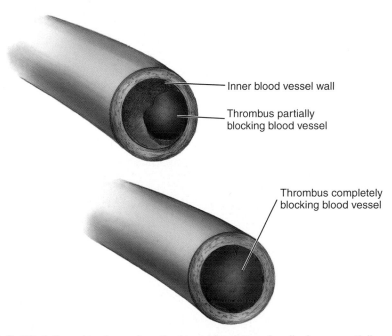

FIGURE 6-16 A thrombus formed on the inner blood vessel wall, shown partially and completely blocking the blood vessel.

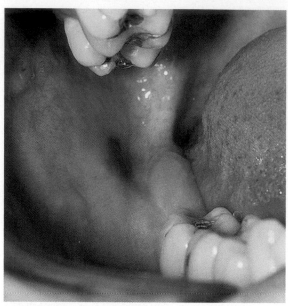

FIGURE 6-18 An intraoral hematoma on the medial surface of the soft tissues overlying the mandibular ramus after an inferior alveolar nerve block.

9). Other blocks such as an infraorbital block or inferior alveolar block may result in intraoral hematomas. These hematomas can vary in extent from minor lesions to major disfiguring lesions. Thus a dental professional needs to be aware of the location of the larger blood vessels to prevent major injury during the dental treatment.

Studies now show a link between periodontal disease and CVD. Several theories exist to explain this link. One theory is that oral bacteria can affect the heart when they enter the blood stream, attaching to fatty plaques in the coronary arteries and contributing to clot formation (see later discussion). Another possibility is that the inflammation caused by periodontal disease increases plaque buildup, which may contribute to swelling of the arteries. Researchers have found that people with periodontal disease are almost twice as likely to suffer from CVD as those without periodontal disease. Periodontal disease can also exacerbate existing heart conditions. Patients at risk for infective endocarditis may require antibiotics before dental procedures (see Chapter 12).

Identification Exercises

Identify the structures on the following diagrams by filling in each blank with the correct anatomical term. You can check your answers by looking back at the figure indicated in parentheses for each identification diagram.

1. (Figure 6-1)

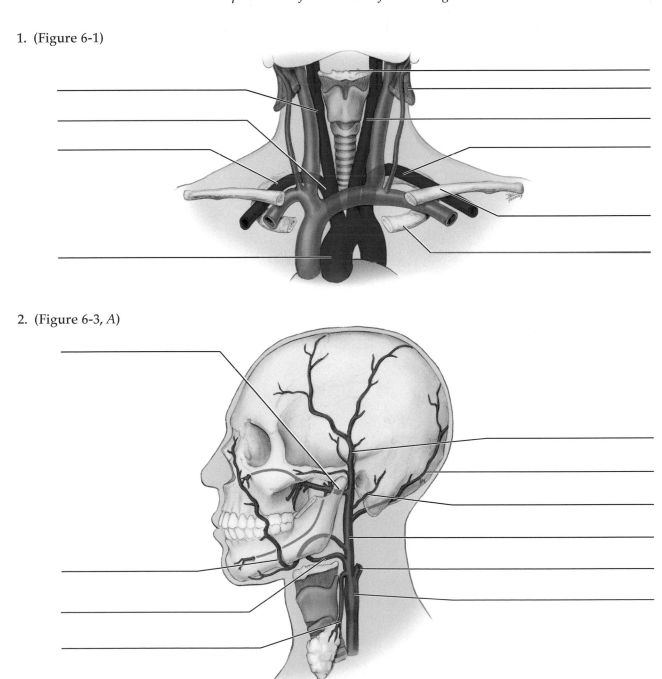

2. (Figure 6-3, *A*)

3. (Figure 6-5)

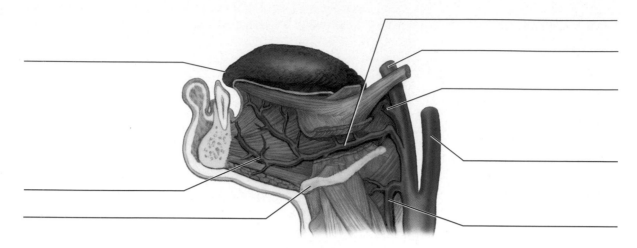

4. (Figure 6-6)

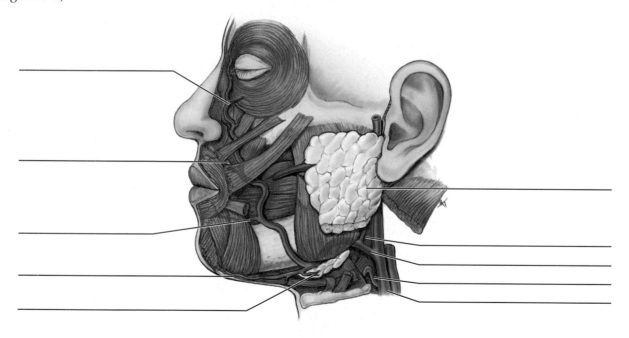

5. (Figure 6-8)

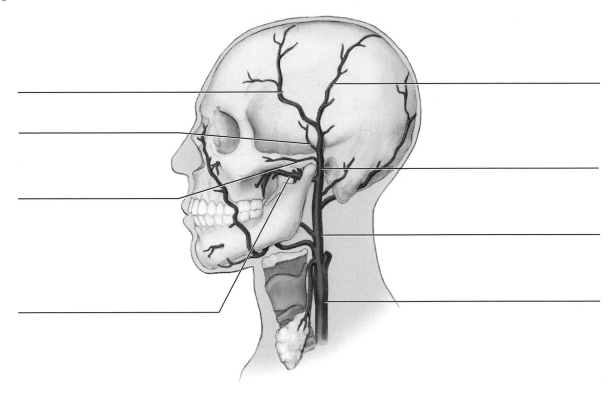

6. (Figure 6-9)

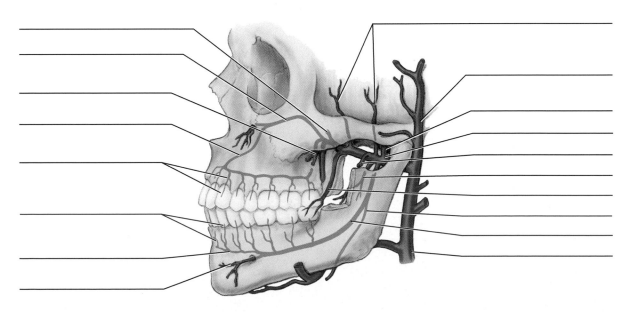

7. (Figure 6-11)

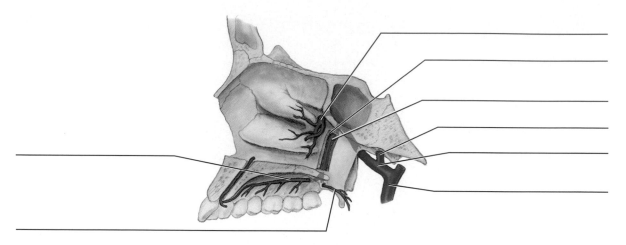

8. (Figure 6-12)

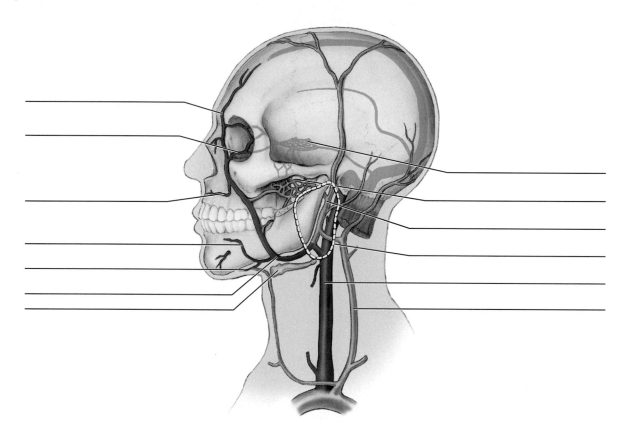

9. (Figure 6-13)

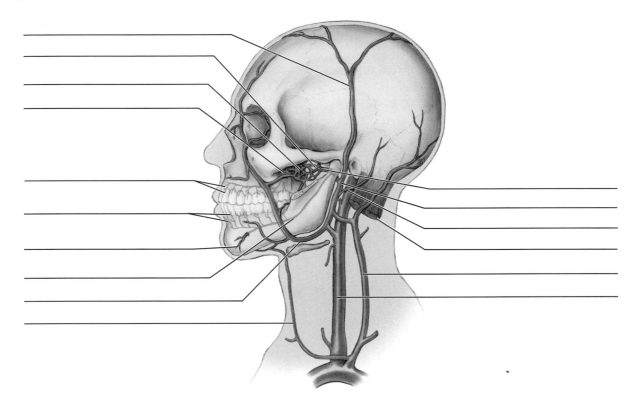

10. (Figure 6-14)

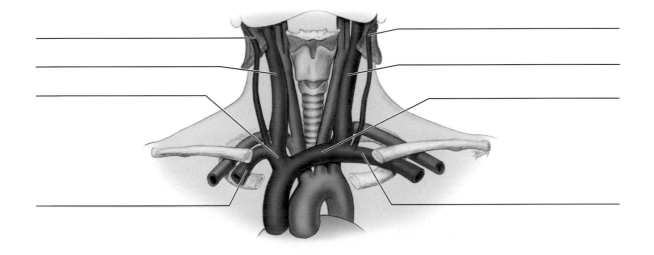

■ REVIEW QUESTIONS

1. The posterior superior alveolar artery and its branches supply the:
   A. Maxillary posterior teeth and periodontium
   B. Mandibular posterior teeth and periodontium
   C. Sternocleidomastoid muscle and thyroid gland
   D. Temporalis muscle and parotid salivary gland

2. Which of the following descriptions concerning the pterygoid plexus is correct?
   A. It is located around the infrahyoid muscles.
   B. It protects the superficial temporal artery.
   C. It drains the maxillary and mandibular dental tissues.
   D. It contains valves to prevent backflow of blood.

3. Which of the following veins results from the merger of the superficial temporal vein and maxillary vein?
   A. Facial vein
   B. Retromandibular vein
   C. Internal jugular vein
   D. External jugular vein
   E. Brachiocephalic vein

4. Which of the following arteries arises from the inferior alveolar artery before the artery enters the mandibular canal?
   A. Mylohyoid artery
   B. Incisive artery
   C. Mental artery
   D. Posterior superior alveolar artery
   E. Submental artery

5. Which of the following artery–foramen pairs below is matched correctly?
   A. Buccal artery–infraorbital foramen
   B. Middle meningeal artery–foramen spinosum
   C. Incisive artery–mental foramen
   D. Inferior labial artery–mandibular foramen
   E. Submental artery–mental foramen

6. Which of the following arteries supply the mucous membranes and glands of the hard and soft palates?
   A. Greater and lesser palatine arteries
   B. Posterior superior alveolar artery
   C. Anterior superior alveolar artery
   D. Infraorbital artery

7. Which of the following vascular lesions may result when a clot on the inner blood vessel wall becomes dislodged and travels in the vessel?
   A. Hematoma
   B. Venous sinus
   C. Embolus
   D. Hemorrhage

8. Which of the following descriptions concerning the maxillary artery is correct?
   A. It arises from the internal carotid artery.
   B. It enters the pterygopalatine fossa and forms terminal branches.
   C. It arises from the zygomaticofacial foramen to emerge on the face.
   D. It has mandibular, maxillary, nasal, palatine, and occipital branches.

9. A venous sinus of the vascular system is a:
   A. Network of blood vessels
   B. Clot on the inner vessel wall
   C. Blood-filled space between two tissue layers
   D. Smaller vein or venule

10. Which of the following is a branch from the facial artery?
    A. Superior labial artery
    B. Ascending pharyngeal artery
    C. Posterior auricular artery
    D. Transverse facial artery

11. Which of the following structures are smaller vessels that branch off an arteriole to supply blood directly to tissue?
    A. Artery
    B. Capillary
    C. Vein
    D. Venule

12. The carotid pulse can be palpated at the level of the:
    A. Thyroid cartilage
    B. Hyoid bone
    C. Angle of the mandible
    D. Supraclavicular fossa

13. The tongue is supplied mainly by a branch from the:
    A. Internal carotid artery
    B. External carotid artery
    C. Sublingual artery
    D. Facial artery

14. Which of the following can sometimes be visible under the skin of the temporal region?
A. Maxillary artery
B. Transverse facial artery
C. Middle temporal artery
D. Superficial temporal artery

15. Which of the following arteries anastomoses with the anterior superior alveolar artery?
A. Mylohyoid artery
B. Posterior superior alveolar artery
C. Facial artery
D. Maxillary artery

16. Which of the following vascular lesions results in a small amount of blood escaping into the surrounding tissue and clotting?
A. Hemorrhage
B. Hematoma
C. Embolus
D. Thrombus

17. For the left side of the body, the common carotid and subclavian arteries arise directly from the:
A. Aorta
B. Brachiocephalic artery
C. Internal carotid artery
D. External carotid artery

18. Which of the following is the larger terminal branch of the external carotid artery?
A. Superficial temporal artery
B. Ascending palatine artery
C. Facial artery
D. Maxillary artery
E. Lingual artery

19. The brachiocephalic veins unite to form the:
A. Subclavian veins
B. External jugular veins
C. Internal jugular veins
D. Superior vena cava
E. Aorta

20. Which of the following is contained in the carotid sheath?
A. Facial nerve
B. Internal jugular vein
C. Aorta
D. Superficial lymph nodes

Glandular Tissue

LEARNING OBJECTIVES

After studying this chapter, the reader should be able to do the following:

1. Define and pronounce all the key terms and anatomical terms in this chapter.
2. Locate and identify all the glandular tissue and associated structures in the head and neck region on a diagram, skull, and patient.
3. Correctly complete the review questions and activities for this chapter.
4. Integrate the knowledge about the head and neck glands during clinical dental practice.

KEY TERMS

Duct Passageway to carry the secretion from the exocrine gland to the location where it will be used.

Endocrine Gland (**en**-dah-krin) Type of gland without a duct, with the secretion being poured directly into the vascular system, which then carries the secretion to the region in which it is to be used.

Exocrine Gland (**ek**-sah-krin) Type of gland with an associated duct that serves as a passageway for the secretion so that it can be emptied directly into the location where the secretion is to be used.

Gland Structure that produces a chemical secretion necessary for normal body functioning.

Goiter (**goit**-er) Enlarged thyroid gland due to a disease process.

OVERVIEW OF THE GLANDULAR TISSUE

The glandular tissue in the head and neck area includes the lacrimal, salivary, thyroid, parathyroid, and thymus glands. A dental professional needs to be able to locate and identify these glands and their innervation, lymphatic drainage, and vascular supply (Table 7-1). This information will help the dental professional determine if the glands are involved in a disease process and, if so, the extent of the involvement.

A **gland** is a structure that produces a chemical secretion necessary for normal body functioning. An **exocrine gland** is a gland that has a duct associated with it. A **duct** is a passageway that allows the secretion to be emptied directly into the location where the secretion is to be used. An **endocrine gland** is a ductless gland, with the secretion being poured directly into the vascular system, which then carries the secretion to the region in which it is to be used. Motor nerves associated with both types of glands help regulate the flow of the secretion, and sensory nerves are also present.

LACRIMAL GLANDS

The **lacrimal glands** (lak-ri-mal) are paired exocrine glands that secrete **lacrimal fluid** or tears (see Chapter 2). Lacrimal fluid is a watery fluid that lubricates the conjunctiva lining the inside of the eyelids and the front of the eyeball. The fluid leaves the gland through 8 to 12 fine tubules. After passing over the eyeball, the lacrimal fluid is drained through a small hole in each eyelid, ending in the **nasolacrimal sac** (nay-so-lak-rim-al), a thin-walled structure behind the medial canthus.

From the nasolacrimal sac, the lacrimal fluid continues into the **nasolacrimal duct,** ultimately draining into the inferior nasal meatus. This connection explains why crying leads to a runny nose. Persistent dryness, scratching, and burning in the eyes are signs of dry eye syndrome. A thin strip of filter paper placed at the edge of the eye, the Schirmer test, can determine the level of dryness of the eye. Treatment varies according to etiology. Many medications or diseases that cause dry eye syndrome can also cause dry mouth (xerostomia).

Location. Each gland is located in the lacrimal fossa of the frontal bone (see Chapter 3). The lacrimal fossa is located just inside the lateral portion of the supraorbital ridge inside the orbit. The nasolacrimal duct is formed at the junction of the lacrimal and maxillary bones.

Innervation. The glands are innervated by parasympathetic fibers from the greater petrosal nerve, a branch of the seventh cranial or facial nerve. These preganglionic fibers synapse at the pterygopalatine ganglion, and postganglionic fibers reach the gland through branches of the trigeminal nerve. The lacrimal nerve serves as an afferent nerve for the lacrimal gland.

Lymphatics. The glands drain into the superficial parotid lymph nodes.

Blood Supply. The glands are supplied by the lacrimal artery, a branch of the ophthalmic artery of the internal carotid artery.

SALIVARY GLANDS

The **salivary glands** (sal-i-ver-ee) produce **saliva** (sah-li-vah), which is part of the immune system. Saliva lubricates and cleanses the oral cavity and helps in digestion. These glands are controlled by the autonomic nervous system. The glands are divided by size into major and minor glands. Both the major and minor salivary glands are exocrine glands and thus have ducts associated with them. These ducts help drain the saliva directly into the oral cavity, where the saliva can function. The salivary glands should be palpated during an extraoral examination (see Appendix B). New research shows that saliva may have many biomarkers for various systematic, and even periodontal, diseases.

Salivary Gland Lesions

Salivary glands may become enlarged, tender, and possibly firmer due to various disease processes. Salivary glands may also become involved in salivary stone (sialolith) formation, blocking the drainage of saliva from the duct and causing gland enlargement and tenderness in the major glands (ranula) or minor glands (mucocele) (Figures 7-1 and 7-2). Salivary duct stones are uncomfortable but not dangerous. An examination demonstrates one or more enlarged, tender salivary glands. The clinician may also be able to feel the stone during examination or facial radiographs, or a computed tomography (CT) scan can be taken to confirm the diagnosis.

The stone is usually removed with only minimal discomfort. If the patient has repeated stones or infections, the affected salivary gland may need to be surgically removed. Certain medications and disease processes may result in decreased (xerostomia) or increased production of saliva by these glands.

Major Salivary Glands

The **major salivary glands** are large paired glands and have named ducts associated with them. The three major salivary glands are the parotid, submandibular, and sublingual glands.

TABLE 7-1

GLANDULAR TISSUE: LOCATION, INNERVATION, LYMPHATIC DRAINAGE, AND BLOOD SUPPLY

Glandular Tissue	Location	Innervation	Lymphatics	Blood Supply
Lacrimal gland with nasolacrimal duct	Lacrimal fossa of frontal bone	Greater petrosal and lacrimal nerves	Superficial parotid nodes	Lacrimal and ophthalmic arteries
Parotid gland with parotid duct	Parotid space posterior to the mandibular ramus, anterior and inferior to ear	Ninth and fifth cranial nerves	Deep parotid nodes	Branches of external carotid artery
Submandibular gland with submandibular duct	Submandibular space: inferior and posterior to the body of mandible	Chorda tympani nerve and seventh cranial nerve	Submandibular nodes	Facial and lingual arteries
Sublingual gland with sublingual duct(s)	Sublingual space: floor of mouth, medial to body of mandible	Chorda tympani nerve and seventh cranial nerve	Submandibular nodes	Sublingual and submental arteries
Minor salivary glands with ducts	Buccal, labial, and lingual mucosa; soft and hard palate; floor of mouth; and base of circumvallate lingual papillae	Seventh cranial nerve	Various nodes, depending on location	Various arteries, depending on location
Thyroid gland	Inferior to hyoid bone, junction of larynx and trachea	Cervical ganglion nodes	Superior deep cervical	Superior and inferior thyroid arteries
Parathyroid gland	Close to or within thyroid	Cervical ganglion	Superior deep cervical nodes	Inferior thyroid artery
Thymus gland	In thorax, inferior to hyoid bone, deep to sternum and superficial and lateral to trachea	Tenth cranial and cervical nerves	Within substance of gland	Inferior thyroid and internal thoracic arteries

PAROTID SALIVARY GLAND

The **parotid salivary gland** (pah-**rot**-id) is the largest encapsulated major salivary gland but provides only 25% of the total salivary volume. The salivary product from the parotid is a purely serous type of secretion. The gland is divided into two lobes—a superficial lobe and a deep lobe.

The duct associated with the gland is the **parotid duct** or Stensen's duct. This long duct emerges from the anterior border of the gland, superficial to the masseter muscle. The duct pierces the buccinator muscle. The duct then opens up into the oral cavity on the inner surface of the cheek, usually opposite the second maxillary molar. The **parotid papilla** (pah-**pil**-ah) is a small elevation of tissue that marks the opening of the parotid duct on the inner surface of the cheek.

Location. The gland occupies the parotid fascial space, an area posterior to the mandibular ramus, anterior and inferior to the ear (Figure 7-3; see Figure 7-8). The gland extends irregularly from the zygomatic arch to the angle of the mandible. This gland is effectively palpated bilaterally. Start anterior to each

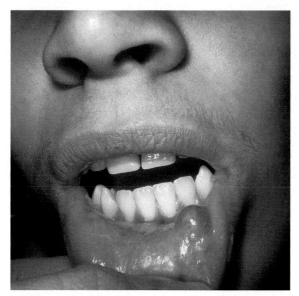

FIGURE 7-1 Mucocele of a minor salivary gland due to severance of the duct from trauma (lip bite) and then blockage of saliva.

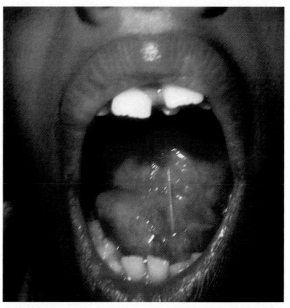

FIGURE 7-2 Ranula of the submandibular salivary gland due to blockage of saliva in a major salivary gland resulting from stone formation.

ear and move to the cheek area and then inferior to the angle of the mandible (Figure 7-4).

Innervation. The gland is innervated by the motor or efferent (parasympathetic) nerves of the otic ganglion of the ninth cranial or glossopharyngeal nerve, as well as by the afferent nerves from the auriculotemporal branch of the fifth cranial or trigeminal nerve. However, the seventh cranial or facial nerve and its branches travel through the gland between its lobes but are not involved in its innervation.

Lymphatics. The gland drains into the deep parotid lymph nodes.

Blood Supply. The gland is supplied by branches of the external carotid artery.

Parotid Gland Lesions.
The parotid gland becomes enlarged and tender when a patient has mumps. This viral infection usually involves the gland bilaterally, first one side and then the other side. The infection is rarely seen now because it is being prevented by childhood vaccination (Figure

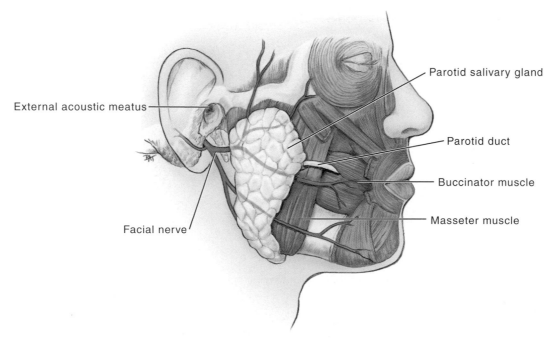

External acoustic meatus

Facial nerve

Parotid salivary gland

Parotid duct

Buccinator muscle

Masseter muscle

FIGURE 7-3 The parotid salivary gland and associated structures.

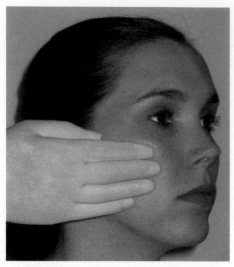

FIGURE 7-4 Palpating the parotid salivary gland by starting in front of each ear and then moving to the cheek area and then inferior to the angle of the mandible.

7-5). The gland can also be involved in tumorous growth that can also change the consistency of the gland and cause unilateral facial pain on the involved side because the facial nerve travels through the gland (see Chapter 8).

SUBMANDIBULAR SALIVARY GLAND

The **submandibular salivary gland** (sub-man-**dib**-you-lar) is the second largest encapsulated major salivary gland yet provides 60% to 65% of total salivary volume. The saliva from the submandibular gland is a mixed salivary product that has both serous and mucous secretions.

The duct associated with the gland is the submandibular duct or Wharton's duct. This long duct

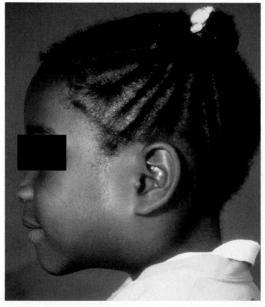

FIGURE 7-5 Enlarged parotid glands noted with mumps. From Reynolds PA, Abrahams PH: McMinn's interactive clinical anatomy: head and neck, ed 2, London, 2001, Mosby Ltd.

travels along the anterior floor of the mouth. The duct then opens into the oral cavity at the **sublingual caruncle** (sub-**ling**-gwal **kar**-unk-el), a small papilla near the midline of the mouth floor on each side of the lingual frenum (see Chapter 2). The duct's tortuous travel for a considerable upward distance in its course may be the reason the gland is the most common salivary gland to be involved in salivary stone formation.

Location. The gland occupies the submandibular fossa in the submandibular fascial space, mainly in its posterior portion (Figure 7-6). Most of the gland is a larger lobe superficial to the mylohyoid muscle, but a smaller and deeper lobe wraps around the posterior border of the muscle. The duct arises from this deep lobe and remains medial to the mylohyoid muscle.

The duct lies close to the large lingual nerve, a branch of the fifth cranial or trigeminal nerve, which is sometimes injured in surgery performed to remove salivary stones from the duct. The submandibular gland is posterior to the sublingual gland. The gland is effectively bilaterally palpated inferior and posterior to the body of the mandible, moving inward from the inferior border of the mandible near its angle as the patient lowers the head (Figures 7-7 and 7-8).

Innervation. The gland is innervated by the efferent (parasympathetic) fibers of the chorda tympani and the submandibular ganglion of the seventh cranial or facial nerve.

Lymphatics. The gland drains into the submandibular lymph nodes.

Blood Supply. The gland is supplied by branches of the facial and lingual arteries.

SUBLINGUAL SALIVARY GLAND

The **sublingual salivary gland** is the smallest, most diffuse, and only unencapsulated major salivary gland, providing only 10% of the total salivary volume. The saliva from the sublingual gland is a mixed salivary product, but with the mucous secretion predominating.

The short ducts associated with the gland sometimes combine to form the **sublingual duct** or Bartholin's duct. The sublingual duct then opens directly into the oral cavity through the same opening as the submandibular duct, the sublingual caruncle. The sublingual caruncle is a small papilla near the midline of the floor of the mouth on each side of the lingual frenum. The other small ducts of the gland open along the **sublingual fold,** a fold of tissue on each side of the mouth floor (see Chapter 2).

Location. The sublingual salivary gland is located in the sublingual fossa in the sublingual fascial space at the floor of the mouth (see Figure 7-8). This gland is superior to the mylohyoid muscle and medial to the body of the mandible. The sublingual gland is also located anterior to the submandibular gland. The

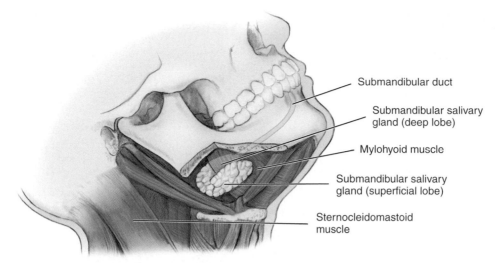

FIGURE 7-6 The submandibular salivary gland and associated structures.

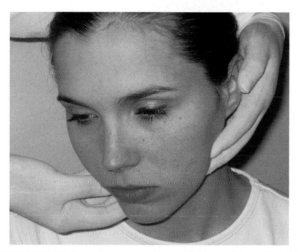

FIGURE 7-7 Palpating the submandibular salivary gland by palpating inward from the inferior border of the mandible near its angle as the patient lowers the head.

gland is effectively palpated on the floor of the mouth posterior to each mandibular canine. Placing one index finger intraorally and the fingertips of the opposite hand extraorally, the compressed gland is manually palpated between (Figure 7-9).

Innervation. The gland is innervated by the efferent (parasympathetic) fibers of the chorda tympani nerve and the submandibular ganglion of the seventh cranial or facial nerve.

Lymphatics. The gland drains into the submandibular lymph nodes.

Blood Supply. The gland is supplied by the sublingual and submental arteries.

Minor Salivary Glands

The **minor salivary glands** are smaller than the larger major salivary glands but are more numerous in number. The minor salivary glands are also exocrine glands, but their unnamed ducts are shorter than those of the major salivary glands.

Location. These minor salivary glands are scattered in the tissues of the buccal, labial, and lingual mucosa, the soft palate, the lateral portions of the hard palate, and the floor of the mouth. In addition, minor salivary glands, **von Ebner's glands** (eeb-ners), are associated with the large circumvallate lingual papillae on the posterior portion of the tongue's dorsal surface (see Chapter 2). Most minor salivary glands secrete a mainly mucous type of salivary product, with some serous secretion. The exception is von Ebner's glands, which secrete only a serous type of salivary product.

Innervation. The minor salivary glands are innervated by the seventh cranial or facial nerve.

Lymphatics and Blood Supply. The minor salivary glands drain into various lymph nodes and are supplied by various arteries depending on the area where they are located.

THYROID GLAND

The **thyroid gland** (**thy**-roid) is the largest endocrine gland. Because it is ductless, the gland produces and secretes **thyroxine** (thy-**rok**-sin) directly into the vascular system. Thyroxine is a hormone that stimulates the metabolic rate.

The gland consists of two lateral lobes. The right and left lobes are connected anteriorly by an isthmus. In a healthy patient the gland is not visible yet can be palpated as a soft mass. In a healthy state the gland is mobile when swallowing occurs. Thus when the patient swallows, the gland moves up, as does the whole larynx. This is because the gland is encased in visceral or pretracheal fascia, which is firmly adherent to the upper part of the trachea (see Chapter 11).

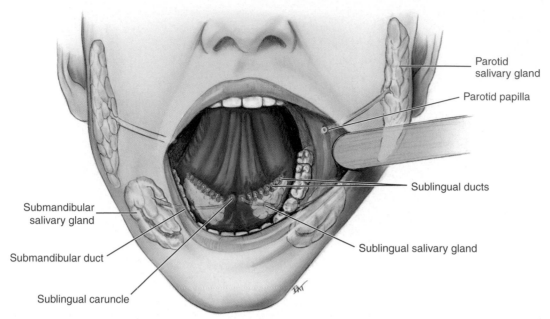

FIGURE 7-8 The salivary major glands and associated structures.

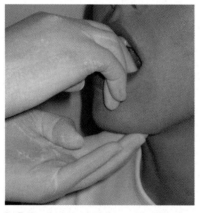

FIGURE 7-9 Palpating the sublingual salivary gland by palpating the floor of the mouth behind each mandibular canine, with one hand placed intraorally and one hand placed extraorally.

Location. The gland is located in the anterior and lateral regions of the neck. The gland is inferior to the thyroid cartilage, at the junction between the larynx and trachea (Figure 7-10). Examination of the thyroid gland is carried out by locating the thyroid cartilage and passing the fingers inferolaterally, examining for abnormal masses or overall thyroid size. Then, place one hand on each of the trachea and gently displace the thyroid tissue to the other side of the neck while the other hand manually palpates the displaced gland tissue (Figure 7-11).

Then, the two lobes of the gland should be compared using visual inspection, as well as bimanual or manual palpation. Finally, ask the patient to swallow; check for mobility of the gland. Many clinicians find that having the patient swallow water helps the examination for mobility, as well as having the patient flex the neck slightly to the side when being palpated.

Innervation. The gland is innervated by sympathetic nerves through the cervical ganglia.

Lymphatics. The gland drains into the superior deep cervical lymph nodes.

Blood Supply. The gland is supplied by the superior and inferior thyroid arteries.

Thyroid Gland Lesions

During a disease process involving the gland, the gland may become enlarged and possibly may be visible in portions during an extraoral examination. This enlarged thyroid gland is called a **goiter** (Figure 7-12). A goiter may be firm and tender when palpated and may contain hard masses. The diseased gland may also lose its mobility and not move upward when the patient swallows, indicating a tumorous growth. The gland may also be partially or fully removed surgically for various disease processes. The patient should be referred to a physician if there are any undiagnosed changes in the gland. Finding out whether the patient had the thymus gland irradiated as an infant is also important. This outdated procedure can cause thyroid cancer (discussed later).

PARATHYROID GLANDS

The **parathyroid glands** (par-ah-**thy**-roid) typically consist of four small endocrine glands, two on each side. Because the glands are ductless, they produce

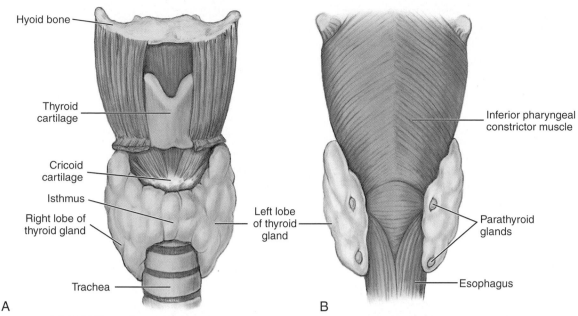

FIGURE 7-10 **A,** Anterior view of the thyroid gland and associated structures. **B,** Posterior view of the parathyroid glands within the thyroid gland and associated structures.

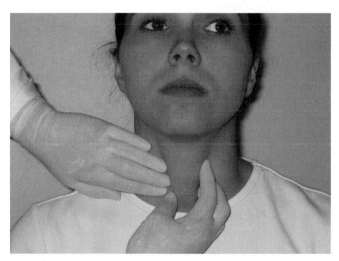

FIGURE 7-11 Palpating the thyroid gland by placing one hand on one side of the trachea and gently displacing the thyroid tissue to the other side of the neck, while the other hand palpates the displaced gland tissue.

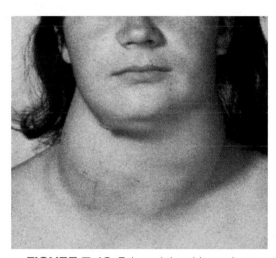

FIGURE 7-12 Enlarged thyroid or goiter.

and secrete **parathyroid hormone** directly into the vascular system to regulate calcium and phosphorus levels. The glands are not visible or palpable during an extraoral examination of a patient. However, the glands may alter the function of the thyroid gland if they are involved in a disease process.

Location. The glands are usually close to or even inside the thyroid gland on its posterior surface (see Figure 7-10, *B*).

Innervation. The glands are innervated by the same nerves that innervate the thyroid gland: sympathetic nerves through the cervical ganglia.

Lymphatics. The glands drain into the superior deep cervical lymph nodes.

Blood Supply. The glands are supplied primarily by the inferior thyroid arteries.

THYMUS GLAND

The **thymus gland** (**thy**-mus) is an endocrine gland and therefore is ductless. The gland is a portion of the immune system that fights disease processes. The **T-cell lymphocytes**, white blood cells of the immune system, mature in the gland in response to stimulation by thymus hormones. The gland grows in size from birth to puberty while performing this task. After puberty, the gland stops growing and starts to shrink, undergoing involution. Thus by adulthood, the gland has almost disappeared. And by the age of 40, it has returned to its weight at birth, making it mainly a temporary structure. The adult gland consists of two lateral lobes in close contact at the midline. The gland is not easily palpated.

Location. The gland is located in the thorax and the anterior region of the base of the neck, inferior to the thyroid gland (Figure 7-13). The gland is deep to the sternum and the sternohyoid and sternothyroid muscles. The gland is also superficial and lateral to the trachea.

Innervation. The gland is innervated by branches of the tenth cranial or vagus nerve and cervical nerves.

Lymphatics. The lymphatics of the gland arise within the substance of the gland and terminate in the internal jugular vein.

Blood Supply. The gland is supplied by the inferior thyroid and internal thoracic arteries.

Thymus Gland Lesions

The thymus gland may not be easily palpated, and it may only be a temporary gland, but its involvement in various disease processes may alter the health of the patient while it is present. Older patients may have had radiation therapy to the gland in childhood to shrink the gland. Now it is known that the larger gland of a child is not related to suffocation and thus sudden infant death. The radiation levels used on these patients in the past may result in future cases of thyroid cancer.

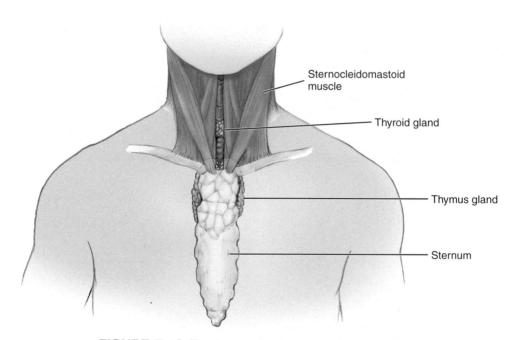

Sternocleidomastoid muscle

Thyroid gland

Thymus gland

Sternum

FIGURE 7-13 The thymus gland and associated structures.

Identification Exercises

Identify the structures on the following diagrams by filling in each blank with the correct anatomical term. You can check your answers by looking back at the figure indicated in parentheses for each identification diagram.

1. (Figure 7-3)

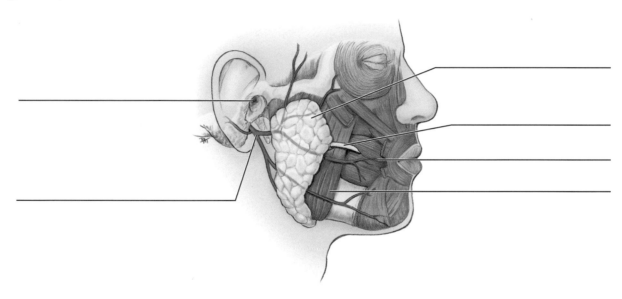

2. (Figure 7-6)

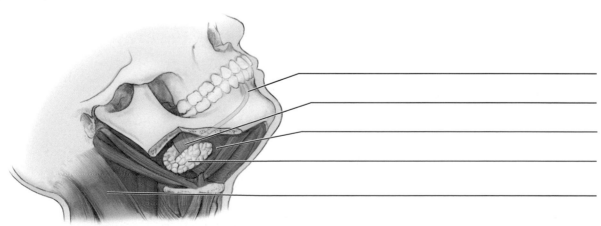

3. (Figure 7-8)

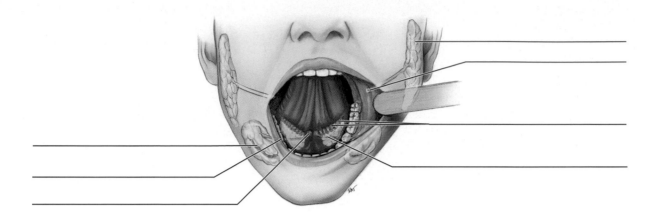

4. (Figure 7-10, *A*)

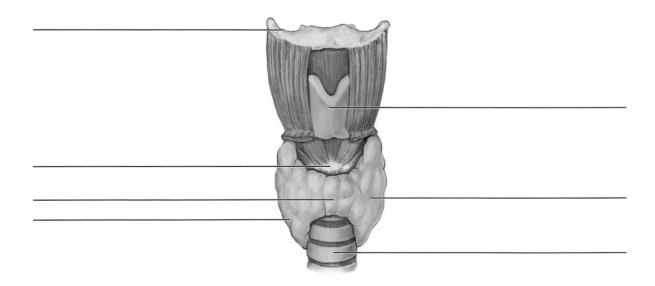

5. (Figure 7-13)

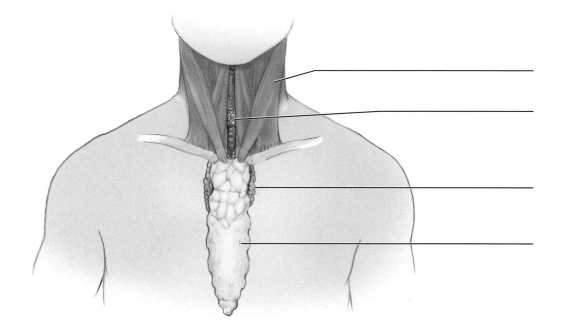

■ REVIEW QUESTIONS

1. The sublingual salivary gland is located:
   A. Anterior to the submandibular gland
   B. Inferior to the mylohyoid muscle
   C. Lateral to the body of the mandible
   D. In the mandibular vestibule area

2. Which of the following glands has both a superficial and deep lobe?
   A. Thymus gland
   B. Parotid gland
   C. Thyroid gland
   D. Sublingual gland
   E. Lacrimal gland

3. Which of the following nerves innervates both the submandibular and sublingual salivary glands?
   A. Trigeminal nerve
   B. Chorda tympani
   C. Hypoglossal nerve
   D. Vagus nerve

4. Which of the following nerves travels through the parotid salivary gland but is not involved in its innervation?
   A. Trigeminal nerve
   B. Facial nerve
   C. Vagus nerve
   D. Glossopharyngeal nerve

5. Which of the following glands shrinks as a person matures?
   A. Thymus gland
   B. Parotid gland
   C. Thyroid gland
   D. Sublingual gland
   E. Submandibular gland

6. Which gland has a duct that usually opens on the inner surface of the cheek, opposite the second maxillary molar?
   A. Thymus gland
   B. Parotid gland
   C. Thyroid gland
   D. Sublingual gland
   E. Submandibular gland

7. Which oral landmark marks the opening of the submandibular duct?
   A. Parotid raphe
   B. Lingual frenum
   C. Parotid papilla
   D. Sublingual caruncle
   E. Nasolacrimal duct

8. The thyroid gland is located:
   A. Anterior to the larynx
   B. Superior to the hyoid bone
   C. Posterior to the surrounding pharynx
   D. In the posterior and medial neck region

9. Which of the following blood vessels supplies the parotid salivary gland?
   A. Facial artery
   B. Lingual artery
   C. Internal carotid artery
   D. External carotid artery

10. As endocrine glands, the parathyroid glands are known to:
    A. Have one primary duct
    B. Have multiple secondary ducts
    C. Drain directly into blood vessels
    D. Drain directly into the thyroid gland

11. The lacrimal gland ultimately drains into the:
    A. Lacrimal fossa
    B. Inferior nasal meatus
    C. Parotid salivary gland
    D. Internal carotid artery

12. Which of the following can block the drainage of saliva from the duct?
    A. Excessive amounts of secretion
    B. Stone formation
    C. Lacrimal gland drainage
    D. Inflammation of blood vessels

13. Which of the following statements concerning minor salivary glands is correct?
    A. Minor glands are smaller and less numerous than the major glands.
    B. Minor glands secrete only mucous saliva.
    C. Minor glands have longer ducts than major glands.
    D. Minor glands are located in the buccal, labial, and lingual mucosa.

14. In a healthy patient, the thyroid gland:
    A. Consists of two lobes that are connected by an isthmus
    B. Does not move with the thyroid cartilage when swallowing
    C. Secretes thyroxine, which slows down the metabolic rate
    D. Is clearly visible and easily palpated

15. When examining the thyroid gland:
    A. Ask the patient to swallow
    B. Ask the patient to cough
    C. Palpate the tissue directly over the trachea
    D. Move the gland superiorly and then inferiorly

16. Into which structure does the lacrimal fluid initially drain into after passing over the eyelid?
A. Sublingual caruncle
B. Nasolacrimal sac
C. Nasolacrimal duct
D. Parathyroid glands

17. Which of the following is a significant feature of the thymus gland?
A. Maturation of immune system T cells
B. Regulation of calcium and phosphorus levels
C. Stimulation of metabolic rate
D. Cleansing of oral cavity and helping in digestion

18. Which of the following oral tissues contain minor salivary glands?
A. Palatine rugae
B. Attached gingiva
C. Hard palate
D. Ventral tongue surface

19. Which of the following lesions is due to an enlarged thyroid gland?
A. Mucocele
B. Ranula
C. Goiter
D. Mumps

20. The initial lymphatic drainage of the sublingual salivary gland is by the:
A. Submental nodes
B. Malar nodes
C. Superior deep cervical nodes
D. Submandibular nodes

Nervous System

OUTLINE

- Overview of the Nervous System
  - Central Nervous System
  - Peripheral Nervous System
  - Cranial Nerves
- Nerves to the Oral Cavity and Associated Structures
  - Trigeminal Nerve
  - Facial Nerve
- Nerve Lesions of the Head and Neck

LEARNING OBJECTIVES

After studying this chapter, the reader should be able to do the following:

1. Define and pronounce all the key terms and anatomical terms in this chapter.
2. Describe the components of the nervous system and outline the actions of nerves.
3. Discuss in general the major divisions of the central and peripheral nervous systems.
4. Identify and trace the routes of the cranial nerves from the skull on a series of diagrams.
5. Briefly discuss the general function of each of the cranial nerves.
6. Identify and trace the routes of the nerves to the oral cavity and associated structures of the head and neck on a diagram, skull, and patient.
7. Describe the tissues innervated by each of the nerves of the head and neck.
8. Discuss certain nerve lesions associated with the head and neck region.
9. Correctly complete the review questions and activities for this chapter.
10. Integrate the knowledge about head and neck nerves into clinical dental practice.

KEY TERMS

Action Potential (po-**ten**-shal) Rapid depolarization of the cell membrane that results in propagation of the nerve impulse along the membrane.

Afferent Nerve (**af**-er-ent) Sensory nerve that carries information from the periphery of the body to the brain or spinal cord.

Anesthesia (ann-es-**thee**-zee-ah) The loss of feeling or sensation resulting from the use of certain drugs or gases that serve as inhibitory neurotransmitters.

Bell's Palsy (**pawl**-ze) Type of unilateral facial paralysis involving the facial nerve.

Continued

KEY TERMS (continued)

Efferent Nerve (**ef**-er-ent) Motor nerve that carries information away from the brain or spinal cord to the periphery of the body.

Facial Paralysis (pah-**ral**-i-sis) Loss of action of the facial muscles.

Ganglion/Ganglia (**gang**-gle-in, **gang**-gle-ah) Accumulation of neuron cell bodies outside the central nervous system.

Innervation (in-er-**vay**-shin) Supply of nerves to tissues or organs.

Neuron (**noor**-on) Cellular component of the nervous system that is individually composed of a cell body and neural processes.

Neurotransmitter (**nu**-ro-**tranz**-mitt-er) Chemical agent from the neuron that is discharged with the arrival of the action potential, diffuses across the synapse, and binds to receptors on another cell's membrane.

Nerve Bundle of neural processes outside the central nervous system; a portion of the peripheral nervous system.

Nervous System The extensive, intricate network of structures that activates, coordinates, and controls all functions of the body.

Resting Potential Charge difference between the fluid outside and inside a cell that results in differences in the distribution of ions.

Synapse (**sin**-aps) Junction between two neurons or between a neuron and an effector organ, where neural impulses are transmitted by electrical or chemical means.

Trigeminal Neuralgia (try-**jem**-i-nal noor-**al**-je-ah) Type of lesion of the trigeminal nerve involving facial pain.

OVERVIEW OF THE NERVOUS SYSTEM

The **nervous system** causes muscles to contract, resulting in facial expressions and joint movements such as those involved in mastication and speech. The system stimulates glands to secrete and regulates many other systems of the body such as the vascular system. The nervous system also allows for sensation to be perceived, such as pain and touch.

Knowledge of the nervous system and its components is important to the dental professional because this system allows for the function of the muscles, temporomandibular joint, and glands of the head and neck (see Chapters 4, 5, and 7). A thorough understanding of certain nerves is important in pain management that involves administering local anesthesia during dental treatment (see Chapter 9). Finally, there are certain related nervous system disorders of the head and neck that need to be known by the dental professional (discussed later).

The nervous system has two main divisions, the central nervous system and the peripheral nervous system (Figures 8-1 and 8-2). These two divisions of the nervous system are constantly interacting. The **neuron** is the cellular component of the nervous system and is composed of a cell body and neural processes. A **nerve** is a bundle of neural processes outside the central nervous system and in the peripheral nervous system. A **synapse** is the junction between two neurons or between a neuron and an effector organ, where neural impulses are transmitted.

In order to function, most tissues and organs have **innervation,** a supply of nerves to the body portion. A nerve allows information to be carried to and from the brain, which is the central informational center. An accumulation of neuron cell bodies outside the central nervous system is termed a **ganglion** (plural, **ganglia**).

Nerves are of two types, afferent and efferent (see Figure 8-1). An **afferent nerve** or sensory nerve carries information from the periphery of the body to the brain (or spinal cord). Thus an afferent nerve carries sensory information such as taste, pain, and proprioception to the brain. Proprioception is information concerning the movement and position of the body. This information is sent on to the brain to be analyzed, acted on, associated with other information, and stored as memory.

An **efferent nerve** or motor nerve carries information away from the brain (or spinal cord) to the periphery of the body. Thus an efferent nerve carries information to the muscles in order to activate them, often in response to information received by way of the afferent nerves. One motor neuron with its branching process may control hundreds of muscle fibers.

The plasma membrane of a neuron, like all other cells, has an unequal distribution of ions and electrical charges between the two sides of the membrane. The fluid outside of the membrane has a positive charge; the fluid inside has a negative charge. This charge difference is a **resting potential** and is measured in millivolts. Resting potential results in part from differences in the distribution of positively charged ions (sodium and potassium) and negatively charged ions in the cytoplasm and extracellular fluid. Sodium ions are more heavily concentrated outside the membrane, while potassium ions are more heavily concentrated inside the membrane. This imbalance is maintained by the active transport of ions against their concentration gradients by the sodium-potassium pump.

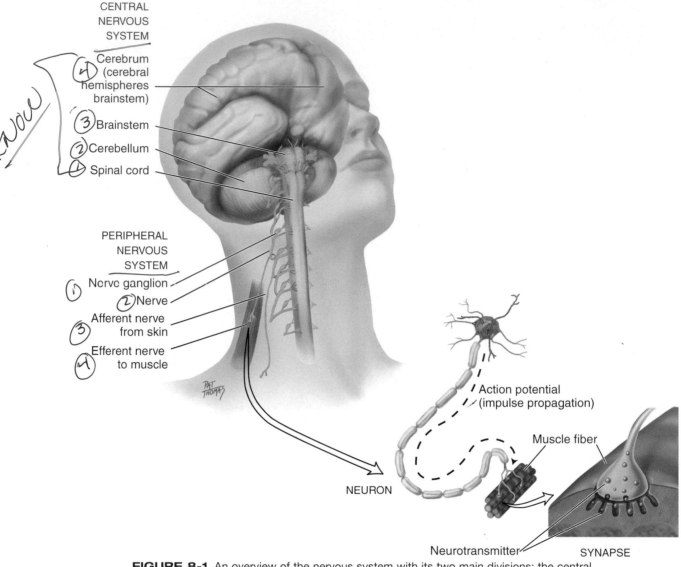

FIGURE 8-1 An overview of the nervous system with its two main divisions: the central nervous and peripheral nervous systems.

The rapid depolarization of the cell membrane, called the **action potential,** results in the propagation of the nerve impulse along the membrane (see Figure 8-1). An action potential is a temporary reversal of the electrical potential along the membrane for a brief period (less than a millisecond). Sodium gates suddenly open in the membrane to allow sodium ions to pour in, bringing their positive charge. At the height of the membrane potential reversal, sodium gates close and potassium channels open to allow potassium ions to pass to the outside of the membrane, reestablishing the resting potential. The changed ionic distributions must be reset by the continuously running sodium-potassium pump.

The action potential begins at one spot on the membrane but spreads to adjacent areas of the membrane, propagating the impulse along the length of the cell membrane. After passage of the action potential, there

is a brief period—the refractory period—during which the membrane cannot be stimulated. This prevents the impulse from being transmitted backward along the membrane. By means of the action potential, nerve impulses travel the length of the neuron.

To have the impulse cross the synapse to another cell requires the actions of chemical agents or **neurotransmitters** from the neuron, which are discharged with the arrival of the action potential. Released neurotransmitters diffuse across the synapse and bind to receptors on the membrane of the other cell. Neurotransmitters cause ion channels to open or close in the second cell, prompting changes in the excitability of that cell's membrane. Excitatory neurotransmitters such as acetylcholine and norepinephrine (in most organs) make it more likely that an action potential will be triggered in the second cell. Inhibitory neurotransmitters such as dopamine and serotonin

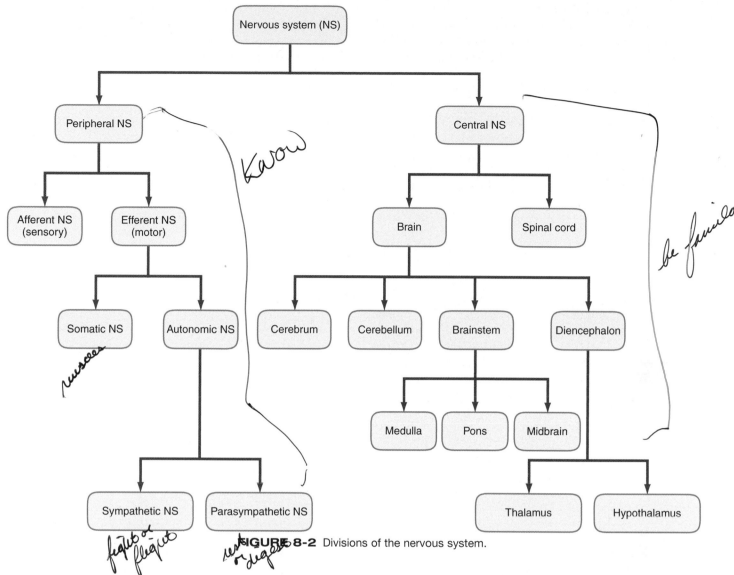

FIGURE 8-2 Divisions of the nervous system.

make an action potential in the second cell less likely. Neurotransmitters are either destroyed by specific enzymes, diffuse away, or are reabsorbed by the neuron.

Neurotransmitters tend to be small molecules; some are even hormones. Some neurological diseases (e.g., Parkinson's disease, Huntington's chorea) are associated with imbalances of neurotransmitters. Some symptoms of Parkinson's disease (e.g., rigidity) are due to a dopamine deficiency. Some symptoms of Huntington's chorea are thought to be caused by loss of a different inhibitory neurotransmitter. Alzheimer's disease is accompanied by a loss of acetylcholine-producing neurons, which may explain the memory problems that result. In addition, depression can sometimes be linked to low levels of excitatory neurotransmitters, and drug therapy for depression alters those levels. Among the drugs that affect neurotransmitter function is cocaine, which blocks the uptake of norepinephrine while stimulating the uptake of dopamine.

Special neurotransmitters involved with the sensation of pain in the central nervous system are endorphins, natural opioids that produce elation and reduction of pain, as do unnatural neurotransmitting chemicals such as opium and heroin. Many local anesthetic agents such as lidocaine, as used in dentistry, mimic inhibitory neurotransmitters by decreasing sensory neurons' ability to generate an action potential, thus producing localized anesthesia. **Anesthesia** is the loss of feeling or sensation resulting from the use of certain drugs or gases that serve as inhibitory neurotransmitters. With damage to the nerves, there can be abnormal sensation or paresthesia to an area such as infection (see Chapter 12) or other trauma or agent toxicity (see Chapter 9).

Central Nervous System

One of the major divisions of the nervous system, the **central nervous system (CNS),** is composed of the brain and spinal cord. The CNS is surrounded by bone, either the skull or vertebrae, with fluid and tissue serving as further protection. The major divisions of the **brain** include the cerebrum, the cerebellum, the brainstem, and the diencephalon (Figure 8-3).

The **cerebrum** (ser-e-brum) is the largest division of the brain and consists of two cerebral hemispheres (see Figure 8-3). The cerebrum coordinates sensory data and motor functions and governs many aspects of intelligence and reasoning, learning, and memory. The **cerebellum** (ser-e-**bel**-um) is the second largest division of the brain, after the cerebrum. It functions to produce muscle coordination and maintains normal muscle tone and posture, as well as coordinating balance.

The **brainstem** has a number of divisions including the medulla, pons, and midbrain (Figure 8-4). The **medulla** (me-**dul**-ah) is closest to the spinal cord and is involved with the regulation of heartbeat, breathing, vasoconstriction (blood pressure), and reflex centers for vomiting, coughing, sneezing, swallowing, and hiccupping. The cell bodies of the motor neurons for the tongue are located in the medulla. The **pons** (ponz) connects the medulla with the cerebellum and with higher brain centers. Cell bodies for cranial nerves V and VII are found in the pons. The **midbrain** includes relay stations for hearing, vision, and motor pathways.

Superior to the brainstem, the **diencephalon** (di-en-**sef**-a-lon) consists primarily of the thalamus and hypothalamus (see Figure 8-4). The **thalamus** (**thal**-a-mus) serves as a central relay point for incoming nerve impulses, and the **hypothalamus** (hi-po-**thal**-a-mus) regulates homeostasis. It has regulatory areas for thirst, hunger, body temperature, water balance, and blood pressure and links the nervous system to the endocrine system.

The **spinal cord** runs along the dorsal side of the body and links the brain to the rest of the body (see Figure 8-4). The spinal cord in adults is encased in a series of bony vertebrae that make up the vertebral column. The gray matter of the spinal cord consists mostly of unmyelinized cell bodies and dendrites. The surrounding white matter is made up of tracts of axons, insulated in sheaths of myelin, a combination of lipids and proteins. Some tracts are ascending (carrying messages to the brain), and others are descending (carrying messages from the brain). The spinal cord is also involved in reflexes that do not immediately involve the brain.

Peripheral Nervous System

The other major division of the nervous system, the **peripheral nervous system (PNS),** is composed of all the nerves stretching among the CNS and the receptors, muscles, and glands of the body. The PNS is further divided into the **afferent nervous system** or sensory, which carries information from receptors to the brain or spinal cord, and the **efferent nervous system** or motor, which carries information from the brain or spinal cord to muscles or glands. A nerve cell leading from the eye to the brain and carrying visual information is a portion of the afferent nervous system. A nerve cell leading from the brain to muscles controlling the eye's movement is a portion of the efferent nervous system. The efferent division of the PNS is further subdivided into the somatic nervous system and autonomic nervous system.

SOMATIC NERVOUS SYSTEM

The **somatic nervous system (SNS)** is a subdivision of the efferent division of the peripheral nervous system and includes all nerves controlling the muscular system and external sensory receptors. External sense organs (including skin) are receptors. Muscle fibers and gland cells are effectors. Sensory input from the PNS is processed by the CNS, and responses are sent by the PNS from the CNS to the organs of the body. The motor neurons of the somatic system are distinct from those of the autonomic system. Inhibitory signals cannot be sent through the motor neurons of the somatic system.

AUTONOMIC NERVOUS SYSTEM

The **autonomic nervous system** (awt-o-**nom**-ik) **(ANS)** is the other subdivision of the efferent division of the peripheral nervous system. This system operates

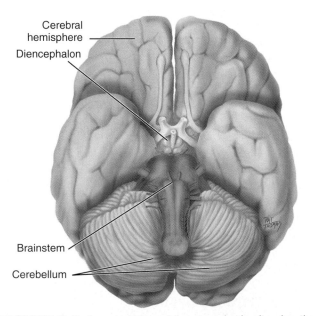

Cerebral hemisphere

Diencephalon

Brainstem

Cerebellum

FIGURE 8-3 A ventral view of the gross brain showing the cerebellum, cerebral hemisphere, and diencephalon, with the brainstem highlighted.

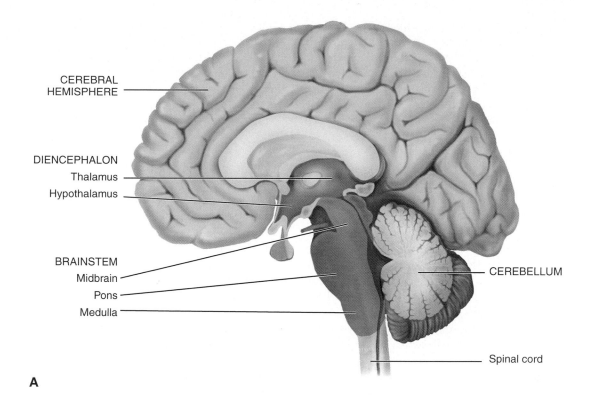

A

CEREBRAL HEMISPHERE

DIENCEPHALON
Thalamus
Hypothalamus

BRAINSTEM
Midbrain
Pons
Medulla

CEREBELLUM

Spinal cord

B

Cerebral hemisphere

DIENCEPHALON
Thalamus

Hypothalamus

BRAINSTEM
Midbrain

Pons

Medulla

CEREBELLUM

Spinal cord

FIGURE 8-4 A, A lateral sagittal section of the gross brain showing the brainstem highlighted with its midbrain, medulla, and pons, and the diencephalon with its thalamus and hypothalamus, as well as the spinal cord, cerebellum, and cerebral hemisphere. **B,** Gross specimen. (**B,** From Reynolds PA, Abrahams PH: *McMinn's interactive clinical anatomy: head and neck,* ed 2, London, 2001, Mosby Ltd.)

without conscious control as the caretaker of the body. Autonomic fibers are efferent nerves, and they always occur in two-nerve chains. The first nerve carries autonomic fibers to a ganglion, where they end near the cell bodies of the second nerve. The ANS itself has two subdivisions: the sympathetic system and the parasympathetic system. Most tissues and organ systems are supplied by both divisions of the ANS. However, the sympathetic and parasympathetic systems generally work in opposition to each other: one stimulates an organ, while the other inhibits it.

The **sympathetic nervous system** (sim-pah-**thet**-ik) is involved in "fight-or-flight responses" such as the shutdown of salivary gland secretion. Thus such a response by the sympathetic system leads to a dry mouth (xerostomia). Sympathetic nerves arise in the spinal cord and relay in ganglia arranged like a chain running up the neck close to the vertebral column on both sides. Therefore all the sympathetic neurons in the head have already relayed in a ganglion. Sympathetic fibers reach the cranial tissues they supply by traveling with the arteries.

The **parasympathetic nervous system** (pare-ah-sim-pah-**thet**-ik) is involved in "rest-or-digest" responses such as the stimulation of salivary gland secretions. Thus such a response by the parasympathetic system leads to salivary flow to aid in digestion.

Parasympathetic fibers associated with the glands of the head and neck region are carried in various cranial nerves and are briefly described here, as well as in greater detail later. Their ganglia are located in the head, and therefore parasympathetic neurons in this region may be either preganglionic neurons (before relaying in the ganglion) or postganglionic neurons (after relaying in the ganglion).

The principal parasympathetic outflow for glands in the head and neck is carried in the seventh and ninth cranial nerves. The seventh cranial or facial nerve has two branches involved in glandular secretion. The greater petrosal nerve is associated with the pterygopalatine ganglion, and the lacrimal gland is the major target organ. The chorda tympani nerve is associated with the submandibular ganglion, and the target organs are the submandibular and sublingual salivary glands. The lesser petrosal nerve, a branch of the ninth cranial or glossopharyngeal nerve, is associated with the otic ganglion, and the target organ is the parotid salivary gland.

Cranial Nerves

The **cranial nerves** (**kray**-nee-al) are an important portion of the peripheral nervous system. All 12 paired cranial nerves are connected to the brain at its base and pass through the skull by way of fissures or foramina (Figures 8-5 and 8-6 and Table 8-1) (see Chapter 3).

Some cranial nerves are either afferent or efferent, and others have both types of neural processes. A general background of all 12 cranial nerves is discussed later. Both Roman numerals (I-VII) and anatomical terms are used to designate the cranial nerves.

CRANIAL NERVE I

The first (I) cranial or **olfactory nerve** (ol-**fak**-ter-ee) transmits smell from the nasal mucosa to the brain and thus functions as an afferent nerve. The nerve enters the skull through the perforations in the cribriform plate of the ethmoid bone to join the olfactory bulb in the brain.

CRANIAL NERVE II

The second (II) cranial or **optic nerve** (**op**-tik) transmits sight from the retina of the eye to the brain and thus functions as an afferent nerve. The nerve enters the skull through the optic canal of the sphenoid bone on its way from the retina. In the skull, the right and left optic nerves join at the optic chiasma, where many of the fibers cross to the opposite side before continuing into the brain as the optic tracts.

CRANIAL NERVE III

The third (III) cranial or **oculomotor nerve** (ok-yule-oh-**mote**-er) serves as an efferent nerve to some of the eye muscles that move the eyeball. The nerve also carries preganglionic parasympathetic fibers to the ciliary ganglion near the eyeball. The postganglionic fibers innervate small muscles inside the eyeball. The nerve lies in the lateral wall of the cavernous sinus and exits the skull through the superior orbital fissure of the sphenoid bone on its way to the orbit.

CRANIAL NERVE IV

The small fourth (IV) cranial or **trochlear nerve** (**trok**-lere) also serves as an efferent nerve for one eye muscle, as well as proprioception, similar to the oculomotor nerve but without any parasympathetic fibers. Similar to the oculomotor nerve, the trochlear nerve runs in the lateral wall of the cavernous sinus and exits the skull through the superior orbital fissure of the sphenoid bone on its way to the orbit.

CRANIAL NERVE V

The fifth (V) cranial or **trigeminal nerve** (try-**jem**-i-nal) has both an efferent component for the muscles of mastication, as well as some other cranial muscles, and an afferent component for the teeth, tongue, and oral cavity, as well as most of the skin of the face and head. Although the trigeminal nerve has no preganglionic parasympathetic fibers, many postganglionic parasympathetic fibers travel along with its branches.

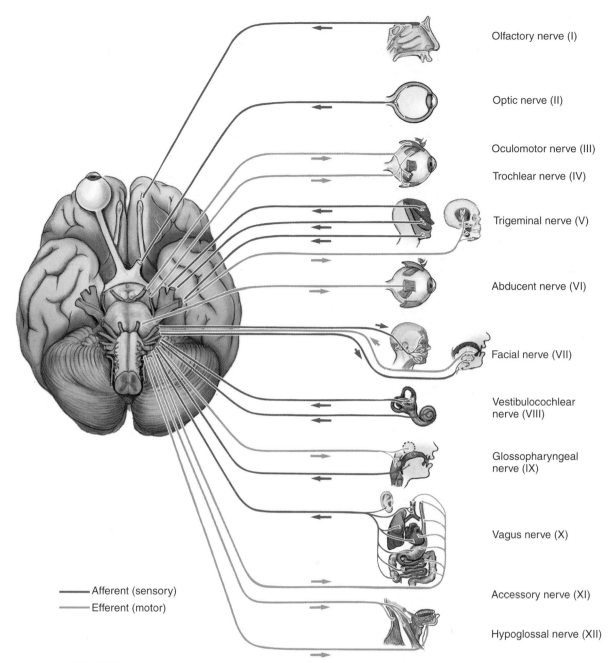

FIGURE 8-5 Inferior view of the brain showing cranial nerves and the organs and tissues they innervate.

Olfactory nerve (I)

Optic nerve (II)

Oculomotor nerve (III)

Trochlear nerve (IV)

Trigeminal nerve (V)

Abducent nerve (VI)

Facial nerve (VII)

Vestibulocochlear nerve (VIII)

Glossopharyngeal nerve (IX)

Vagus nerve (X)

Accessory nerve (XI)

Hypoglossal nerve (XII)

——— Afferent (sensory)
——— Efferent (motor)

The trigeminal nerve is the largest cranial nerve and has two roots, sensory and motor roots (see Figure 8-5). The **sensory root of the trigeminal nerve** has three divisions: the ophthalmic, maxillary, and mandibular nerves. The ophthalmic nerve provides sensation to the upper face and scalp. The maxillary and mandibular nerves provide sensation to the middle and lower face, respectively.

Each division of the sensory root of the nerve enters the skull in a different location in the sphenoid bone.

The ophthalmic nerve enters through the superior orbital fissure. The maxillary nerve enters by way of the foramen rotundum. The mandibular nerve passes through the skull by way of the foramen ovale.

The **motor root of the trigeminal nerve** accompanies the mandibular nerve of the sensory root and also exits the skull through the foramen ovale of the sphenoid bone.

The trigeminal nerve is the most important cranial nerve to the dental professional because it innervates

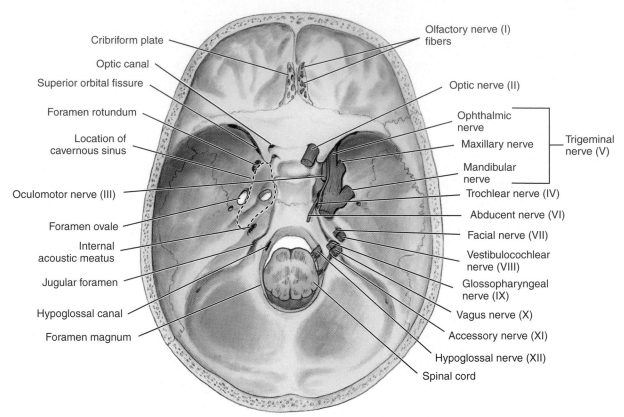

FIGURE 8-6 Internal view of the base of the skull showing cranial nerves exiting or entering the skull.

many relevant tissues of the head and neck (Table 8-2). The trigeminal nerve is discussed in greater detail later, and local anesthesia of its nerve branches is discussed in Chapter 9.

CRANIAL NERVE VI

The sixth (VI) cranial or abducent nerve or **abducens** (ab-**doo**-senz) serves as an efferent nerve to one of the muscles that moves the eyeball, similar to the oculomotor and trochlear nerves. Similar to both of those cranial nerves, the nerve exits the skull through the superior orbital fissure of the sphenoid bone on its way to the orbit.

However, the nerve has a somewhat different intracranial course. Rather than lying in the wall of the cavernous sinus, the nerve runs through the sinus, close to the internal carotid artery, and is often the first nerve affected by infection of the sinus (see Chapter 12).

CRANIAL NERVE VII

The seventh (VII) cranial or **facial nerve** carries both efferent and afferent components. The nerve carries an efferent component for the muscles of facial expression and for the preganglionic parasympathetic innervation of the lacrimal gland (relaying in the pterygopalatine ganglion) and submandibular and sublingual salivary glands (relaying in the submandibular ganglion). The afferent component serves a tiny patch of skin behind the ear, taste sensation, and the body of the tongue.

The facial nerve leaves the cranial cavity by passing through the internal acoustic meatus, which leads to the facial canal inside the temporal bone. Finally, the nerve exits the skull by way of the stylomastoid foramen of the temporal bone. The facial nerve is also important to dental professionals because it innervates many relevant tissues of the head and neck (see Table 8-2). The facial nerve can also be involved in a complication with the administration of local anesthesia (see Chapters 7 and 9). The facial nerve is discussed in greater detail later.

CRANIAL NERVE VIII

The eighth (VIII) cranial or **vestibulocochlear nerve** (ves-tib-you-lo-**kok**-lere) serves as an afferent nerve for hearing and balance. This nerve conveys signals from the inner ear to the brain. The inner ear is located within the temporal bone. The nerve enters the cranial cavity through the internal acoustic meatus of the temporal bone.

The nerve supplies the two major portions of the inner ear. The first portion, the cochlea, serves the function of hearing and is supplied by the cochlear

TABLE 8-1

THE 12 CRANIAL NERVES AND THE NERVE TYPES AND TISSUES INNERVATED

	Nerve	Nerve Types and Tissues Innervated
I:	Olfactory	Afferent: nasal mucosa
II:	Optic	Afferent: retina of the eye
III:	Oculomotor	Efferent: eye muscles
IV:	Trochlear	Efferent: eye muscles
V:	Trigeminal	Efferent: muscles of mastication and other cranial muscles Afferent: face and head skin, teeth, oral cavity, parotid gland, and tongue (general sensation)
VI:	Abducens	Efferent: eye muscles
VII:	Facial	Efferent: muscles of facial expression, other cranial muscles, and lacrimal, submandibular, sublingual, and minor glands (parasympathetic) Afferent: skin around ear and tongue (taste sensation)
VIII:	Vestibulocochlear	Afferent: inner ear
IX:	Glossopharyngeal	Efferent: stylopharyngeus muscle and parotid gland (parasympathetic) Afferent: skin around ear and tongue (taste and general sensation)
X:	Vagus	Efferent: muscles of soft palate, pharynx, and larynx and thorax and abdominal organs (parasympathetic) Afferent: skin around ear and epiglottis (taste sensation)
XI:	Accessory	Efferent: muscles of neck, soft palate, and pharynx
XII:	Hypoglossal	Efferent: tongue muscles

part of the vestibulocochlear nerve. The second portion, the semicircular canals, serves the function of balance and is supplied by the vestibular portion of the semicircular canals.

CRANIAL NERVE IX

The ninth (IX) cranial or **glossopharyngeal nerve** (gloss-oh-fah-**rin**-je-al) carries an efferent component for a pharyngeal muscle, the stylopharyngeus muscle, and preganglionic gland parasympathetic innervation for the parotid salivary gland (relaying the otic ganglion). The nerve also carries an afferent component for the pharynx and for taste and general sensation from the base of the tongue.

The nerve passes through the skull by way of the jugular foramen, between the occipital and temporal bones. The tympanic branch, with sensory fibers for the middle ear and preganglionic parasympathetic fibers for the parotid gland, arises here and reenters the skull.

After supplying the ear, parasympathetic fibers leave the skull through the foramen ovale of the sphenoid bone as the **lesser petrosal nerve** (peh-**troh**-sil). These preganglionic fibers then end in the **otic ganglion** (**ot**-ik). The otic ganglion is located near the medial surface of the mandibular nerve of the trigeminal or fifth cranial nerve, just inferior to the foramen ovale. Inferior branches of the nerve supply the carotid artery, pharynx, and base of the tongue (afferent component), as well as the stylopharyngeus muscle. The glossopharyngeal nerve is important to dental professionals because it innervates many relevant tissues of the head and neck (see Table 8-2).

CRANIAL NERVE X

The tenth (X) cranial or **vagus nerve** (**vay**-gus) carries a large efferent component for the muscles of the soft palate, pharynx, and larynx and for parasympathetic fibers to many organs in the thorax and abdomen including the thymus gland, heart, and stomach. The nerve carries a smaller afferent component for a small amount of skin around the ear and for taste sensation for the epiglottis.

The nerve passes through the skull by way of the jugular foramen, between the occipital and temporal bones. The vagus nerve is important to dental professionals because it innervates many relevant tissues of the head and neck (see Table 8-2).

CRANIAL NERVE XI

The eleventh (XI) cranial or **accessory nerve** (ak-**ses**-o-re) functions as an efferent nerve for the trapezius and sternocleidomastoid muscles, as well as for muscles of the soft palate and pharynx. This nerve is only partly a cranial nerve and consists of two roots, one arising from the brain and one from the spinal cord. The accessory nerve exits the skull through the jugular foramen, between the occipital and temporal bones. The accessory nerve is important to dental professionals because it innervates many relevant tissues of the head and neck (see Table 8-2).

TABLE 8-2

TISSUES OF THE HEAD AND NECK AND THEIR ASSOCIATED NERVES AND TYPE

Head and Neck Tissues	Nerves and Type
Maxillary anterior lingual gingiva and anterior hard palate	Nasopalatine of V_2: afferent
Maxillary posterior lingual gingiva and posterior hard palate	Greater palatine of V_2: afferent
Soft palate and palatine tonsillar tissue	Lesser palatine of V_2, glossopharyngeal (IX); afferent branches of V_3, accessory (XI), and vagus (X): efferent
Maxillary anterior teeth, maxillary anterior facial gingiva	ASA of V_2: afferent and anterior labial mucosa
Maxillary posterior teeth, maxillary posterior buccal gingiva, posterior labial mucosa, and maxillary sinus	MSA and PSA of V_2: afferent
Mandibular teeth and facial gingiva of mandibular anterior teeth and premolars	IA of V_3: afferent
Mandibular buccal gingiva and buccal mucosa	Buccal of V_3: afferent
Mandibular labial mucosa	Mental of V_3: afferent
Floor of mouth and mandibular lingual gingiva	Lingual of V_3: afferent
Tongue muscles	Hypoglossal (III): efferent
Tongue—general sensation	Body, lingual of V_3: afferent base; glossopharyngeal (IX): afferent
Tongue—taste sensation	Body, chorda tympani of facial (VII): afferent base; glossopharyngeal (IX): afferent
Parotid gland	Lesser petrosal of glossopharyngeal (IX): efferent (parasympathetic) and auriculotemperal of V_3: afferent
Submandibular and sublingual glands	Chorda tympani of facial (VII): efferent (parasympathetic)
Muscles of facial expression	Branches of facial (VII): efferent
Muscles of mastication	Medial pterygoid, deep temporal, masseteric, and lateral pterygoid of V_3: efferent
Trapezius and sternocleidomastoid muscles	Accessory (XI): efferent

ASA, Anterior superior alveolar; *IA,* inferior alveolar; *MSA,* middle superior alveolar; *PSA,* posterior superior alveolar; V_2, maxillary nerve; V_3, mandibular nerve.

CRANIAL NERVE XII

The twelfth (XII) cranial or **hypoglossal nerve** (hi-poh-**gloss**-al) functions as an efferent nerve for the intrinsic and extrinsic muscles of the tongue. The nerve exits the skull through the hypoglossal canal in the occipital bone. The hypoglossal nerve is important to dental professionals because it innervates the tongue (see Table 8-2).

NERVES TO THE ORAL CAVITY AND ASSOCIATED STRUCTURES

The dental professional must understand the basic components of the nervous system, as well as the location of the major nerves of the head and neck. Knowledge of the nervous system is important because it adds to the general background of certain

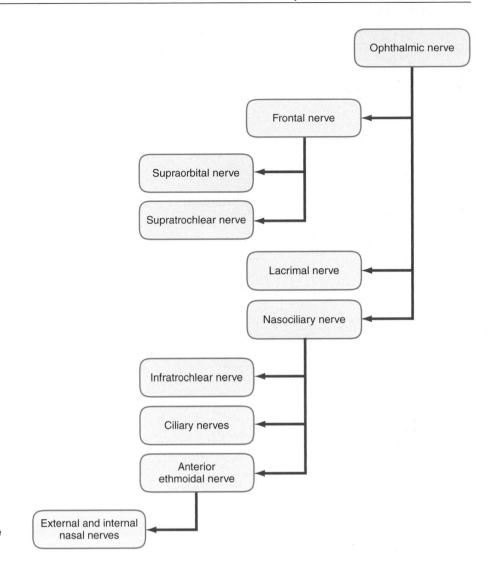

FIGURE 8-10 The ophthalmic nerve (V$_1$) to the facial region.

Lacrimal Nerve.

The **lacrimal nerve** (**lak**-ri-mal) serves as an afferent nerve for the lateral portion of the upper eyelid, conjunctiva, and lacrimal gland. The nerve also delivers the postganglionic parasympathetic nerves to the lacrimal gland. These nerves are responsible for the production of lacrimal fluid or tears. The nerve runs posteriorly along the lateral roof of the orbit and then joins the frontal and nasociliary nerves near the superior orbital fissure of the sphenoid bone to form V$_1$.

Nasociliary Nerve.

Several afferent nerve branches converge to form the **nasociliary nerve** (nay-zo-**sil**-ee-a-re). These branches include the **infratrochlear nerve** (in-frah-**trok**-lere) from the skin of the medial portion of the eyelids and the side of the nose, **ciliary nerves** (**sil**-ee-a-re) to and from the eyeball, and **anterior ethmoidal nerve** (eth-**moy**-dal) from the nasal cavity and paranasal sinuses. The anterior ethmoidal nerve is formed by the **external**

nasal nerve (**nay**-zil) from the skin of the ala and apex of the nose and the **internal nasal nerves** from the anterior portion of the nasal septum and lateral wall of the nasal cavity.

The nasociliary nerve is an afferent nerve that runs within the orbit, superior to the second cranial or optic nerve, to join the frontal and lacrimal nerves near the superior orbital fissure of the sphenoid bone to form V$_1$.

MAXILLARY NERVE

The second division (V$_2$) from the sensory root of the trigeminal nerve is the **maxillary nerve** (**mak**-sil-ar-ee) (Figures 8-11 and 8-12). The afferent nerve branches of the maxillary nerve carry sensory information for the maxilla and overlying skin, maxillary sinuses, nasal cavity, palate, and nasopharynx and a portion of the dura mater.

The maxillary nerve is a nerve trunk formed in the pterygopalatine fossa by the convergence of many nerves. The largest contributor is the infraorbital

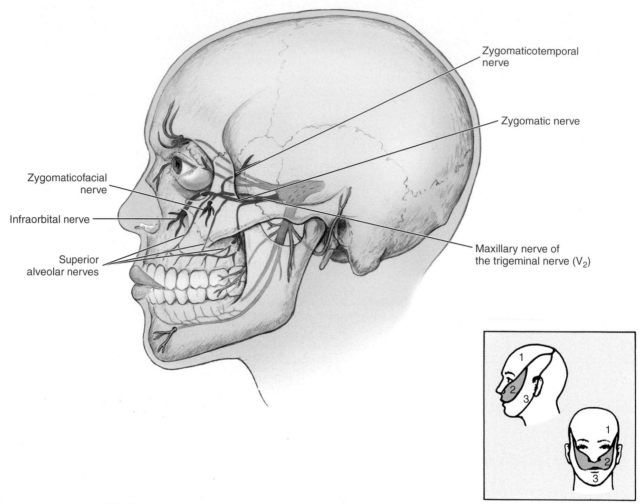

FIGURE 8-11 The pathway of the maxillary nerve of the trigeminal nerve is highlighted.

nerve. Tributaries of the infraorbital nerve or maxillary nerve trunk include the zygomatic, anterior, middle and posterior superior alveolar, greater and lesser palatine, and nasopalatine nerves.

After all these branches come together in the pterygopalatine fossa to form the maxillary nerve, the nerve enters the skull through the foramen rotundum of the sphenoid bone (see Chapter 3). Small afferent meningeal branches (me-**nin**-je-al) from portions of the dura mater join the maxillary nerve as it enters the trigeminal ganglion.

Another ganglion, the **pterygopalatine ganglion** (teh-ri-go-**pal**-ah-tine), lies just inferior to the maxillary nerve in the pterygopalatine fossa. This ganglion serves as a relay station for parasympathetic nerves that arise in the facial nerve (described later). Fibers from the ganglion (postganglionic) are then distributed to various tissues such as the minor salivary glands by the nerves of V_2. Because the pterygopalatine ganglion lies between the maxillary nerve and its tributaries from the palate, the sensory fibers actually pass through the ganglion. However, unlike the

parasympathetic fibers, the sensory fibers do not synapse in the ganglion.

Zygomatic Nerve.

The **zygomatic nerve** (zy-go-**mat**-ik) is an afferent nerve composed of the merger of the zygomaticofacial nerve and the zygomaticotemporal nerve in the orbit (see Figure 8-11). This nerve also conveys the post-ganglionic parasympathetic fibers for the lacrimal gland to the lacrimal nerve. The zygomatic nerve courses posteriorly along the lateral orbit floor; enters the pterygopalatine fossa through the inferior orbital fissure, between the sphenoid bone and maxilla; and finally joins V_2.

The rather small **zygomaticofacial nerve** (zygo-mat-i-ko-**fay**-shal) serves as an afferent nerve for the skin of the cheek. This nerve pierces the frontal process of the zygomatic bone and enters the orbit through its lateral wall. The zygomaticofacial nerve then turns posteriorly to join with the zygomaticotemporal nerve.

The other nerve, the **zygomaticotemporal nerve** (zy-go-mat-i-ko-**tem**-poh-ral), serves as an afferent

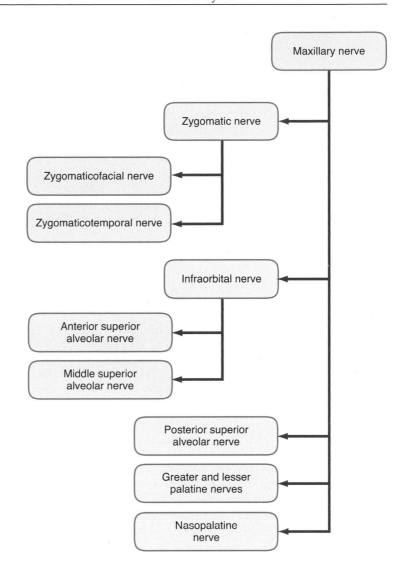

FIGURE 8-12 The maxillary nerve (V₂) to the oral cavity.

nerve for the skin of the temporal region, pierces the temporal surface of the zygomatic bone; and traverses the lateral wall of the orbit to join the zygomaticofacial nerve, forming the zygomatic nerve.

Infraorbital Nerve.

The **infraorbital nerve** (in-frah-**or**-bit-al) or **IO nerve** is an afferent nerve formed from the merger of cutaneous branches from the upper lip, medial portion of the cheek, lower eyelid, and side of the nose (Figure 8-13). The IO nerve then passes into the infraorbital foramen of the maxilla and travels posteriorly through the infraorbital canal, along with the infraorbital blood vessels, where it is joined by the anterior superior alveolar nerve.

From the infraorbital canal and groove, the IO nerve passes into the pterygopalatine fossa through the inferior orbital fissure. After it leaves the infraorbital groove and within the pterygopalatine fossa, the IO nerve receives the posterior superior alveolar nerve.

Anterior Superior Alveolar Nerve.

The **anterior superior alveolar nerve** (al-ve-o-lar) or **ASA nerve** serves as an afferent nerve of sensation (including pain) for the maxillary central incisors, lateral incisors, and canine, as well as their associated tissues.

The ASA nerve originates from dental branches in the pulp tissue of these teeth that exit through the apical foramina (see Figure 8-13). The ASA nerve also receives interdental branches from the surrounding periodontium, forming a dental plexus or nerve network in the maxilla for the region. The ASA nerve also innervates the overlying facial gingiva. The ASA nerve then ascends along the anterior wall of the maxillary sinus to join the IO nerve in the infraorbital canal.

Many times the ASA nerve crosses over the midline to the opposite side in a patient. This is important to consider when administering local anesthesia for the maxillary anterior teeth and associated tissues (see Chapter 9).

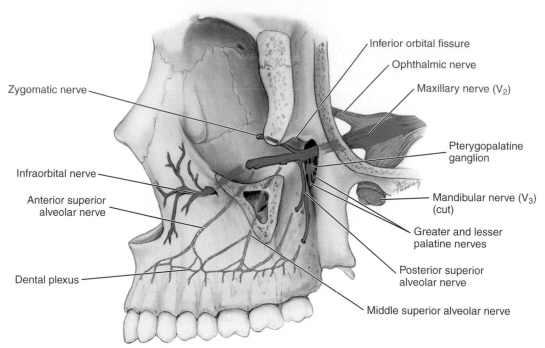

FIGURE 8-13 Lateral view of the skull (*a portion of the lateral wall of the orbit has been removed*) with the branches of the maxillary nerve highlighted.

Middle Superior Alveolar Nerve.

The **middle superior alveolar nerve** or **MSA nerve** serves as an afferent nerve of sensation (including pain), typically for the maxillary premolar teeth and mesiobuccal root of the maxillary first molar and their associated periodontium and overlying buccal gingiva.

The MSA nerve originates from dental branches in the pulp tissue that exit the teeth through the apical foramina, as well as interdental and interradicular branches from the periodontium (see Figure 8-13). The MSA nerve, like the posterior superior alveolar and ASA nerves, forms the dental plexus or nerve network in the maxilla. The MSA nerve then ascends to join the IO nerve by running in the lateral wall of the maxillary sinus.

The MSA nerve is not present in all patients. If this nerve is not present, the area is innervated by both the ASA and posterior superior alveolar nerves, but mainly by the ASA nerve. If the MSA nerve is present, there is communication between the MSA nerve and both the ASA and posterior superior alveolar nerves. These considerations are important when administering local anesthesia for the maxillary posterior teeth and associated tissues (see Chapter 9).

Posterior Superior Alveolar Nerve

The **posterior superior alveolar nerve** or **PSA nerve** joins the IO nerve (or the maxillary nerve directly) in the pterygopalatine fossa (see Figure 8-13). The PSA nerve

serves as an afferent nerve of sensation (including pain) for most portions of the maxillary molar teeth and their periodontium and buccal gingiva, as well as the maxillary sinus.

Some branches of the PSA nerve remain external to the posterior surface of the maxilla. These external branches provide afferent innervation for the buccal gingiva that overlies the maxillary molars.

Other afferent nerve branches of the PSA nerve originate from dental branches in the pulp tissue of each of the maxillary molar teeth that exit the teeth by way of the apical foramina. These dental branches are then joined by interdental branches and interradicular branches from the periodontium, forming a dental plexus or a nerve network in the maxilla for the region.

All these internal branches of the PSA nerve exit from several posterior superior alveolar foramina on the maxillary tuberosity of the maxilla. The posterior superior alveolar arteries (from the maxillary artery) enter the maxillary tuberosity through these same foramina.

Both the external and internal branches of the PSA nerve then ascend together along the maxillary tuberosity, which forms the posterolateral wall of the maxillary sinus, to join either the IO nerve or maxillary nerve. The PSA nerve typically provides afferent innervation for the maxillary second and third molars and the palatal and distal buccal root of the maxillary first molar, as well as the mucous membranes of the maxillary sinus.

Greater and Lesser Palatine Nerves.

Both palatine nerves join with the maxillary nerve from the palate (Figure 8-14). The **greater palatine nerve (pal**-ah-tine) or **GP nerve,** also called the *anterior palatine nerve,* is located between the mucoperiosteum and bone of the anterior hard palate. This nerve serves as an afferent nerve for the posterior hard palate and posterior lingual gingiva. Communication occurs with the terminal fibers of the nasopalatine nerve in the hard palate area, lingual to the maxillary canines.

Posteriorly, the GP nerve enters the greater palatine foramen in the palatine bone near the maxillary second or third molar to travel in the pterygopalatine canal, along with the greater palatine blood vessels.

The **lesser palatine nerve,** also called the *posterior palatine nerve,* serves as an afferent nerve for the soft palate and palatine tonsillar tissues. The lesser palatine nerve enters the lesser palatine foramen in the palatine bone near its junction with the pterygoid process of the sphenoid bone, along with the lesser palatine blood vessels (see Figure 8-14). The lesser palatine nerve then joins the GP nerve in the pterygopalatine canal.

Both palatine nerves ascend through the pterygopalatine canal, toward the maxillary nerve in the pterygopalatine fossa. On the way, the palatine nerves are joined by lateral nasal branches (**nay**-zil), which are afferent nerves from the posterior nasal cavity.

Nasopalatine Nerve.

The **nasopalatine nerve** (nay-zo-**pal**-ah-tine) or **NP nerve** originates in the mucosa of the anterior hard palate, lingual to the maxillary anterior teeth (see Figure 8-14). The right and left NP nerves enter the incisive canal by way of the incisive foramen, beneath the incisive papilla, thus exiting the oral cavity. The nerve then travels along the nasal septum. The NP nerve serves as an afferent nerve for the anterior hard palate and the lingual gingiva of the maxillary anterior teeth, as well as the nasal septal tissues. Communication also occurs with the GP nerve in the area that is located lingual to the maxillary canines.

MANDIBULAR NERVE

The third division (V_3) of the trigeminal nerve is the **mandibular nerve** (man-**dib**-you-lar), which is a short main trunk formed by the merger of a smaller anterior trunk and a larger posterior trunk in the infratemporal fossa, before the nerve passes through the foramen ovale of the sphenoid bone (Figures 8-15, 8-16, and 8-17). The mandibular nerve then joins with the ophthalmic and maxillary nerves to form the trigeminal ganglion of the trigeminal nerve. The mandibular nerve is the largest of the three divisions that form the trigeminal nerve.

A few small branches arise from the V_3 trunk before its separation into the anterior and posterior trunks (see Figure 8-20). These branches from the undivided

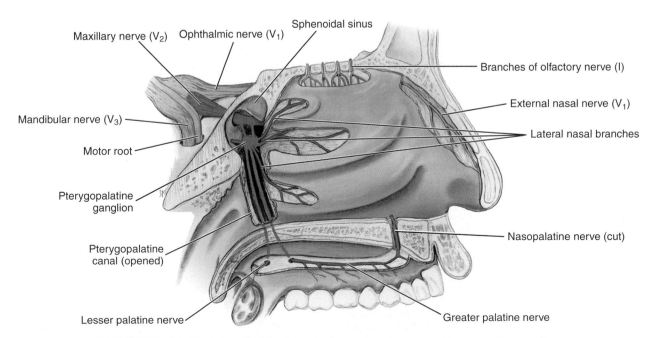

FIGURE 8-14 Medial view of the lateral nasal wall and opened pterygopalatine canal highlighting the maxillary nerve and its palatine branches. The nasal septum has been removed, thus severing the nasopalatine nerve.

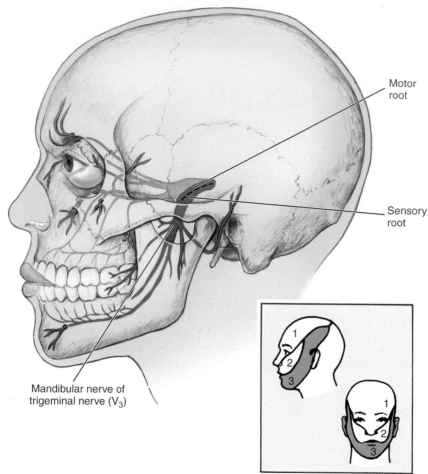

FIGURE 8-15 The pathway of the mandibular nerve of the trigeminal nerve is highlighted.

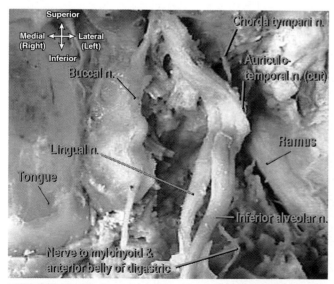

FIGURE 8-16 Gross anatomy of the mandibular nerve of the trigeminal nerve. (Reprinted with permission of Jeremy S. Melker, MD, 1999.)

mandibular nerve include the **meningeal branches** (me-**nin**-je-al), which are afferent nerves for portions of the dura mater. Also from the undivided mandibular nerve are muscular branches, which are efferent nerves for the medial pterygoid, tensor tympani, and tensor veli palatini muscles.

The anterior trunk of the mandibular nerve is formed by the merger of the buccal nerve and additional muscular nerve branches (Figure 8-18). The posterior trunk of the mandibular nerve is formed by the merger of the auriculotemporal, lingual, and inferior alveolar nerves (Figure 8-19).

Buccal Nerve.

The **buccal nerve** or long buccal nerve serves as an afferent nerve for the skin of the cheek, buccal mucous membranes, and buccal gingiva of the mandibular posterior teeth. The nerve is located on the surface of the buccinator muscle (see Figure 8-17). The buccal nerve then travels posteriorly in the cheek, deep to the masseter muscle.

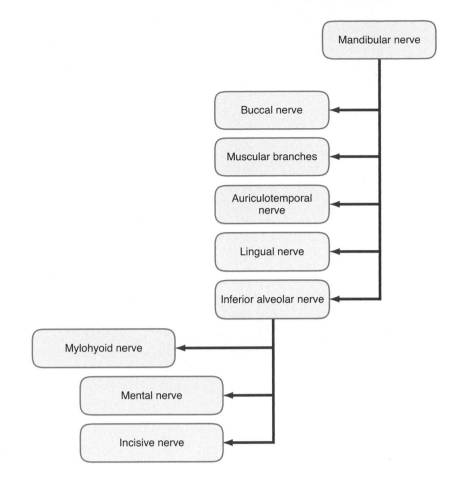

FIGURE 8-17 Mandibular nerve (V₃) to the oral cavity.

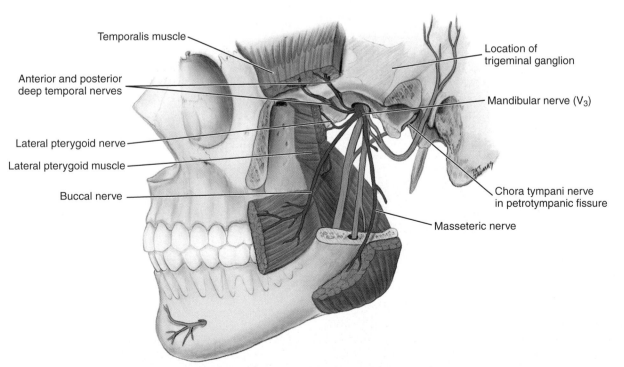

FIGURE 8-18 The pathway of the anterior trunk of the mandibular nerve of the trigeminal nerve is highlighted.

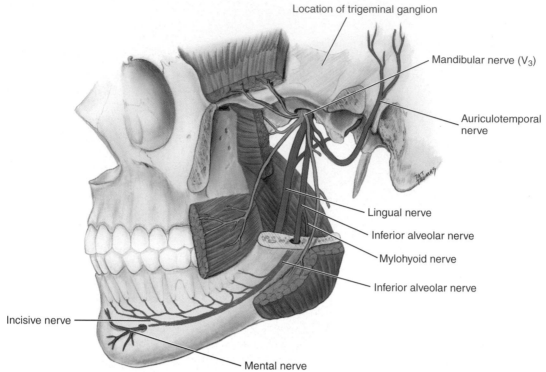

FIGURE 8-19 The pathway of the posterior trunk of the mandibular nerve of the trigeminal nerve is highlighted.

At the level of the occlusal plane of the last mandibular molar, the nerve crosses in front of the anterior border of the ramus and goes between the two heads of the lateral pterygoid muscle to join the anterior trunk of V$_3$. This nerve must not be confused with the buccal nerve, which innervates the buccinator muscle and is an efferent nerve branch from the facial nerve.

Muscular Branches.

Several muscular branches are part of the anterior trunk of V$_3$ (see Figure 8-18). They arise from the motor root of the trigeminal nerve. The **deep temporal nerves** (**tem**-poh-ral), usually two in number, anterior and posterior, are efferent nerves that pass between the sphenoid bone and the superior border of the lateral pterygoid muscle and turn around the infratemporal crest of the sphenoid bone to end in the deep surface of the temporal muscle that they innervate. The posterior temporal nerve may arise in common with the masseteric nerve, and the anterior temporal nerve may be associated at its origin with the buccal nerve.

The **masseteric nerve** (mass-et-**tehr**-ik) is also an efferent nerve that passes between the sphenoid bone and the superior border of the lateral pterygoid muscle. The nerve then accompanies the masseteric blood vessels through the mandibular notch to innervate the masseter muscle. A small sensory branch also

goes to the temporomandibular joint. The **lateral pterygoid nerve** (**teh**-ri-goid), after a short course, enters the deep surface of the lateral pterygoid muscle between the muscle's two heads of origin and serves as an efferent nerve for that muscle.

Auriculotemporal Nerve.

The nerve known as the **auriculotemporal nerve** (aw-rik-yule-lo-**tem**-poh-ral) travels with the superficial temporal artery and vein and serves as an afferent nerve for the external ear and scalp (Figure 8-20; see Figure 8-19). The nerve also carries postganglionic parasympathetic nerve fibers to the parotid salivary gland. Important to note is that these parasympathetic fibers arise from the lesser petrosal branch of the glossopharyngeal or ninth cranial nerve, joining the auriculotemporal nerve only after relaying in the otic ganglion near the foramen ovale.

Communication of the auriculotemporal nerve with the facial nerve near the ear also occurs. The nerve courses deep to the lateral pterygoid muscle and neck of the mandible, then splits to encircle the middle meningeal artery, and finally joins the posterior trunk of V$_3$.

Lingual Nerve.

The **lingual nerve** is formed from afferent branches from the body of the tongue that travel along the lateral surface of the tongue (see Figures 8-17, 8-18,

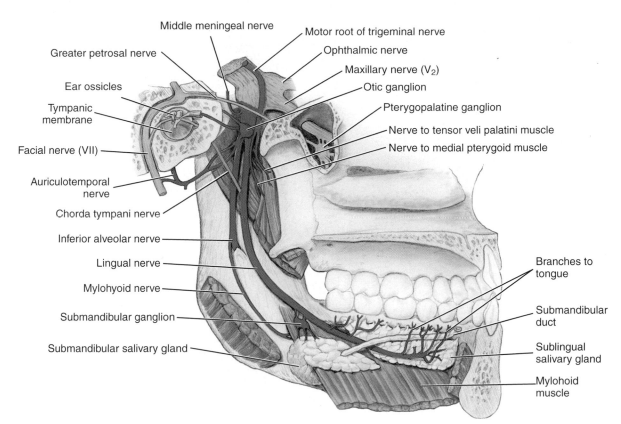

FIGURE 8-20 Medial view of the mandible with the motor and sensory branches of the mandibular nerve highlighted.

and 8-19). The nerve then passes posteriorly, passing from the medial to the lateral side of the duct of the submandibular salivary gland by going under the duct.

The lingual nerve communicates with the **submandibular ganglion** (sub-man-**dib**-you-lar) located superior to the deep lobe of the submandibular salivary gland (Figure 8-21). The submandibular ganglion is a portion of the parasympathetic system. Parasympathetic efferent innervation for the sublingual and submandibular salivary glands arises from the facial nerve (specifically, a branch of the facial nerve, the chorda tympani, which is discussed later) but travels along with the lingual nerve.

At the base of the tongue, the lingual nerve ascends and runs between the medial pterygoid muscle and the mandible, anterior and slightly medial to the inferior alveolar nerve. Thus the lingual nerve is also anesthetized when administering an inferior alveolar local anesthetic nerve block through diffusion of the local anesthetic agent. Because the nerve is only a short distance posterior to the roots of the last mandibular molar tooth and is covered only by a thin layer of oral mucosa, its location is sometimes visible clinically. Thus the lingual nerve can be endangered by dental procedures in this region such as the extraction of permanent mandibular third molars.

The lingual nerve then continues to travel upward to join the posterior trunk of V_3. Thus the lingual nerve

serves as an afferent nerve for general sensation for the body of the tongue, floor of the mouth, and lingual gingiva of the mandibular teeth.

Inferior Alveolar Nerve.

The **inferior alveolar nerve** or **IA nerve** is an afferent nerve formed from the merger of the mental and incisive nerves (see Figure 8-19). The mental and incisive nerves are discussed later in this section.

After forming, the IA nerve continues to travel posteriorly through the mandibular canal, along with the inferior alveolar artery and vein. The IA nerve is joined by dental branches and interdental and interradicular branches from the mandibular posterior teeth, forming a dental plexus or nerve network in the region. The IA nerve then exits the mandible through the mandibular foramen, where it is joined by the mylohyoid nerve (discussed later). The mandibular foramen is a central opening on the internal surface of the ramus, three-fourths the distance from the coronoid notch to the posterior border of the ramus.

The IA nerve then travels lateral to the medial pterygoid muscle, between the sphenomandibular ligament and ramus of the mandible within the pterygomandibular space. This is posterior and slightly lateral to the lingual nerve. The IA nerve then joins the posterior trunk of V_3 (see Figures 8-19

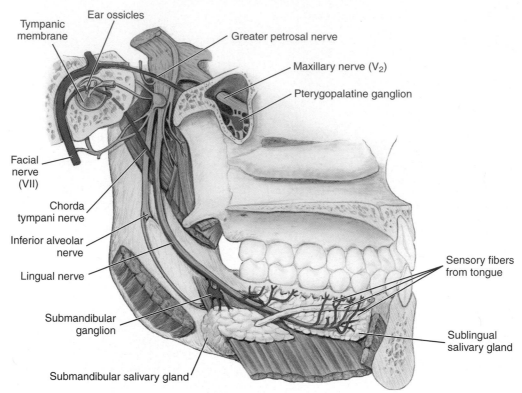

FIGURE 8-21 The pathway of the trunk of the facial nerve, greater petrosal nerve, and chorda tympani nerve (*note relationship with lingual nerve*) is highlighted.

and 8-20). The IA nerve carries afferent innervation for the mandibular teeth.

In some cases there are two nerves present on the same side, creating bifid IA nerves. This situation can occur unilaterally or bilaterally and can be detected on a radiograph by the presence of a double mandibular canal. As discussed in Chapter 3, there can be more than one mandibular foramen, usually inferiorly placed, either unilaterally or bilaterally, along with the bifid IA nerves. These considerations must be kept in mind when administering local anesthesia for the mandibular teeth and associated tissues (see Chapter 9).

Mental Nerve.

The **mental nerve** (**ment**-il) is composed of external branches that serve as an afferent nerve for the chin, lower lip, and labial mucosa of the mandibular premolars and anterior teeth (see Figure 8-19). The mental nerve then enters the mental foramen on the anterolateral surface of the mandible, usually between the apices of the mandibular first and second premolars, and merges with the incisive nerve to form the IA nerve in the mandibular canal.

Incisive Nerve.

The **incisive nerve** (in-**sy**-ziv) is an afferent nerve composed of dental branches from the mandibular premolar and anterior teeth that originate in the

pulp tissue, exit the teeth through the apical foramina, and join with interdental branches from the surrounding periodontium, forming a dental plexus in the region (see Figure 8-19). The incisive nerve then merges with the mental nerve, just posterior to the mental foramen, to form the IA nerve in the mandibular canal. The incisive nerve serves as an afferent nerve for the mandibular premolars and anterior teeth.

Crossover from the opposite incisive nerve sometimes occurs, which is an important consideration when administering local anesthesia for the mandibular premolars and anterior teeth and associated tissues (see Chapter 9).

Mylohyoid Nerve.

After the inferior alveolar nerve exits the mandibular foramen, a small branch occurs, called the **mylohyoid nerve** (my-lo-**hi**-oid) (see Figures 8-19 and 8-20). This nerve pierces the sphenomandibular ligament and runs inferiorly and anteriorly in the mylohyoid groove and then onto the inferior surface of the mylohyoid muscle. The mylohyoid nerve serves as an efferent nerve to the mylohyoid muscle and anterior belly of the digastric muscle (the posterior belly of the digastric muscle is innervated by a branch from the facial nerve). This nerve may in some cases also serve as an afferent nerve for the mandibular first molar, which needs to be considered when there is failure

2. (Figure 8-5)

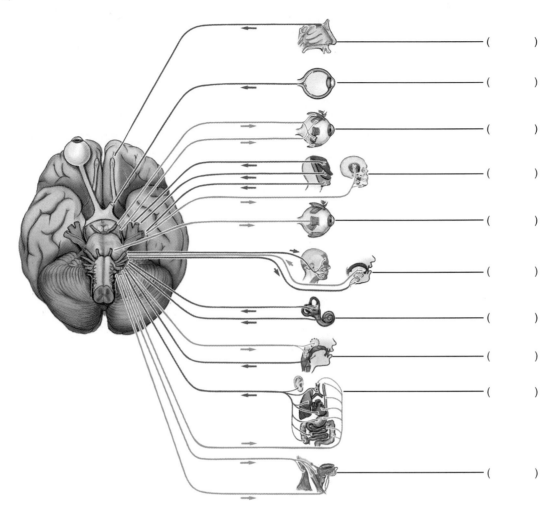

3. (Figure 8-6)

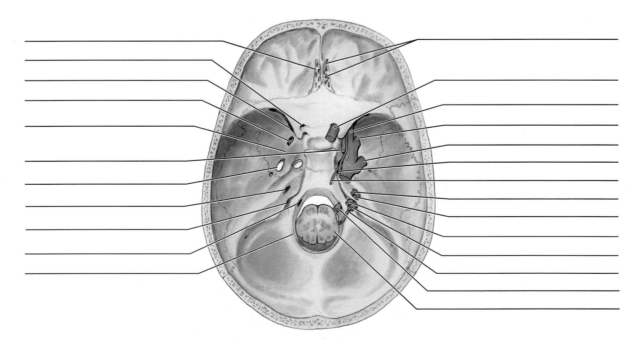

4. (Figures 8-8 and 8-11)

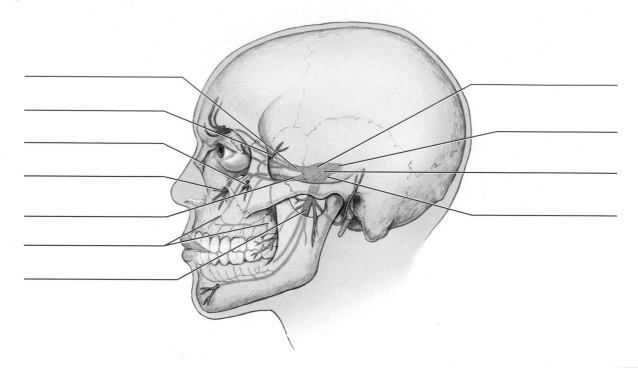

5. (Figure 8-13)

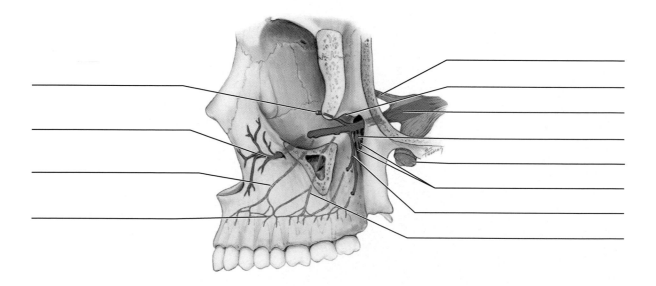

6. (Figure 8-14)

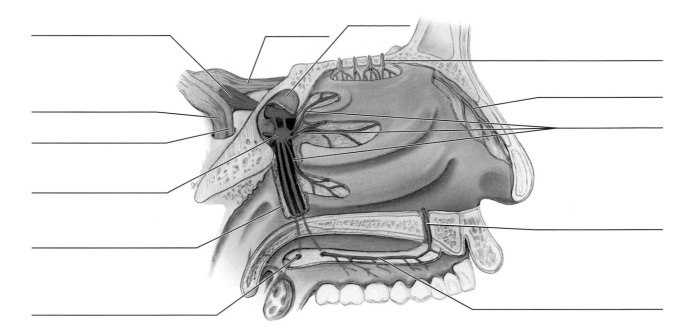

7. (Figure 8-18)

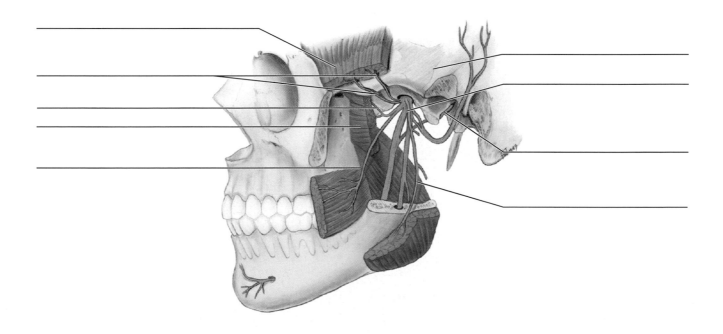

8. (Figure 8-19)

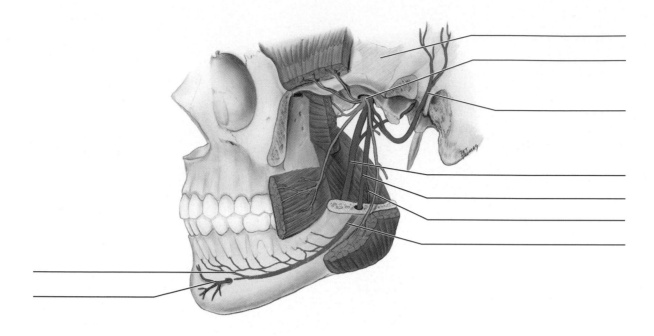

9. (Figure 8-20)

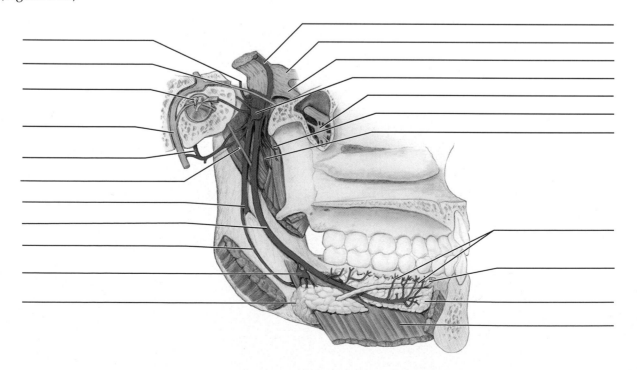

10. (Figure 8-21)

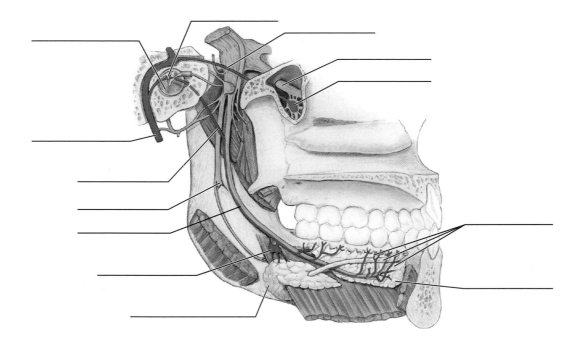

■ REVIEW QUESTIONS

1. The brainstem consists of which structures?
   A. Cerebrum, cerebellum, pons, and medulla
   B. Medulla, cerebrum, midbrain, and pons
   C. Medulla, pons, and midbrain
   D. Midbrain, ganglia, and nerves

2. The central nervous system consists of which structures?
   A. Spinal cord and peripheral nervous system
   B. Brain and spinal cord
   C. Autonomic and somatic nervous systems
   D. Brain and autonomic nervous system

3. Which of the following is a correct statement concerning neurotransmitters?
   A. They are discharged with the arrival of the action potential.
   B. They bind to red blood cells so as to prompt transmission of impulses.
   C. Inhibitory ones initiate an action potential in an adjacent cell.
   D. They are destroyed by specific white blood cells while still active.

4. To which division of the nervous system does a nerve cell belong if it leads from the eye to the brain and carries visual information?
   A. Central nervous system
   B. Medulla and pons
   C. Afferent nervous system
   D. Efferent nervous system

5. An efferent nerve carries information:
   A. From the periphery of the body to the brain (or spinal cord)
   B. Such as taste or pain to the spinal cord
   C. Such as proprioception to the brain
   D. Away from the brain (or spinal cord) to the periphery of the body

6. Which of the following does the posterior superior alveolar nerve and its branches supply?
   A. Frontal sinus
   B. Maxillary posterior teeth
   C. Parotid salivary gland
   D. Temporalis muscle

7. Through which of the following foramina does the facial nerve pass through the skull?
   A. Foramen rotundum
   B. Foramen ovale
   C. Jugular foramen
   D. Stylomastoid foramen

8. Which of the following cranial nerves is involved in Bell's palsy?
   A. Trigeminal nerve
   B. Facial nerve
   C. Glossopharyngeal nerve
   D. Vagus nerve

9. Which of the following nerve and muscle pairs is correctly matched?
   A. Long buccal nerve, buccinator muscle
   B. Accessory nerve, platysma muscle
   C. Hypoglossal nerve, intrinsic tongue muscles
   D. Auriculotemporal nerve, temporalis muscle

10. Which of the following nerve and tissue pairs are correctly matched?
    A. Facial nerve, parotid salivary gland
    B. Chorda tympani, sublingual salivary gland
    C. Vagus nerve, temporomandibular joint
    D. Lingual nerve, base of tongue

11. Which of the following cranial nerves has fibers that cross to the opposite side in the skull before continuing into the brain?
    A. Facial nerve
    B. Optic nerve
    C. Trochlear nerve
    D. Vestibulocochlear nerve

12. Which of the following cranial nerves carries taste sensation for the base of the tongue?
    A. Trigeminal nerve
    B. Facial nerve
    C. Vagus nerve
    D. Glossopharyngeal nerve

13. In which of the following areas is the trigeminal ganglion located?
    A. Superior to the deep lobe of the submandibular salivary gland
    B. Anterior surface of the petrous portion of the temporal bone
    C. Posterior surface of the maxillary tuberosity of the maxilla
    D. Anterior to the infraorbital foramen of the maxilla

14. Sensory information is supplied for the soft palate by which of the following?
    A. Greater palatine nerve
    B. Lesser palatine nerve
    C. Nasopalatine nerve
    D. Posterior alveolar nerve

15. The posterior belly of the digastric muscle is innervated by branches from which of the following?
    A. Facial nerve
    B. Mylohyoid nerve
    C. Buccal nerve
    D. Maxillary nerve

16. Which of the following nerves may show crossover from the opposite side in a patient?
    A. Posterior superior alveolar nerve
    B. Anterior superior alveolar nerve
    C. Posterior auricular nerve
    D. Buccal nerve

17. Which of the following nerves is a portion of the ophthalmic nerve?
    A. Nasociliary nerve
    B. Maxillary nerve
    C. Zygomaticotemporal nerve
    D. Zygomaticofacial nerve

18. Which of the following anatomical names is also used for cranial nerve X?
    A. Hypoglossal nerve
    B. Vagus nerve
    C. Glossopharyngeal nerve
    D. Accessory nerve

19. Which of the following nerves is located in the mandibular canal?
    A. Lingual nerve
    B. Mylohyoid nerve
    C. Inferior alveolar nerve
    D. Masseteric nerve

20. Which of the following nerves exits the foramen ovale of the sphenoid bone?
    A. Chorda tympani of the facial nerve
    B. Greater petrosal nerve of the facial nerve
    C. Ophthalmic nerve of the trigeminal nerve
    D. Motor root of the trigeminal nerve

21. Which of the motor functions of the following cranial nerves is involved when a patient protrudes the tongue and a deviation to the right side is noted?
    A. V
    B. VII
    C. X
    D. XII

22. Which of the following nerves exits the skull through the foramen ovale?
    A. Facial nerve
    B. Ophthalmic nerve
    C. Maxillary nerve
    D. Mandibular nerve
    E. Glossopharyngeal nerve

23. Which of the following nerves serves the pulpal tissues of the mandibular molars?
    A. Lingual nerve
    B. Buccal nerve (long buccal)
    C. Mental nerve
    D. Incisive nerve
    E. Inferior alveolar nerve

24. Which of the following is the loss of feeling or sensation resulting from the use of certain drugs or gases that serve as inhibitory neurotransmitters?
    A. Paresthesia
    B. Bell's palsy
    C. Trigeminal neuralgia
    D. Anesthesia

25. Which nerve may in some cases also serve as an afferent nerve for the mandibular first molar, which needs to be considered when there is failure of the inferior alveolar local anesthetic block?
    A. Mylohyoid nerve
    B. Posterior superior alveolar nerve
    C. Anterior middle superior alveolar nerve
    D. Glossopharyngeal nerve

Anatomy of Local Anesthesia

LEARNING OBJECTIVES

After studying this chapter, the reader should be able to do the following:

1. Define and pronounce all the key terms and anatomical terms in this chapter.
2. List the tissues anesthetized by each type of injection and describe the target areas.
3. Locate and identify the anatomical structures used to determine the local anesthetic needle's penetration site for each type of injection on a skull and a patient.
4. Demonstrate the correct placement of the local anesthetic needle for each type of injection on a skull and a patient.
5. Identify the correct tissues penetrated by the local anesthetic needle for each type of injection.
6. Discuss the complications of local anesthesia of the oral cavity associated with anatomical considerations for each type of injection.
7. Correctly complete the review questions and activities for this chapter.
8. Integrate the knowledge about the anatomy of the nerves and their associated tissues into clinical dental practice.

KEY TERMS

Local Infiltration (in-fil-**tray**-shun) Type of injection that anesthetizes a small area—one or two teeth and associated structures—when the local anesthetic agent is deposited near terminal nerve endings.

Nerve Block Type of injection that anesthetizes a larger area than the local infiltration because the

local anesthetic agent is deposited near large nerve trunks.

Paresthesia (par-es-**the**-ze-ah) Abnormal sensation from an area such as burning or prickling.

OVERVIEW OF ANATOMICAL CONSIDERATIONS FOR LOCAL ANESTHESIA

The management of pain through local anesthesia by dental professionals requires a thorough knowledge of the anatomy of the skull, trigeminal nerve, and related tissues. This text discusses the anatomical considerations for local anesthesia. Dental professionals will also want to refer to a current textbook on local anesthesia in dentistry for more information on this topic.

The skull bones involved in the local anesthetic administration are the maxilla, palatine bone, and mandible (see Chapter 3). Soft tissues of the face and oral cavity may serve the dental professional as initial landmarks to visualize and palpate for local anesthesia (see Chapter 2). However, there are many variations in soft tissue topographical anatomy among patients. Thus to increase the reliability of the local anesthesia, the dental professional must learn to rely mainly on the visualization and palpation of hard tissues for landmarks while injecting patients.

The dental professional must also know the location of certain adjacent soft tissue structures, such as major blood vessels and glandular tissue, so as to avoid inadvertently injecting these structures (see Chapters 6 and 7). If certain soft tissue structures are accidentally injected with local anesthetic agent, complications may occur. Infections may also be spread to deeper tissues by needle-tract contamination (see Chapter 12).

The fifth cranial or trigeminal nerve provides sensory information for the teeth and associated tissues (see Chapter 8). Thus branches of the trigeminal nerve are those anesthetized before most dental procedures. Knowledge of the location of these nerve branches in relationship to the facial skull bones, as well as soft tissues, also increases the reliability of each injection.

Two types of local anesthetic injections are used commonly in dentistry: the local infiltration and nerve block. The type of injection used for a given dental procedure is determined by the type and length of the procedure.

The **local infiltration** anesthetizes a small area, including one or two teeth and associated tissues, by injection near their apices. For this type of local anes-

thetic injection, the local anesthetic agent is deposited near terminal nerve endings. This localized deposition has varying degrees of success depending on the anatomy of the region.

The **nerve block** affects a larger area than the local infiltration and thus, more teeth. With a nerve block, the local anesthetic agent is deposited near large nerve trunks. This generalized deposition has more degrees of success than that of infiltration. This type of injection is discussed in this chapter.

The clinician must never inject through an area with an abscess, cellulitis, or osteomyelitis so as to prevent the spread of dental infection (see Chapter 12). Also, the effectiveness of local anesthetic agents is greatly reduced when administered in areas of infection, so additional amounts may be needed keeping the maximal recommended dosage always in mind for each patient. In addition, the clinician must use the proper amount of local anesthetic agent because there will be possible failure of the anesthesia if too little agent is used. This is commonly noted in the patient who may have large teeth with unusually long roots. The bone surrounding the roots may also be excessively thick in a patient needing more agent.

The clinician also must be careful to not start the dental treatment before the local anesthetic can take effect. This is a particular problem with injections for mandibular teeth. In addition, when working in quadrant dentistry, the injections should be administered from posterior to anterior, with the dental work commencing in the same direction, from posterior to anterior.

MAXILLARY NERVE ANESTHESIA

The **maxillary nerve** (**mak**-sil-lare-ee) and its branches can be anesthetized in a number of ways depending on the tissues requiring local anesthesia (Figure 9-1, Table 9-1). Most local anesthesia of the maxilla is more successful than that of the mandible because the bone over the facial surface of the maxillary teeth is less dense than that of the mandible over similar teeth (see Chapter 3). Less variation also exists in the anatomy of the maxillary and palatine bones and associated nerves with respect to local anesthetic landmarks as compared with similar mandibular structures.

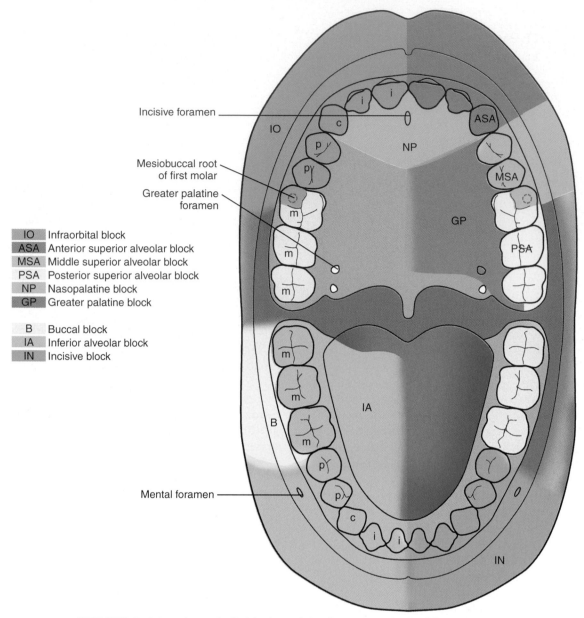

Incisive foramen

Mesiobuccal root
of first molar

Greater palatine
foramen

IO	Infraorbital block
ASA	Anterior superior alveolar block
MSA	Middle superior alveolar block
PSA	Posterior superior alveolar block
NP	Nasopalatine block
GP	Greater palatine block

B	Buccal block
IA	Inferior alveolar block
IN	Incisive block

Mental foramen

FIGURE 9-1 Local anesthetic blocks and the tissues anesthetized (note that the anterior middle superior alveolar, mental, or Gow-Gates mandibular blocks are not included. See associated figures for more clarification of these blocks).

Pulpal anesthesia is achieved through anesthesia of each tooth's dental branches as they extend into the pulp tissue by way of the apical foramen. The hard and soft tissues of the periodontium are anesthetized by way of the interdental and interradicular branches for each tooth.

The posterior superior alveolar block is generally recommended for anesthesia of the maxillary molar teeth and associated buccal tissues in one quadrant. The middle superior alveolar block is generally recommended for anesthesia of the maxillary premolars and associated buccal tissues in one quadrant. The anterior superior alveolar block is recommended for anesthesia

of the maxillary canine and incisors and their associated facial tissues in one quadrant. The infraorbital block is generally recommended for anesthesia of the maxillary anterior and premolar teeth and associated facial tissues in one quadrant.

Palatal anesthesia usually involves anesthesia of the soft and hard tissues of the periodontium of the palatal area such as the gingiva, periodontal ligament, and alveolar bone. Palatal anesthesia usually does not provide any pulpal anesthesia to the maxillary teeth or associated facial or buccal tissues. The greater palatine block is generally recommended for anesthesia of the palatal tissues distal to the maxillary canine in one

SUMMARY OF MAXILLARY LOCAL ANESTHESIA OF THE TEETH AND ASSOCIATED TISSUES

Maxillary Tooth and Tissues	ASA Block	PSA Block	MSA Block	IO Block	NP Block	GP Block	AMSA Block
Central Incisor							
Facial/pulpal	X			X			X
Lingual					X		X
Lateral Incisor							
Facial/pulpal	X			X			X
Lingual					X		X
Canine							
Facial/pulpal	X			X			X
Lingual					X		X
First Premolar							
Buccal/pulpal			X	X			X
Lingual						X	X
Second Premolar							
Buccal/pulpal			X	X			X
Lingual						X	X
First Molar							
Buccal/pulpal		X					
Lingual						X	
Second Molar							
Buccal/pulpal		X					
Lingual						X	
Third Molar							
Buccal/pulpal		X					
Lingual						X	

The anesthesia is not included for the mesiobuccal root of the first molar nor for anatomical variants.

AMSA, Anterior middle superior alveolar; *ASA*, anterior superior alveolar; *GP*, greater palatine; *IO*, infraorbital; *MSA*, middle superior alveolar; *NP*, nasopalatine; *PSA*, posterior superior alveolar.

quadrant. The nasopalatine block is generally recommended for anesthesia of the palatal tissues between the right and left maxillary canines.

Separate from these palatal blocks that only provide palatal tissue anesthesia is another block administered on the palate, the anterior middle superior alveolar block. This block is generally recommended for anesthesia of most of the maxillary teeth and their

associated tissues in one quadrant, except for those innervated by the posterior superior alveolar nerve.

Posterior Superior Alveolar Block

The **posterior superior alveolar block** (al-ve-o-lar) or **PSA block** is used to achieve pulpal anesthesia in the maxillary third, second, and first molars in most patients. Thus the PSA block is indicated when the dental procedure involves two or more maxillary molars or their associated buccal tissues.

In some patients the mesiobuccal root of the maxillary first molar is not innervated by the PSA nerve but by the MSA nerve. Therefore a second injection to anesthetize the MSA nerve may be necessary to achieve pulpal anesthesia of all the roots of the maxillary first molar.

The PSA block also anesthetizes the buccal periodontium overlying the maxillary third, second, and first molars including the associated gingiva, periodontal ligament, and alveolar bone. If anesthesia of the lingual tissues is desired, the greater palatine block also may be necessary.

TARGET AREA AND INJECTION SITE FOR PSA BLOCK

The target area for the PSA block is the PSA nerve as it enters the maxilla through the posterior superior alveolar foramina on the maxilla's infratemporal surface (Figures 9-2 and 9-3). This area is posterosuperior and medial on the maxillary tuberosity.

The injection site for the PSA block is into the tissues at the height of the mucobuccal fold at the apex of the maxillary second molar, distal to the zygomatic process of the maxilla (Figures 9-4 and 9-5). The needle is inserted into the mucobuccal fold tissues in a distal and medial direction to the tooth and maxilla without touching the maxillary bone in order to reduce trauma, and then the injection is administered (Figure 9-6).

A certain angulation of the needle to the injection site must be maintained. The angulation of the needle

should be upward or superiorly at a 45-degree angle to the occlusal plane, inward or medially at a 45-degree angle to the occlusal plane, and backward or posteriorly at a 45-degree angle to the long axis of the second maxillary molar. The syringe should be extended from the ipsilateral labial commissure.

If bone is contacted too early or resistance is felt, the angle of the needle toward the midline is too great (more than a 45-degree angle) and the syringe barrel needs to be closer to the occlusal plane, thereby reducing the angle (to less than 45 degrees). A conservative insertion technique should be used so as to reduce possible complications (discussed next).

SYMPTOMS AND POSSIBLE COMPLICATIONS OF PSA BLOCK

Usually no symptoms result from soft tissue anesthesia with a PSA block. Thus the patient frequently has difficulty determining the extent of anesthesia because a lip or the tongue is not anesthetized. Instead, the patient will state that the teeth in the area feel dull when gently tapped, and there will be an absence of discomfort during dental procedures. It may be necessary to inform the patient of this before starting the procedure so as to allay fears that the anesthetic has not worked.

Complications can occur if the needle is advanced too far distally into the tissues during a PSA block (Figure 9-7). The needle may penetrate the pterygoid plexus of veins and the maxillary artery if overinserted, possibly causing a hematoma in the infratemporal fossa (see Chapter 6). This results in a bluish-reddish extraoral swelling of hemorrhaging blood in the tissues on the affected side of the face a few minutes

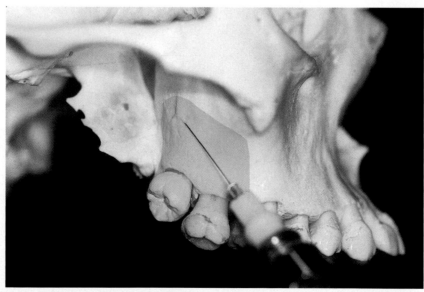

FIGURE 9-2 Target area for the **posterior superior alveolar block** is the PSA nerve located at the posterior superior alveolar foramina on the infratemporal surface of the maxilla, posterosuperior and medial to the maxillary tuberosity. Area anesthetized is highlighted.

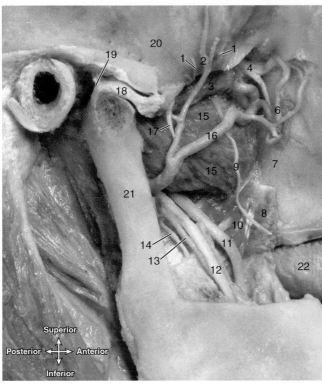

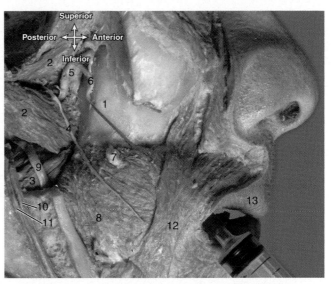

FIGURE 9-4 Dissection showing the needle at the injection site for a **posterior superior alveolar block**. *1*, Posterior surface of maxilla; *2*, lateral pterygoid muscle; *3*, medical pterygoid muscle; *4*, buccal nerve; *5*, maxillary artery; *6*, posterior superior alveolar nerve and vessels; *7*, parotid salivary duct; *8*, buccinator muscle; *9*, lingual nerve; *10*, inferior alveolar nerve; *11*, inferior alveolar artery; *12*, labial commissure; *13*, upper lip. (From Logan BM, Reynold PA, Hutching RT: *McMinn's color atlas of head and neck anatomy*, ed 3, London, 2004, Mosby Ltd.)

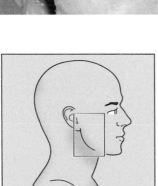

FIGURE 9-3 Deep dissection of the face demonstrating the right infratemporal fossa (with the zygomatic arch and mandible removed) showing the nerves and other structures in the area where the **posterior superior alveolar block** is given (as well as the **inferior alveolar block** discussed later). *1*, Deep temporal nerve; *2*, deep temporal artery; *3*, lateral pterygoid muscle; *4*, maxillary nerve; *5*, posterior superior alveolar nerve; *6*, posterior superior alveolar artery; *7*, infratemporal surface of maxilla; *8*, buccinator muscle; *9*, buccal nerve; *10*, medial pterygoid muscle; *11*, lingual nerve; *12*, inferior alveolar nerve; *13*, inferior alveolar artery; *14*, nerve to mylohyoid muscle; *15*, lateral pterygoid muscle; *16*, maxillary artery; *17*, masseteric nerve; *18*, disc of the joint and mandibular condyle; *19*, joint capsule; *20*, temporal bone; *21*, mandibular ramus; *22*, tongue. (From Logan BM, Reynold PA, Hutching RT: *McMinn's color atlas of head and neck anatomy*, ed 3, London, 2004, Mosby Ltd.)

after the injection, progressing over time inferiorly and anteriorly toward the lower anterior region of the cheek. If the needle is contaminated, there may be a spread of infection to the cavernous venous sinus (see Chapter 12). Aspiration should always be attempted in all injections in order to avoid injection into blood

vessels, and strict standard precautions of infection control should be observed.

Inadvertent and harmless anesthesia of branches of the mandibular nerve may occur with a PSA block because they are located lateral to the PSA nerve. This may result in varying degrees of lingual anesthesia and anesthesia of the lower lip.

Middle Superior Alveolar Block

The **middle superior alveolar block** or **MSA block** is indicated for dental procedures on the maxillary premolars and mesiobuccal root of the maxillary first molar. Most clinicians utilize this block even if the MSA nerve is possibly not present in order for completeness of anesthesia to entire the quadrant or when working only on the maxillary premolars. Where the MSA nerve is absent, the area is innervated by both the PSA AND ASA nerves.

Thus the MSA block anesthetizes the pulp tissue of the maxillary first and second premolars and possibly the mesiobuccal root of the maxillary first molar and the associated buccal periodontal tissues including the gingiva, periodontal ligament, and alveolar bone if the MSA nerve is present. If lingual tissue anesthesia of these teeth is desired, the greater palatine block may also be necessary.

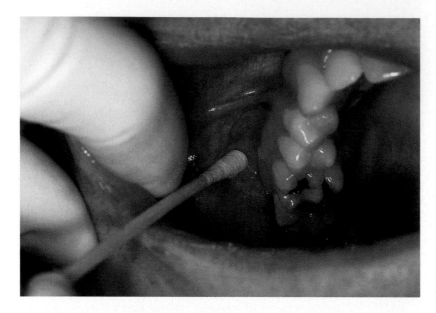

FIGURE 9-5 The injection site for the **posterior superior alveolar block** is probed at the height of the mucobuccal fold at the apex of the maxillary second molar.

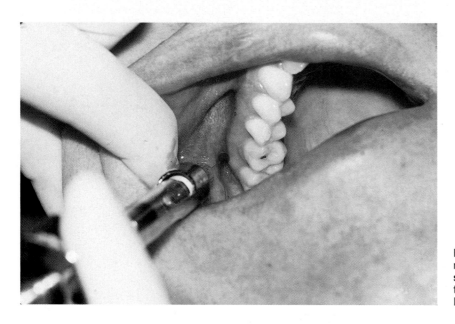

FIGURE 9-6 Needle penetration of the mucobuccal fold tissues for the **posterior superior alveolar block** is demonstrated at the apex of the maxillary second molar. Injection site is highlighted.

TARGET AREA AND INJECTION SITE FOR MSA BLOCK

The target area for the MSA block is the MSA nerve at the apex of the maxillary second premolar (Figures 9-8 and 9-9). Thus the injection site is the tissues at the height of the mucobuccal fold at the apex of the maxillary second premolar (Figure 9-10). The needle is inserted into the mucobuccal fold tissues until its tip is located superior to the apex of the maxillary second premolar without touching the bone in order to reduce trauma, and then the injection is administered (Figure 9-11).

SYMPTOMS AND POSSIBLE COMPLICATIONS OF MSA BLOCK

Symptoms of anesthesia with the MSA block include harmless tingling or numbness of the upper lip and absence of discomfort during dental procedures. Overinsertion with complications such as a hematoma is rare with the MSA block.

Anterior Superior Alveolar Block

The **anterior superior alveolar block** or **ASA block** is commonly used in conjunction with an MSA block

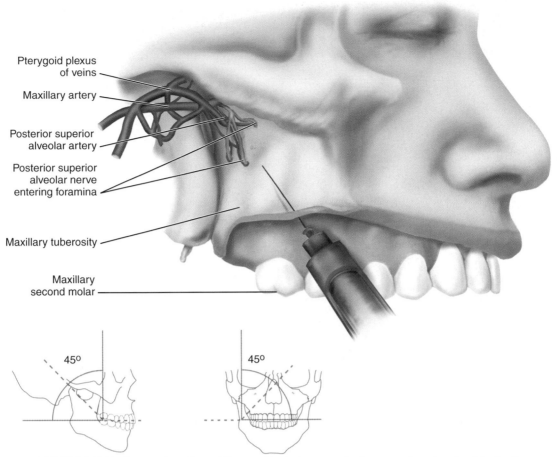

Pterygoid plexus of veins

Maxillary artery

Posterior superior alveolar artery

Posterior superior alveolar nerve entering foramina

Maxillary tuberosity

Maxillary second molar

45°   45°

FIGURE 9-7 Correct insertion of the needle during a **posterior superior alveolar block**. If the needle is overinserted, it can penetrate the pterygoid plexus of the veins and maxillary artery, which may lead to complications such as a hematoma.

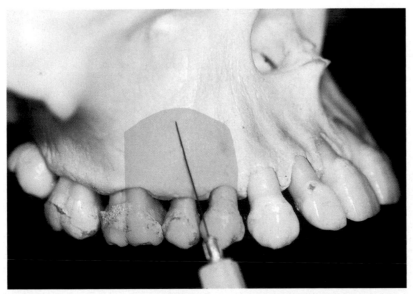

FIGURE 9-8 Target area for the **middle superior alveolar block** is the MSA nerve located at the apex of the maxillary second premolar. Area anesthetized is highlighted.

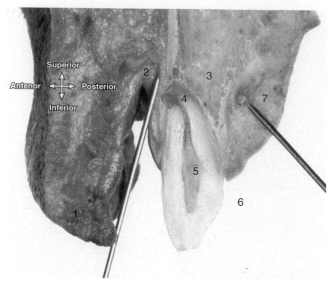

FIGURE 9-9 Coronal section of maxilla and buccal mucosa through the permanent maxillary first premolar tooth, showing one needle at the injection site for **middle superior alveolar block** *(needle to the left)* and the other needle for the **anterior middle superior alveolar block** *(needle to the right).* *1,* Upper lip; *2,* height of mucobuccal fold; *3,* alveolar process of maxilla; *4,* apex of tooth; *5,* pulp cavity; *6,* gingival margin; *7,* mucoperiosteum of hard palate. (From Logan BM, Reynold PA, Hutching RT: *McMinn's color atlas of head and neck anatomy,* ed 3, London, 2004, Mosby Ltd.)

instead of using an infraorbital block. Communication occurs between the ASA nerve and the MSA and PSA nerves. In addition, many times the ASA nerve crosses over the midline to the opposite side in a patient; this may need to be taken into account when using local anesthesia in this area. Bilateral injections of the ASA block or local infiltration over the opposite maxillary central incisor may be indicated.

The ASA block anesthetizes the pulp tissue of the maxillary canine and incisor teeth, as well as the associated facial periodontal tissues including the gingiva, periodontal ligament, and alveolar bone. If lingual tissue anesthesia of these teeth is desired, a nasopalatine block may also be necessary.

TARGET AREA AND INJECTION SITE FOR ASA BLOCK

The target area for the ASA block is the ASA nerve at the apex of the maxillary canine (Figure 9-12). The injection site is the tissues at the height of the mucobuccal fold at the apex of the maxillary canine, just anterior to and parallel with the canine eminence. Note that a slight depression or canine fossa is located anterior to the canine eminence (Figure 9-13). The needle tip is placed superior to the apex of the maxillary canine without touching the bone so as to reduce trauma, and then the injection is administered (Figure 9-14). This is approximately 10 degrees off an imaginary line drawn parallel to the long axis of the canine tooth.

SYMPTOMS AND POSSIBLE COMPLICATIONS OF ASA BLOCK

Symptoms of the ASA block include harmless tingling or numbness of the upper lip and an absence of discomfort during dental procedures. Overinsertion with complications such as a hematoma is rare with ASA block.

Infraorbital Block

The **infraorbital block** (in-frah-**or**-bit-al) or **IO block** is a useful nerve block because it anesthetizes both the MSA and ASA nerves. The IO block is used for anesthesia of the maxillary premolars, maxillary

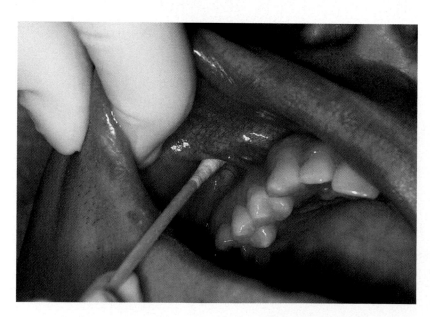

FIGURE 9-10 The injection site for the **middle superior alveolar block** is probed at the height of the mucobuccal fold at the apex of the maxillary second premolar.

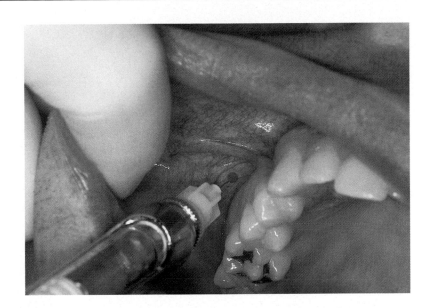

FIGURE 9-11 Needle penetration of the mucobuccal fold tissues for the **middle superior alveolar block** is demonstrated at the apex of the maxillary second premolar. Injection site is highlighted.

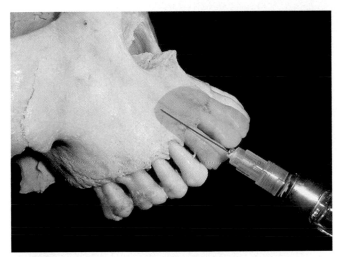

FIGURE 9-12 Target area for the **anterior superior alveolar block** is the ASA nerve located at the apex of the maxillary canine. Area anesthetized is highlighted.

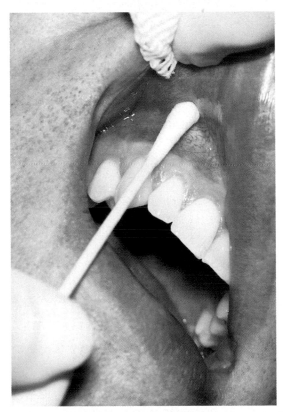

FIGURE 9-13 The injection site for the **anterior superior alveolar block** is probed at the height of the mucobuccal fold at the apex of the maxillary canine.

canine, and maxillary incisors. The IO block is indicated when the dental procedures involve more than two maxillary premolars or anterior teeth and the overlying facial periodontium including the gingiva, periodontal ligament, and alveolar bone. Many clinicians feel that this block should be referred to as the *anterior superior nerve* block due to the tissues it anesthetizes, but the name comes from the foramen where the injection is administered. If lingual tissue anesthesia is necessary, a nasopalatine block may also be necessary.

In many patients the ASA nerve crosses over the midline from the opposite side, so bilateral injections of the IO block or local infiltration over the opposite maxillary central incisor may be indicated.

TARGET AREA AND INJECTION SITE FOR IO BLOCK

The target area for the IO block is the ASA and MSA nerves as they ascend to join the IO nerve after it enters the infraorbital foramen (Figure 9-15). Branches of the IO nerve to the lower eyelid, side of

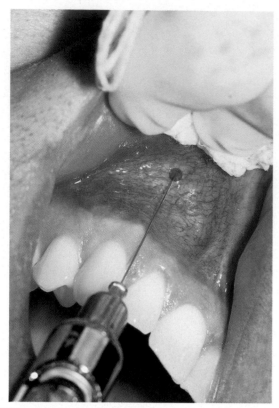

FIGURE 9-14 Needle penetration at the height of the mucobuccal fold tissues for the **anterior superior alveolar block** is demonstrated at the apex of the maxillary canine. Injection site is highlighted.

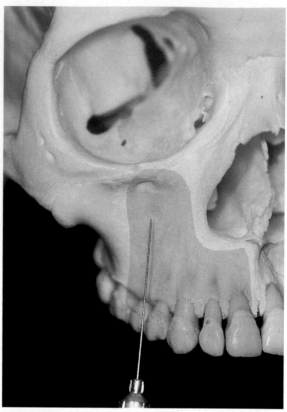

FIGURE 9-15 Target area for the **infraorbital block** is the anterior superior alveolar and middle superior alveolar nerves located at the infraorbital foramen. Note the position of the infraorbital rim. Area anesthetized is highlighted.

the nose, and upper lip are also inadvertently anesthetized.

To locate the infraorbital foramen, palpate extraorally the patient's infraorbital rim and then move slightly downward about 10 mm, applying pressure until the depression created by the infraorbital foramen is located (Figure 9-16). The patient may feel a dull aching sensation when pressure is applied to the nerves in the region. The infraorbital foramen is about 1 to 4 mm medial to the pupil of the eye if the patient looks straightforward.

The injection site for the IO block is the tissues at the height of the mucobuccal fold at the apex of the maxillary first premolar. A preinjection approximation of the depth of needle penetration for the IO block can be made by placing one finger on the infraorbital foramen and the other one on the injection site and estimating the distance between them (Figure 9-17). The approximate depth of needle penetration for the IO block may vary. In a patient with a high or deep mucobuccal fold or low infraorbital foramen, less tissue penetration will be required than in a patient with a shallow mucobuccal fold or high infraorbital foramen.

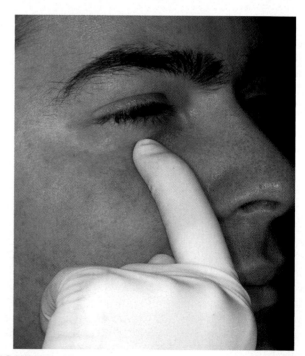

FIGURE 9-16 Palpation of the depression created by the infraorbital foramen for the **infraorbital block** is demonstrated by moving slightly downward on the face from the infraorbital rim.

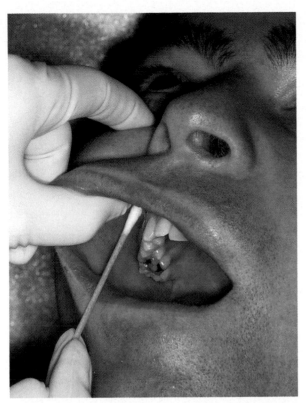

FIGURE 9-17 The injection site for the **infraorbital block** is probed at the height of the mucobuccal fold at the apex of the maxillary first premolar. The palpation over the infraorbital foramen is maintained.

The needle is inserted for the IO block into the mucobuccal fold tissues while keeping the finger of the other hand on the infraorbital foramen during the injection to help keep the syringe toward the foramen (Figure 9-18). The needle is advanced while keeping it parallel with the long axis of the tooth to avoid premature contact with the maxillary bone. The point of contact of the needle with the maxillary bone should be the upper rim of the infraorbital foramen. Keeping the needle in contact with the bone at the roof of the infraorbital foramen prevents overinsertion and possible puncture of the orbit.

SYMPTOMS AND POSSIBLE COMPLICATIONS OF IO BLOCK

Symptoms of the IO block include harmless tingling and numbness of the eyelid, side of the nose, and upper lip because there is inadvertent anesthesia of the branches of the IO nerve. Additionally, there is numbness in the teeth and associated tissue along the distribution of the ASA and MSA nerves and absence of discomfort during dental procedures. Rarely the complication of a hematoma may develop across the lower eyelid and the tissues between it and the infraorbital foramen.

Greater Palatine Block

The **greater palatine block** (pal-ah-tine) or **GP block** is used during dental procedures that involve more than two maxillary posterior teeth or palatal soft tissues distal to the maxillary canine. This maxillary block anesthetizes the posterior portion of the hard palate, anteriorly as far as the maxillary first premolar and medially to the midline.

Because the GP block does not provide pulpal anesthesia of the area teeth, the use of the ASA, PSA, and MSA blocks or the IO block may also be indicated. In addition, soft tissue anesthesia in the palatal area of the maxillary first premolar may prove inadequate because of overlapping nerve fibers from the nasopalatine nerve. This lack of anesthesia may be corrected by additional administration of the nasopalatine block.

Because the overlying palatal tissues are dense and adhere firmly to the underlying palatal bone, the use of pressure anesthesia posterior to the injection site before and during the injection to blanch the tissues will reduce patient discomfort. This pressure anesthesia of the tissues produces a dull ache that blocks pain impulses that arise from needle penetration. The slow deposition of the local anesthetic agent will also reduce patient discomfort.

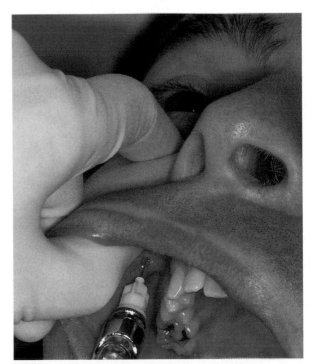

FIGURE 9-18 Needle penetration at the height of the mucobuccal fold tissues for the **infraorbital block** is demonstrated at the apex of the maxillary first premolar. The palpation over the infraorbital foramen is maintained. Injection site is highlighted.

TARGET AREA AND INJECTION SITE FOR GP BLOCK

The target area for the GP block is anterior to where the GP nerve enters the greater palatine foramen from its location between the mucoperiosteum and bone of the hard palate (Figures 9-19 and 9-20). The greater palatine foramen is located at the junction of the maxillary alveolar process and posterior hard palate, at the apex of the maxillary second (in children) or third molar, about 10 mm medial and directly superior to the lingual gingival margin. In patients who have a vaulted palate, the foramen will appear closer to the dentition. Conversely, in patients with a more shallow palate, the foramen will appear closer to the midline.

The site of injection is in palatal tissues anterior to the depression created by the greater palatine foramen (Figure 9-21). This depression can be palpated about midway between the median palatine raphe and lingual gingival margin of the molar tooth. The needle for the GP block is inserted into the previously blanched palatal tissues at a 90-degree angle to the palate (Figure 9-22). The needle is advanced during the GP block until the palatine bone is contacted, and then the injection is administered. There is no need to enter the greater palatine canal. Although such an entrance is not potentially hazardous, it is not necessary for this block.

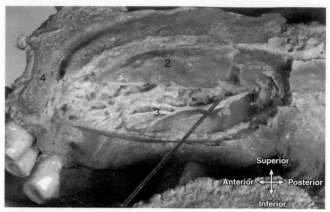

FIGURE 9-20 Dissection of palatal mucoperiosteum showing the needle at the injection site for the **greater palatine block**, anterior to the greater palatine foramen so that it can anesthetize the GP nerve. *1 (and arrow),* Greater palatine foramen; *2,* mucoperiosteum of the hard palate; *3,* GP nerve traveling horizontally; *4,* incisive foramen. (From Logan BM, Reynold PA, Hutching RT: *McMinn's color atlas of head and neck anatomy,* ed 3, London, 2004, Mosby Ltd.)

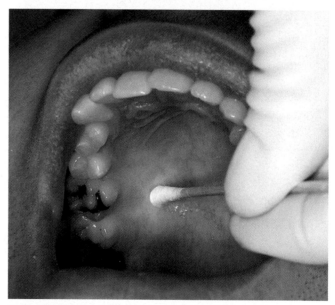

FIGURE 9-21 The depression caused by the greater palatine foramen is probed. The palatal tissues around the greater palatine foramen are blanched to cause pressure anesthesia before the **greater palatine block** is administered.

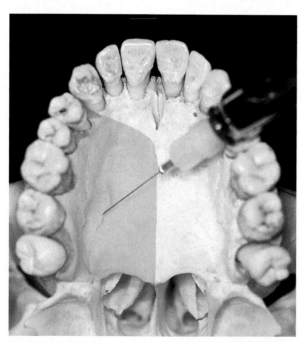

FIGURE 9-19 Target area for the **greater palatine block** is anterior to the greater palatine foramen to anesthetize the GP nerve, which is at the junction of the maxillary alveolar process and the hard palate, at the apex of the maxillary second or third molar. Area anesthetized is highlighted.

SYMPTOMS AND POSSIBLE COMPLICATIONS OF GP BLOCK

Symptoms of the GP block are numbness in the posterior portion of the palate and absence of discomfort during dental procedures. Some patients may become uncomfortable and may gag if the soft palate becomes inadvertently and harmlessly anesthetized, which is a distinct possibility given the proximity of the lesser palatine nerve.

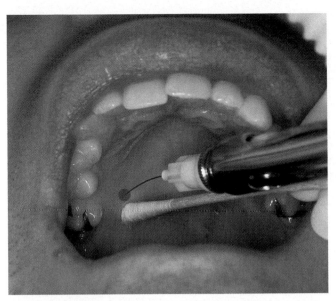

FIGURE 9-22 Needle penetration of the palatal tissues for the **greater palatine block** is demonstrated anterior to the depression created by the greater palatine foramen. The needle may bow slightly, and the tissue blanching is maintained during the injection. Injection site is highlighted.

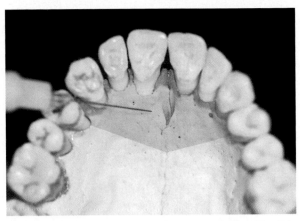

FIGURE 9-23 Target area for the **nasopalatine block** is the right and left NP nerves located at the incisive foramen on the anterior hard palate of the maxilla, lingual to the maxillary central incisors. Area anesthetized is highlighted.

Nasopalatine Block

The **nasopalatine block** (nay-zo-**pal**-ah-tine) or **NP block** is useful for anesthesia of the bilateral anterior portion of the hard palate, from the mesial of the right maxillary first premolar to the mesial of the left maxillary first premolar. Both the right NP nerve and the left NP nerve are anesthetized by this block. The NP block is used when palatal soft tissue anesthesia is required for two or more maxillary anterior teeth.

The NP block does not provide pulpal anesthesia of these teeth, so additional anesthesia such as the MSA and ASA block or the IO block may be indicated.

Because the dense overlying palatal tissues adhere firmly to the underlying maxillary bone, the use of pressure anesthesia on the contralateral side of the injection site of the incisive papilla before and during the injection to blanch the tissues will reduce patient discomfort. This pressure anesthesia to the tissues produces a dull ache to block pain impulses that arise from needle penetration. Slow deposition of the local anesthetic agent will also help reduce patient discomfort.

TARGET AREA AND INJECTION SITE FOR NP BLOCK

The target area for the NP block is both the right and left NP nerves as they enter the incisive foramen from the mucosa of the anterior hard palate, beneath the incisive papilla (Figures 9-23 and 9-24; also see Figure 9-9).

The injection site is the palatal tissues lateral to the incisive papilla, which is located at the midline, about 10 mm lingual to the maxillary central incisor teeth (Figure 9-25). Pressure anesthesia is performed on palatal tissues on the contralateral side of the incisive papilla. The needle is inserted for this block into the previously blanched palatal tissues at a 45-degree angle to the palate (Figure 9-26). The needle is advanced into the tissues until the maxillary bone is contacted, and then the injection is administered.

SYMPTOMS AND POSSIBLE COMPLICATIONS OF NP BLOCK

Symptoms of the NP block include numbness in the anterior portion of the palate and absence of discomfort during dental procedures. Complications such as hematoma are extremely rare.

Anterior Middle Superior Alveolar Block

The **anterior middle superior alveolar block** or **AMSA block** is useful for soft tissue and pulpal anesthesia of the large area covered by the ASA, MSA, GP, and NP blocks in the maxillary arch. Thus the single-site palatal injection of the AMSA can anesthetize multiple teeth (from the second premolar through the central incisor), without causing usual collateral anesthesia to the soft tissues of the patient's lip and face.

This injection is commonly used in aesthetic/cosmetic dentistry because after the procedures are completed, the clinician can immediately and accurately assesses the patient's smile line. The AMSA, together with a traditional PSA block, will anesthetize a maxillary quadrant for other dental procedures. However, recent studies show that due to the extensive anatomy involved, this block may be variable in

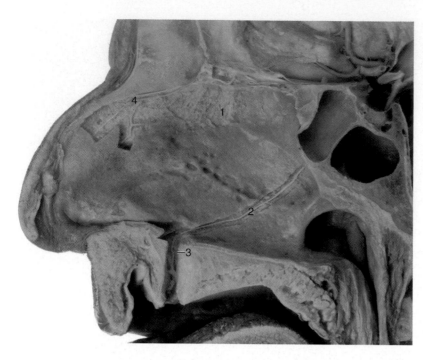

FIGURE 9-24 Sagittal section of nerves of the right side of the nasal septum showing the nerves and other structures in the area where the **nasopalatine block** is given. *1,* Olfactory nerve; *2,* NP nerve; *3,* incisive canal; *4,* anterior ethmoidal nerve. (From Logan BM, Reynold PA, Hutching RT: *McMinn's color atlas of head and neck anatomy,* ed 3, London, 2004, Mosby Ltd.)

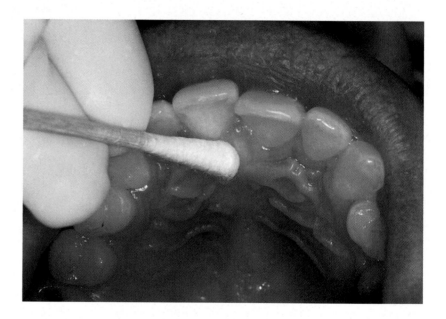

FIGURE 9-25 The injection site for the **nasopalatine block** is probed at the palatal tissues lateral to the incisive papilla on the anterior portion of the palate. The palatal tissues lateral to the incisive papilla on the contralateral side are blanched to cause pressure anesthesia.

depth and duration of anesthesia. Other studies also show that this injection is best accomplished with a computer-controlled delivery device because it regulates the pressure and volume ratio of agent delivered, which is not readily attained with a manual syringe.

The use of pressure anesthesia before and during with this injection near the injection site to blanch the tissues will reduce patient discomfort. This pressure anesthesia to the tissues produces a dull ache to block pain impulses that arise from needle penetration. Slow deposition of the local anesthetic agent will also help reduce patient discomfort.

TARGET AREA AND INJECTION SITE FOR AMSA BLOCK

The target area for the AMSA block is the tissues of the hard palate (Figures 9-9 and 9-27). This block takes advantage of a number of small pores in the maxillary bone in the area and the tight attachment of the palatal tissues. As the agent penetrates the pores, it has access to the anterior to middle portion of the dental plexus, which then anesthetizes the teeth and associated facial tissues as well as the lingual tissues of the surrounding palate.

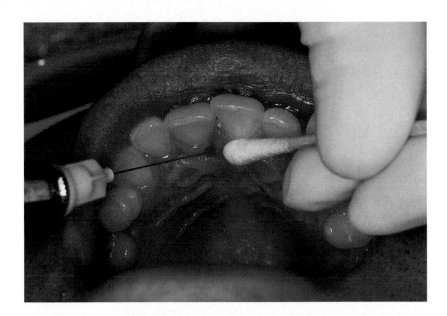

FIGURE 9-26 Needle penetration of the palatal tissues for the **nasopalatine block** is demonstrated lateral to the incisive papilla. Blanching of the palatal tissues on the contralateral side is continued during the injection. Injection site is highlighted.

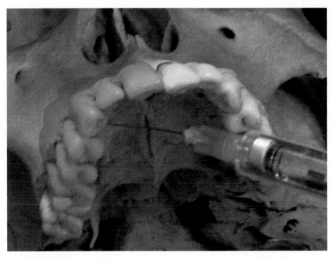

FIGURE 9-27 Target area for the **anterior middle superior alveolar block** is on the hard palate of the maxilla. Area anesthetized is highlighted.

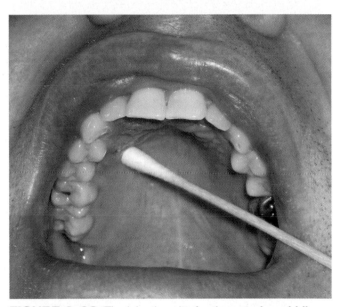

FIGURE 9-28 The injection site for the **anterior middle superior alveolar block** is probed at the palatal, an area bisecting the apex of the maxillary premolars as well as an area that is midway between the lingual gingival margin and the median palatal suture.

The injection site for the AMSA block is an area bisecting the apex of the maxillary premolars, as well as being midway between the lingual gingival margin and the median palatal suture (Figure 9-28). Orientation of the handpiece of the syringe should be from the contralateral premolars. The previously blanched tissue is approached with the needle at a 45-degree angle until the palatal tissues are penetrated and the maxillary bone is contacted, and then the injection is administered (Figure 9-29).

SYMPTOMS AND POSSIBLE COMPLICATIONS OF AMSA BLOCK

Blanching occurs on the palatal and buccal tissues after the AMSA block and, if excessive, may cause postoperative tissue ischemia and sloughing. If excessive blanching is noted, slowing or stopping the injection for a few seconds to let the agent dissipate will diminish the chance of this postoperative event. Other complications are extremely rare.

MANDIBULAR NERVE ANESTHESIA

The **mandibular nerve** (man-**dib**-you-lar) and its branches can be anesthetized in a number of ways depending on the tissues requiring anesthesia (Table 9-2; see Figure 9-1). However, infiltration anesthesia of the mandible is not as successful as that of the

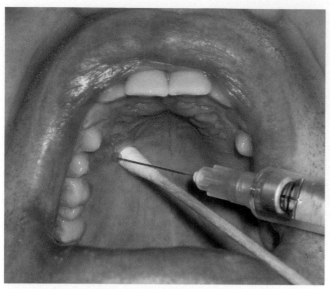

FIGURE 9-29 Needle penetration of the palatal tissues for the **anterior middle superior alveolar block** is demonstrated using a computer-controlled delivery device. Blanching of the nearby palatal tissues is continued during the injection. Injection site is highlighted.

maxilla because overall the mandible is denser than the maxilla over similar teeth, especially in the area of the posterior teeth (see Chapter 3). For this reason, nerve blocks are preferred to local infiltrations in most portions of the mandible.

Substantial variation also exists in the anatomy of local anesthetic landmarks of the mandibular bone and nerves compared with similar structures in the maxilla, complicating mandibular anesthesia. This text covers some of the most common mandibular variations.

Pulpal anesthesia is achieved through anesthesia of each nerve's dental branches as they extend into the pulp tissue by way of each tooth's apical foramen. The hard and soft tissues of the periodontium are anesthetized by way of the interdental and interradicular branches for each tooth.

The inferior alveolar block is generally recommended for anesthesia of the mandibular teeth and their associated lingual tissues to the midline, as well as the facial tissues anterior to the mandibular first molar. The buccal block is generally recommended for anesthesia of the tissues buccal to the mandibular molars. The mental block is generally recommended for anesthesia of the facial tissues anterior to the mental foramen (usually the mandibular premolars and anterior teeth). The incisive block is generally recommended for anesthesia of the teeth and associated facial tissues anterior to the mental foramen (usually the mandibular premolars and anterior teeth). The Gow-Gates mandibular nerve block anesthetizes most of the mandibular nerve and is useful for extensive procedures during quadrant dentistry.

Inferior Alveolar Block

The **inferior alveolar block** also known as the **IA block** or mandibular block, is the most commonly used injection in dentistry. The IA block is used when dental procedures are performed on the mandibular teeth and pulpal anesthesia is necessary. This block also gives anesthesia of the lingual periodontium of all the mandibular teeth, as well as anesthesia of the facial periodontium of the mandibular anterior and premolar teeth.

Additional use of the buccal nerve block may be considered if anesthesia of the buccal periodontium of the mandibular molars is also necessary. Sometimes there is overlap of the left and right incisive nerves. The incisive nerve is a branch of the mandibular nerve that serves the pulp tissue of the mandibular anterior teeth. If this is the case, a bilateral IA block can be used, but it is not recommended. Bilateral IA blocks are usually avoided unless absolutely necessary. This is because bilateral mandibular injections produce complete anesthesia of the body of the tongue and floor of the mouth, which can cause difficulty with swallowing and speech, especially in patients with full or partial removable mandibular dentures, until the effects of the local anesthetic agent wear off. Comprehensive dental treatment planning can usually prevent the need for bilateral IA blocks.

More often, the use of an incisive block or local infiltration at the apices of the mandibular teeth that fail to achieve initial pulpal anesthesia may be indicated. Local infiltrations on the facial surface of the anterior mandible are more successful than more posterior injections but less successful than injections over the maxilla in similar locations. Again, these differences in success rates are due to differences in the density of the facial bones.

Even though the IA block is the most commonly used dental injection, it is not always initially successful. This may mean that the patient must be reinjected to achieve the necessary anesthesia of the tissues. This lack of consistent success is due in part to anatomical variation in the height of the mandibular foramen on the medial side of the ramus and the great depth of soft tissue penetration required to achieve pulpal anesthesia. Other techniques to achieve mandibular anesthesia, such as the Gow-Gates mandibular nerve block, may also be employed with failure of the IA block.

TARGET AREA AND INJECTION SITE FOR IA BLOCK

The target area for the IA block is slightly superior to the entry point of the IA nerve into the mandibular foramen, overhung anteriorly by the lingula (Figures 9-30, 9-31 and 9-32; see Figure 9-3). The local anesthetic

TABLE 9-2

SUMMARY OF MANDIBULAR LOCAL ANESTHESIA OF THE TEETH AND ASSOCIATED TISSUES

Mandibular Tooth and Tissues	IA Block	Buccal Block	Mental Block	Incisive Block
Central Incisor				
Pulpal	X		X	X
Facial	X	X	X	
Lingual	X			
Lateral Incisor				
Pulpal	X		X	X
Facial	X	X	X	X
Lingual	X			
Canine				
Pulpal	X			X
Facial	X		X	X
Lingual	X			
First Premolar				
Pulpal	X			X
Facial	X		X	X
Lingual	X			
Second Premolar				
Pulpal	X			X
Facial	X		X	X
Lingual	X			
First Molar				
Lingual/pulpal	X			
Buccal		X		
Second Molar				
Lingual/pulpal	X			
Buccal		X		
Third Molar				
Lingual/pulpal	X			
Buccal		X		

The anesthesia for anatomical variants is not included.
IA, Inferior alveolar.

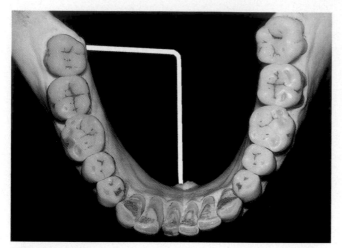

FIGURE 9-30 Area anesthetized by the **inferior alveolar block** is highlighted.

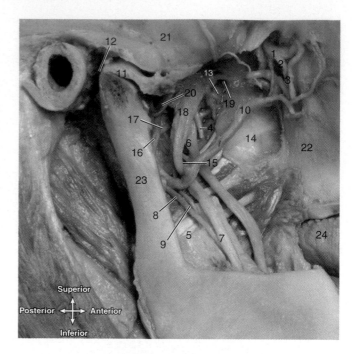

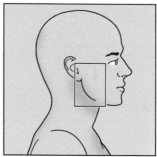

FIGURE 9-31 Deep dissection of the face and right infratemporal fossa (after removal of the lateral pterygoid muscle, zygomatic arch, and portion of mandible) to show the nerves in the area where the **inferior alveolar block** is given (as well as the **posterior superior alveolar block** discussed earlier). *1,* Maxillary nerve; *2,* PSA nerve; *3,* posterior superior alveolar artery; *4,* buccal nerve; *5,* medial pterygoid muscle; *6,* lingual nerve; *7,* IA nerve; *8,* inferior alveolar artery; *9,* nerve to mylohyoid muscle; *10,* maxillary artery; *11,* disc of joint and mandibular condyle; *12,* joint capsule; *13,* nerve to medial pterygoid muscle; *14,* lateral pterygoid plate; *15,* chorda tympani nerve; *16,* middle meningeal artery; *17,* accessory meningeal artery; *18,* mandibular nerve; *19,* nerve to lateral pterygoid muscle; *20,* auriculotemporal nerve; *21,* temporal bone; *22,* maxilla; *23,* mandibular ramus; *24,* tongue. (From Logan BM, Reynold PA, Hutching RT: *McMinn's color atlas of head and neck anatomy,* ed 3, London, 2004, Mosby Ltd.)

agent must be accurately deposited within 1 mm of the target area to achieve anesthesia. The adjacent anteriorly placed lingual nerve will also be anesthetized as the local anesthetic agent diffuses.

The injection site for the IA block is the mandibular tissues on the medial border of the mandibular ramus at the correct height and anteroposterior direction for the injection (Figures 9-33 and 9-34). Mainly hard tissues are used as landmarks to locate the injection site, such as the coronoid notch and the occlusal plane of the mandibular molars, to reduce errors caused by patient soft tissue variance.

The correct height of the injection for the IA block is determined by palpating the coronoid notch, the greatest depression on the anterior border of the ramus. To determine the injection height, it helps to visualize an imaginary horizontal line that extends posteriorly from the coronoid notch to the pterygomandibular fold as it turns upward toward the soft palate, demarcating the posterior border of the ramus (Figure 9-35). The pterygomandibular fold covers the deeper pterygomandibular raphe, which is located between the buccinator and superior pharyngeal constrictor muscles. This fold is accentuated as the patient opens the mouth wider.

This imaginary horizontal line showing the height of IA block injection site is also parallel to and 6 to 10 mm superior to the occlusal plane of the mandibular molar teeth in the majority of adults. In children and small adults, this imaginary horizontal line for the height of the injection should be at the occlusal plane of the mandibular molars (see Figure 9-35). In partially edentulous patients, when the mandibular molars are absent, the mandibular foramen may appear to be more superior than when the dentition is present because the occlusal plane of molars is not present as a guide. The clinician's retracting finger can be kept at this height to help maintain it throughout the injection.

This will also help keep the needle and syringe parallel to the occlusal plane at all times to ensure correct placement of the needle tip near the mandibular foramen.

The correct anteroposterior direction of the IA block injection is achieved at the same time as the determination of the correct height of the injection. To determine this anteroposterior direction, it helps

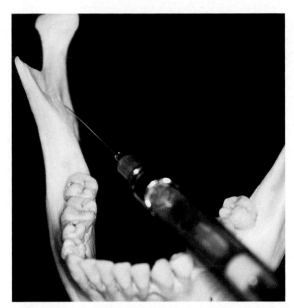

FIGURE 9-32 Target area for the **inferior alveolar block** is the inferior alveolar nerve located at the mandibular foramen on the medial surface of the mandibular ramus, inferior to the lingula.

to visualize an imaginary vertical line, three fourths of the distance between the coronoid notch and the posterior border of the ramus, demarcated by the pterygomandibular fold as it turns upward toward the soft palate (see Figure 9-35).

Thus the injection site of the IA block is determined by the intersection of these two imaginary lines, which is located at the deepest or most posterior portion of the pterygomandibular space, lateral to the pterygomandibular fold and the sphenomandibular ligament (Figure 9-36; see Figure 9-35 and Chapter 11). The syringe barrel is usually over the contralateral mandibu-

lar second premolar (and at the contralateral labial commissure).

The needle is inserted into the tissues of the pterygomandibular space until the mandible is contacted (Figures 9-37 and 9-38). The needle is withdrawn 1 mm from the tissues to protect the periosteum, and then the injection is administered. It is not necessary to deposit small amounts of the local anesthetic agent as the needle enters the tissue for the IA block to anesthetize the adjacent anteriorly placed lingual nerve because anesthesia of the lingual nerve will occur through diffusion of the local anesthetic agent placed near the IA nerve. These small amounts injected early will not reduce any tissue discomfort for the patient.

TROUBLESHOOTING THE IA BLOCK

If bone is contacted too soon when trying to administer an IA block, the needle tip is located too far anterior on the ramus. Correction is made by withdrawing the needle slightly and bringing the syringe barrel more closely over the mandibular anterior teeth. This correction moves the needle tip more posteriorly when it is reinserted.

If bone is not contacted when trying to administer an IA block, the needle tip is located too far posterior on the ramus. Correction is made by withdrawing the needle slightly and bringing the syringe barrel more closely over the mandibular molars. This correction moves the needle tip more anteriorly when it is reinserted.

It is important not to deposit the local anesthetic agent if bone is not contacted on initial insertion of the needle for an IA block. The needle tip may be too posterior and thus resting within the parotid salivary gland near the seventh cranial or facial nerve, resulting

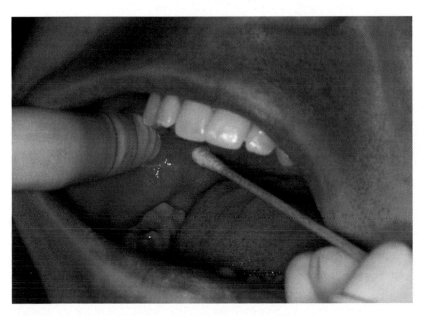

FIGURE 9-33 The injection site for the **inferior alveolar block** is probed at the depth of the pterygomandibular space on the medial surface of the ramus.

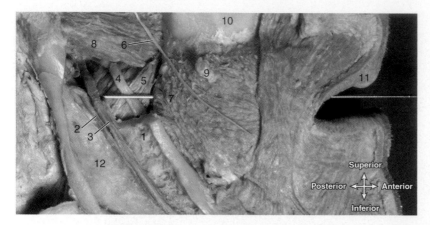

FIGURE 9-34 Dissection of the right infratemporal fossa showing the needle at the injection site for the **inferior alveolar block**. *1,* Lingula; *2,* inferior alveolar artery; *3,* inferior alveolar nerve; *4,* lingual nerve; *5,* medial pterygoid muscle; *6,* buccal nerve; *7,* buccinator muscle; *8,* lateral pterygoid muscle; *9,* parotid salivary duct; *10,* maxilla; *11,* upper lip; *12,* mandibular ramus. (From Logan BM, Reynold PA, Hutching RT: *McMinn's color atlas of head and neck anatomy,* ed 3, London, 2004, Mosby Ltd.)

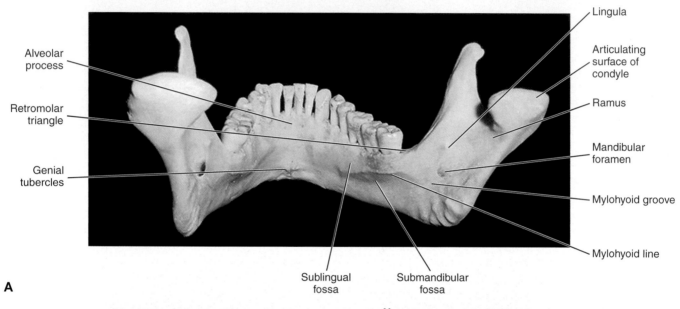

A

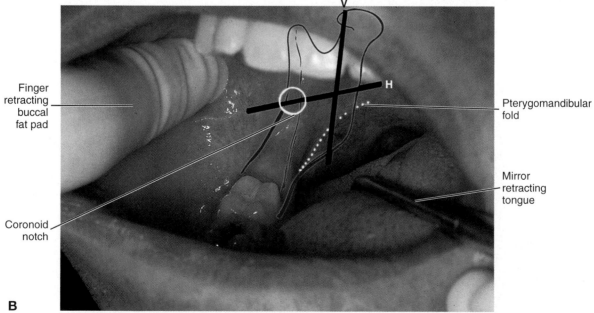

B

FIGURE 9-35 Imaginary horizontal line *(H)* showing the correct height and imaginary vertical line *(V)* showing the correct anteroposterior direction of the injection for the **inferior alveolar block**. The intersection of these two lines is the correct injection site for this block, which is at the depth of the pterygomandibular space. **A,** Posteromedial surface of the mandible. **B,** Oral view of the pterygomandibular space.

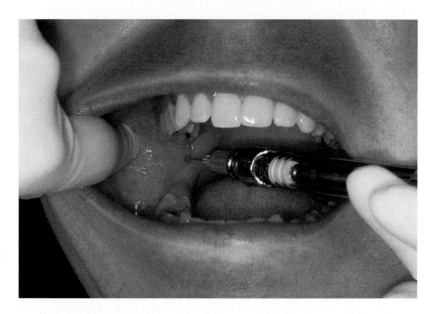

FIGURE 9-36 Needle penetration of the mandibular tissues for the **inferior alveolar block** is demonstrated at the depth of the pterygomandibular space. Injection site is highlighted.

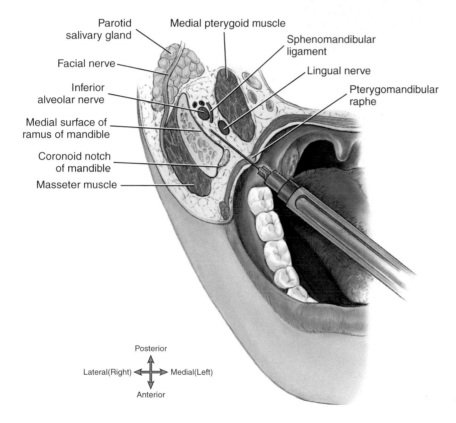

Parotid salivary gland
Medial pterygoid muscle
Sphenomandibular ligament
Facial nerve
Lingual nerve
Inferior alveolar nerve
Pterygomandibular raphe
Medial surface of ramus of mandible
Coronoid notch of mandible
Masseter muscle

Posterior
Lateral(Right) — Medial(Left)
Anterior

FIGURE 9-37 Correct needle penetration into the pterygomandibular space during an **inferior alveolar block** If the needle is inserted too far posteriorly, it may enter the parotid salivary gland containing the facial nerve, causing a complication such as transient facial paralysis.

in complications (discussed later; see Figures 9-37 and 9-38). If the insertion and deposition are too shallow and bone is not contacted, the medially located sphenomandibular ligament can become a physical barrier that stops the important diffusion of the local anesthetic agent to the mandibular foramen and IA nerve.

If there is failure of anesthesia, there may be accessory innervation of the mandibular teeth. Current thinking supports the mylohyoid nerve as the nerve that may be involved in this accessory mandibular innervation. To correct this problem, local anesthesia of the mylohyoid nerve using infiltration technique on the lingual border of the mandible is indicated. This additional anesthetic technique is discussed in most current dental local anesthesia textbooks.

Whenever a bifid IA nerve is detected by noting a doubled mandibular canal on intraoral radiograph (see Chapters 3 and 8), incomplete anesthesia of the mandible may follow an IA block. In many such cases

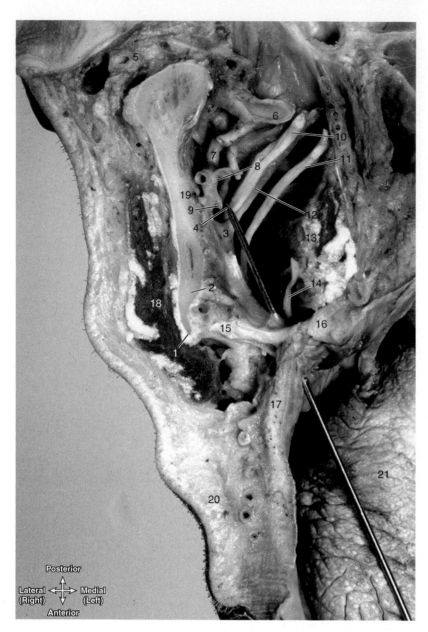

FIGURE 9-38 Dissection of the right infratemporal fossa (on a horizontal section) showing the needle at the injection site for the **inferior alveolar block** *1*, Coronoid notch (superior to the external oblique ridge); *2*, mylohyoid line; *3*, lingula; *4*, mandibular foramen; *5*, parotid salivary gland; *6*, styloid process; *7*, maxillary artery; *8*, IA vein; *9*, inferior alveolar artery; *10*, IA nerve; *11*, lingual nerve; *12*, sphenomandibular ligament; *13*, medial pterygoid muscle; *14*, buccal (long) nerve; *15*, temporalis muscle; *16*, pterygomandibular raphe; *17*, buccinator muscle; *18*, masseter muscle; *19*, mandibular ramus; *20*, buccal fat pad; *21*, tongue. (From Logan BM, Reynold PA, Hutching RT: *McMinn's color atlas of head and neck anatomy*, ed 3, London, 2004, Mosby Ltd.)

a second mandibular foramen, more inferiorly placed, exists. To correct this, the local anesthetic agent is deposited more inferior to the usual anatomical landmarks.

SYMPTOMS AND POSSIBLE COMPLICATIONS OF IA BLOCK

Symptoms of the IA block include harmless numbness or tingling of the lower lip because the mental nerve, a branch of the IA nerve, is anesthetized. This is a good indication that the IA nerve is anesthetized, but it is not a reliable indicator of the depth of anesthesia, especially concerning pulpal anesthesia.

Another symptom is harmless numbness or tingling of the body of the tongue and floor of the mouth, which indicates that the lingual nerve, a branch of the mandibular nerve, is anesthetized. Important to note is that this anesthesia of the tongue may occur without anesthesia of the IA nerve. Possibly the needle was not advanced deeply enough into the tissues to anesthetize the deeper IA nerve. The most reliable indicator of a successful IA nerve block is the absence of discomfort during dental procedures.

Another symptom that can sometimes occur is "lingual shock" as the needle passes by the lingual nerve. The patient may make an involuntary movement, varying from a slight opening of the eyes to jumping in the chair. This symptom is only momentary, and anesthesia will quickly occur.

One complication with an IA block is transient facial paralysis if the facial nerve is mistakenly

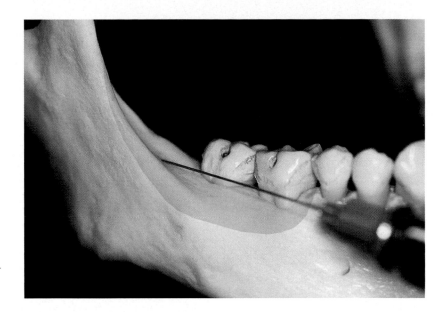

FIGURE 9-39 Target area for the **buccal block** is the buccal nerve located on the anterior border of the mandibular ramus. Area anesthetized is highlighted.

anesthetized. This can occur because of an incorrect administration of anesthetic into the deeper parotid salivary gland (containing the seventh cranial or facial nerve) because the mandibular bone was not contacted (see Figures 9-37 and 9-38). Symptoms of this temporary paralysis include the inability to close the eyelid and the drooping of the lips on the affected side (see Chapter 4).

Other complications such as hematoma can occur (see Chapter 6). Muscle soreness or limited movement of the mandible is rarely seen with this injection. Patient-inflicted trauma such as lip biting and resulting swelling can occur.

Finally, damage can occur after administration of the IA block, causing **paresthesia,** usually from trauma to the lingual nerve. Paresthesia is an abnormal sensation from an area such as burning or prickling, like a "pins-and-needles" feeling. Recent studies demonstrate that this paresthesia may be due to lack of adequate fascia around the lingual nerve or possibly neurotoxicity from the local anesthetic agent. Paresthesia can also occur with the spread of dental infection (see Chapter 12), but it mainly occurs due to surgical extraction of impacted molars.

Buccal Block

The **buccal block** or long buccal block is useful for anesthesia of the buccal periodontium of the mandibular molars including the gingiva, periodontal ligament, and alveolar bone. Many times this block is not necessary, such as when the buccal tissues are not impacted by the dental procedures performed. However, this is a successful dental injection because the buccal nerve is readily located on the surface of the tissue and not within bone.

TARGET AREA AND INJECTION SITE FOR BUCCAL BLOCK

The target area for the buccal block is the buccal nerve (or long buccal nerve) as it passes over the anterior border of the ramus and through the buccinator muscle before it enters the buccal region (Figure 9-39). Thus the injection site is the buccal tissues distal and buccal to the most distal molar tooth in the arch, on the anterior border of the ramus (Figure 9-40). The needle is advanced until it contacts the mandible, and then the injection is administered (Figure 9-41).

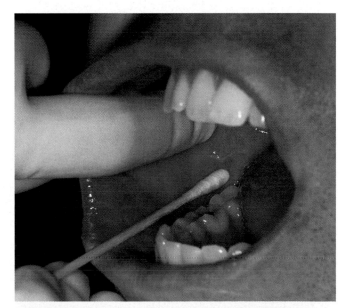

FIGURE 9-40 The injection site for the **buccal block** is probed in the buccal tissues that are distal and buccal to the most distal molar tooth in the arch.

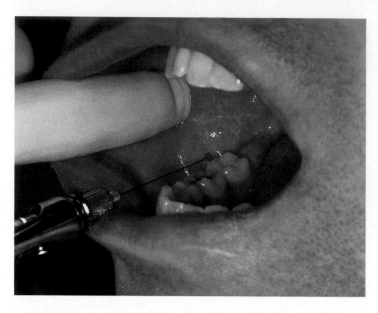

FIGURE 9-41 Needle penetration of the buccal tissues for the **buccal block** is demonstrated distal and buccal to the most distal molar tooth in the arch. Injection site is highlighted.

SYMPTOMS AND POSSIBLE COMPLICATIONS OF BUCCAL BLOCK

The patient rarely feels any symptoms of the buccal nerve block because of the location and small size of the anesthetized area. There is usually only absence of discomfort with dental procedures. Sometimes patient-inflicted trauma such as cheek bites occurs. The complication of a hematoma rarely occurs.

Mental Block

The **mental block** (**ment**-il) is used to anesthetize the facial periodontium of the mandibular premolars and anterior teeth on one side, including the gingiva, periodontal ligament, and other alveolar tissues. If pulpal anesthesia is necessary on the mandibular pre-

molar or anterior teeth, administration of an incisive block (discussed later) or use of the IA block may be considered. This block also does not provide any lingual tissue anesthesia of the involved teeth.

TARGET AREA AND INJECTION SITE FOR MENTAL BLOCK

The target area for the mental block is anterior to where the mental nerve enters the mental foramen to merge with the incisive nerve and form the IA nerve (Figures 9-42 and 9-43).

The mental foramen is usually located on the surface of the mandible between the apices of the first and second mandibular premolars. The mental foramen in adults faces posterosuperiorly. The mental

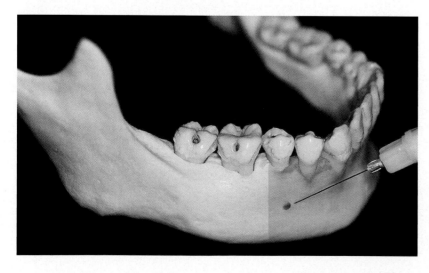

FIGURE 9-42 Target area for the **mental block** is anterior to the mental foramen where the mental nerve enters on the surface of the mandible, usually between the apices of the mandibular first and second premolars. Area anesthetized is highlighted.

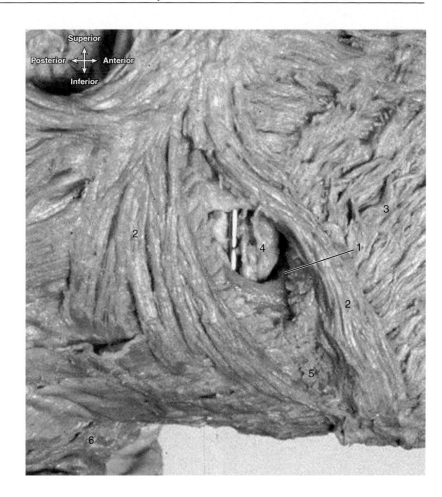

FIGURE 9-43 Dissection showing a probe deep at the injection site for the **mental** and **incisive blocks.** *1,* Mental foramen; *2,* depressor anguli oris muscle; *3,* depressor labii inferioris muscle; *4,* mental nerve and vessels; *5,* lower chin; *6,* neck. (From Logan BM, Reynold PA, Hutching RT: *McMinn's color atlas of head and neck anatomy,* ed 3, London, 2004, Mosby Ltd.)

foramen can be located on a radiograph before performing the injection to allow for a better determination of its position. To locate the mental foramen for the mental block, palpate intraorally the height of the mucobuccal fold between the apices of the mandibular first and second premolars or at a site indicated by a radiograph until a depression is felt on the surface of the skull, surrounded by smoother bone (Figure 9-44). The patient will comment that pressure in this area produces soreness as the mental nerve is compressed against the mandible near the foramen. However, studies show that the mental foramen can be as far posterior as the mandibular first molar or as far anterior as the distal surface of the mandibular canine.

Thus the insertion site for a mental block is anterior to the depression created by the mental foramen at the height of the mucobuccal fold. The needle is advanced without bony contact, and then the injection is administered (Figure 9-45). There is no need to enter the mental foramen to achieve anesthesia.

SYMPTOMS AND POSSIBLE COMPLICATIONS OF MENTAL BLOCK

The symptoms of a mental block are harmless tingling or numbness of the lower lip and absence of dis-

comfort during dental procedures. The complication of a hematoma rarely occurs.

Incisive Block

The **incisive block** (in-**sy**-ziv) anesthetizes the pulp tissue and facial tissues of the mandibular teeth anterior to the mental foramen (usually the mandibular premolars and anterior teeth). If lingual anesthesia is necessary, an IA block would be administered instead because the incisive block does not provide lingual anesthesia. The incisive block has a high success rate because the incisive nerve is readily accessible.

TARGET AREA AND INJECTION SITE FOR INCISIVE BLOCK

The target area for the incisive block is the same as the mental block: it is anterior to where the mental nerve enters the mental foramen to merge with the incisive nerve and form the IA nerve (Figure 9-46; see Figure 9-43).

The mental foramen is usually located on the surface of the mandible between the apices of the first and second mandibular premolars. The mental foramen in

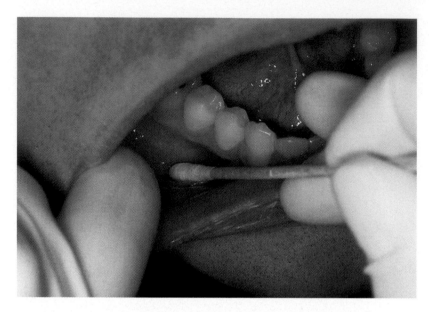

FIGURE 9-44 The injection site for both the **mental block** and **incisive block** is probed anterior to the depression caused by the mental foramen, usually located in the height of the mucobuccal fold between the apices of the mandibular first and second premolars.

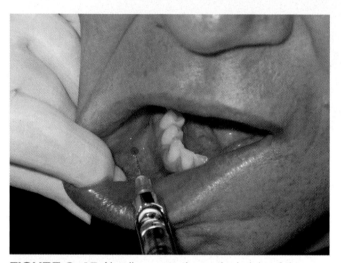

FIGURE 9-45 Needle penetration at the height of the mucobuccal fold tissues for both the **mental block** and **incisive block** is demonstrated anterior to the depression created by the mental foramen. Injection site is highlighted.

adults faces posterosuperiorly. The mental foramen can be located on a radiograph before performing the injection to allow for a better determination of its position. To locate the mental foramen for the mental block, palpate intraorally the height of the mucobuccal fold between the apices of the mandibular first and second premolars or at a site indicated by a radiograph until a depression is felt on the surface of the skull, surrounded by smoother bone (see Figure 9-44). The patient will comment that pressure in this area produces soreness as the mental nerve is compressed against the mandible near the foramen. However, studies show that the mental foramen can be as far posterior as the mandibular first molar or as far anterior as the distal surface of the mandibular canine.

Thus the insertion site for an incisive block is anterior to the depression created by the mental foramen. The needle is advanced without bony contact, and

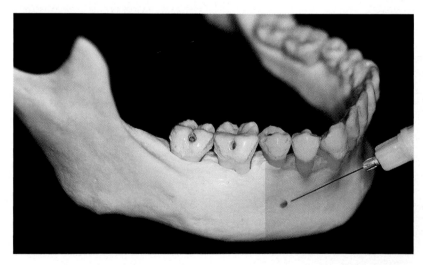

FIGURE 9-46 Target area for the **incisive block** is anterior to where the mental nerve enters the mental foramen on the surface of the mandible, usually between the apices of the mandibular first and second premolars. Area anesthetized is highlighted.

then the injection is administered (see Figure 9-45). Entering the mental foramen to achieve anesthesia is unnecessary. More local anesthetic agent is deposited within the tissue for the incisive block than for the mental block, and pressure is applied after the injection. This pressure forces more local anesthetic agent into the mental foramen, thus anesthetizing first the shallow mental nerve and then the deeper incisive nerve. Thus anesthesia of the tissues innervated by the mental nerve will precede that of the deeper incisive nerve's tissues. It is important to note that it is not necessary to have the needle enter the mental foramen to achieve a successful block.

SYMPTOMS AND POSSIBLE COMPLICATIONS OF INCISIVE BLOCK

The symptoms of an incisive block are the same as the symptoms of a mental block, except that there is pulpal anesthesia of the involved teeth. No discomfort occurs during dental procedures. As with a mental block, a hematoma rarely occurs.

Gow-Gates Mandibular Nerve Block

The nerves anesthetized with a **Gow-Gates mandibular nerve block** are the inferior alveolar, mental, incisive, lingual, mylohyoid, auriculotemporal, and buccal (long) nerves in most patients (Figure 9-47). It is a true mandibular block because it anesthetizes almost the entire V_3.

A Gow-Gates technique is indicated for use in quadrant dentistry in which the buccal soft tissue anesthesia from most distal molar to midline and lingual soft tissue is necessary, and in some cases in which a conventional IA block is unsuccessful. Thus the success rate is higher than that of an IA block.

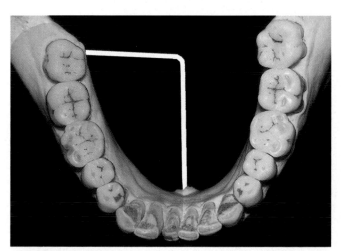

FIGURE 9-47 Area anesthetized by a **Gow-Gates mandibular nerve block** is highlighted and includes almost the entire mandibular nerve.

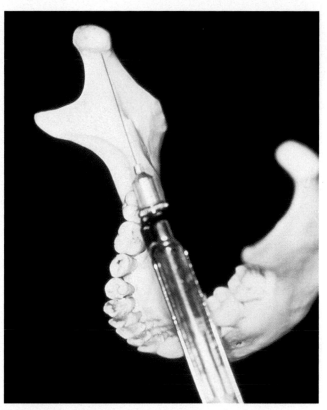

FIGURE 9-48 Target area for the **Gow-Gates mandibular nerve block** is located at the anteromedial border of the mandibular condyle neck, just inferior to the insertion of the lateral pterygoid muscle.

TARGET AREA AND INJECTION SITE FOR GOW-GATES MANDIBULAR NERVE BLOCK

The target area for the Gow-Gates technique is the anteromedial border of the mandibular condylar neck, just inferior to the insertion of the lateral pterygoid muscle (Figure 9-48). The injection site is located intraorally on the oral mucosa on the mesial of the mandibular ramus, just distal to the height of the mesiolingual cusp of the maxillary second molar, following a line extraorally from the ipsilateral intertragic notch of the ear to the ipsilateral labial commissure (Figure 9-49).

The extraoral landmarks of the intertragic notch and labial commissure are first located (Figure 9-50). The condyle assumes a more frontal position with the mouth open, and the injection site is closer to the mandibular nerve trunk. With a more closed mouth, the condyle will move out of the injection site and the soft tissue will become thicker.

Initially the needle is placed just inferior to the mesiolingual cusp of the maxillary second molar to assess the approximate vertical location for the injection site. The needle is then placed distal to the maxillary second molar, maintaining the established height (Figure 9-51). The barrel of the needle is maintained over the contralateral mandibular canine-to-premolar

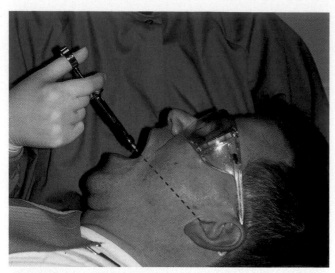

FIGURE 9-49 The extraoral line that is followed for the **Gow-Gates mandibular nerve block.** The line extends from the intertragic notch of the ear to the ipsilateral labial commissure.

region, such that the angulation of the syringe parallels a line connecting the ipsilateral labial commissure and the intertragic notch. The needle is inserted parallel to the determined line until bony contact is made with the neck of the condyle, and the injection is administered (Figure 9-52).

The height of insertion is superior to the mandibular occlusal plane, which is higher than that of an IA block, around 10 to 25 mm, depending on the patient's size. When a maxillary third molar is present, the site of injection will be just distal to that tooth.

SYMPTOMS AND POSSIBLE COMPLICATIONS OF GOW-GATES MANDIBULAR NERVE BLOCK

The mandibular teeth to midline, the buccal mucoperiosteum and mucous membranes, and lingual soft tissues and periosteum will be anesthetized. Inadver-

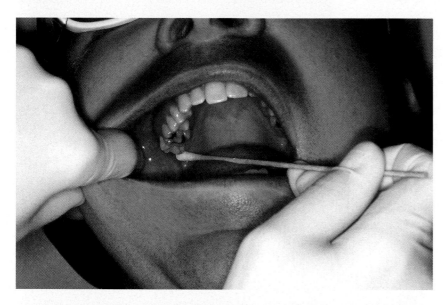

FIGURE 9-50 The injection site for the **Gow-Gates mandibular nerve block** is probed at the soft tissues just distal to the height of the mesiolingual cusp of the maxillary second molar, following a line extraorally from the intertragic notch to the ipsilateral labial commissure.

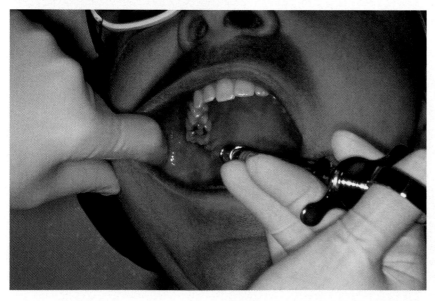

FIGURE 9-51 Using the needle to assess the vertical location for the **Gow-Gates mandibular nerve block** by placing the needle just inferior to the mesiolingual cusp of the maxillary second molar. Note that the barrel of the needle is over the contralateral mandibular canine-to-premolar region.

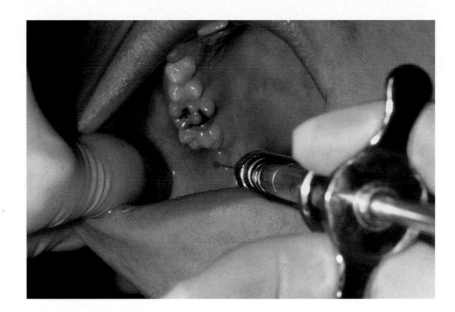

FIGURE 9-52 Needle penetration for the **Gow-Gates mandibular nerve block** is demonstrated at the soft tissues just distal to the maxillary second molar, maintaining the established injection height. Injection site is highlighted.

tently, the anterior two thirds of the tongue, floor of mouth, and body of the mandible and inferior ramus, as well as the skin over the zygoma and the posterior cheek and temporal regions, are anesthetized.

Two disadvantages of the Gow-Gates technique are the anesthesia of the lower lip, as well as the temporal area, and the longer time necessary for the anesthetic to take effect. The increased time is due to the larger size of the nerve trunk being anesthetized and the distance of the trunk from the site of deposition, which is 5 to 10 mm. However, the injection also lasts longer than the IA block because the area of the injection is less vascular and a larger volume of anesthetic may be necessary. The injection is contraindicated in patients with limited ability to open the mouth, but trismus is rarely involved.

Identification Exercises

Identify the structures on the following diagrams by filling in each blank with the correct anatomical term. You can check your answers by looking back at the figure indicated in parentheses for each identification diagram.

1. (Figure 9-7)

2. (Figure 9-37)

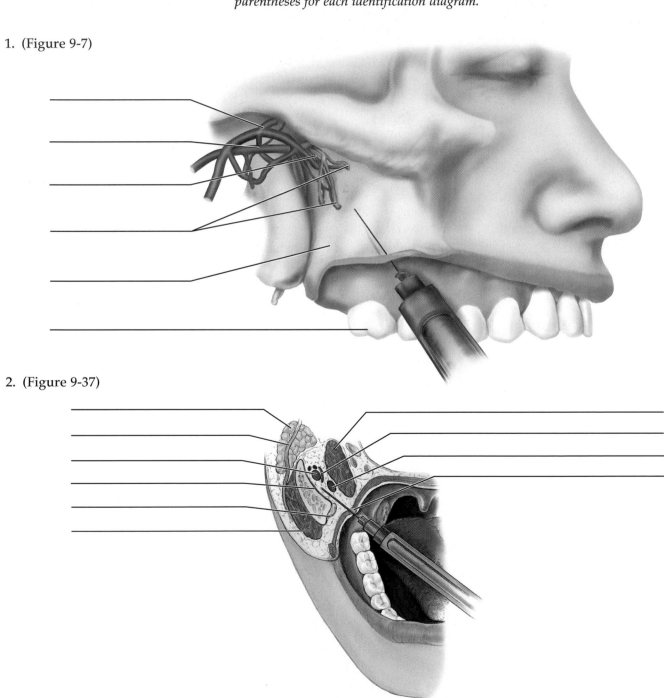

■ REVIEW QUESTIONS

1. An extraoral hematoma can result from an incorrectly administered posterior superior alveolar block because the needle was overinserted and penetrated which of the following?
   A. Parotid salivary gland
   B. Pterygoid plexus of veins
   C. Floor of the nose
   D. Seventh cranial or facial nerve

2. Which of the following local anesthetic blocks has the same injection site as the incisive block?
   A. Nasopalatine block
   B. Greater palatine block
   C. Inferior alveolar block
   D. Buccal block
   E. Mental block

3. Which of the following nerves is *not* anesthetized during an IA block?
   A. Buccal nerve
   B. Lingual nerve
   C. Mental nerve
   D. Incisive nerve

4. Which of the following local anesthetic blocks uses pressure anesthesia of the tissue to reduce patient discomfort?
   A. Posterior superior alveolar block
   B. Infraorbital block
   C. Greater palatine block
   D. Inferior alveolar block
   E. Buccal block

5. Which of the following are usually anesthetized during an infraorbital block?
   A. Bilateral anterior hard palate
   B. Buccal periodontium of maxillary molars
   C. Upper lip, side of nose, and lower eyelid
   D. Lingual periodontium of maxillary anteriors
   E. Side of face, upper eyelid, and bridge of nose

6. If the mesiobuccal root of the maxillary first molar is not anesthetized by a posterior superior alveolar block, what should the dental professional do?
   A. Reinject at the same site as for the posterior superior alveolar block
   B. Perform a buccal block injection
   C. Administer an middle superior alveolar block injection
   D. Perform an nasopalatine block injection

7. Which of the following is an important landmark to locate before performing an inferior alveolar block?
   A. Coronoid notch
   B. Tongue
   C. Buccal fat pad
   D. Mental foramen

8. The injection site for the greater palatine block is usually located on the palate near which of the following?
   A. Maxillary first premolar
   B. Maxillary second or third molar
   C. Incisive papilla
   D. Midline portion

9. If an extraction of a permanent maxillary lateral incisor is scheduled, which of the following local anesthetic blocks can be administered instead of the Infraorbital block?
   A. Posterior superior alveolar block
   B. Middle superior alveolar block
   C. Nasopalatine block
   D. Greater palatine block

10. Transient facial paralysis can occur with which incorrectly administered block?
    A. Posterior superior alveolar block
    B. Middle superior alveolar block
    C. Nasopalatine block
    D. Inferior alveolar block
    E. Mental block

11. Which local anesthetic block anesthetizes the largest intraoral area?
    A. Buccal block
    B. Inferior alveolar block
    C. Mental block
    D. Incisive block

12. Which of these situations can occur if bone is contacted too soon in an Inferior alveolar block?
    A. needle tip is located too far anteriorly on the ramus.
    B. needle tip is located too far posteriorly on the maxillary tuberosity.
    C. syringe barrel is mainly over the maxillary posterior teeth.
    D. syringe barrel is mainly over the mandibular posterior teeth.

13. In which of the following locations is the outcome most successful when using local infiltrations of local anesthetic?
   A. Facial surface of anterior maxilla
   B. Facial surface of posterior maxilla
   C. Facial surface of anterior mandible
   D. Facial surface of posterior mandible

14. If working within the mandibular anterior sextant, which block is most successful and comfortable for the patient?
   A. Unilateral posterior superior alveolar block
   B. Bilateral lingual block
   C. Bilateral inferior alveolar block
   D. Bilateral incisive block

15. Which of the following injections anesthetizes the buccal tissues of the mandibular molars?
   A. Buccal block
   B. Inferior alveolar block
   C. Mental block
   D. Incisive block

16. The mental foramen is usually located between the apices of which of the following mandibular teeth?
   A. First and second molars
   B. Second and third molars
   C. First and second premolars
   D. First premolar and canine

17. To have complete anesthesia of the quadrant, which of the following blocks needs to be administered along with the anterior middle superior alveolar?
   A. Middle superior alveolar block
   B. Nasopalatine block
   C. Posterior superior alveolar block
   D. Anterior superior alveolar block

18. Which of the following can serve as a landmark for the anterior middle superior alveolar block?
   A. Incisive papilla
   B. Premolar teeth
   C. Lesser palatine foramen
   D. Canine eminence

19. Which of the following is considered a true mandibular block because it anesthetizes most of the mandibular nerve?
   A. Posterior superior alveolar block
   B. Mental block
   C. Inferior alveolar block
   D. Gow-Gates block
   E. Buccal block

20. Which of the following landmarks are noted when administering a Gow-Gates block?
   A. Maxillary second molar
   B. Contralateral labial commissure
   C. Coronoid notch
   D. Pterygomandibular space

Lymphatic System

LEARNING OBJECTIVES

After studying this chapter, the reader should be able to do the following:

1. Define and pronounce all the key terms and anatomical terms in this chapter.
2. List and discuss the lymphatic system and its components.
3. Locate and identify all the major groups of lymph nodes of the head and neck on a diagram and extraorally on a patient.
4. Locate and identify all the tonsillar tissues of the head and neck on a diagram and intraorally on a patient.
5. Identify the patterns of lymph drainage for each head and neck tissue or region.
6. Describe and discuss lymphadenopathy of lymphoid tissue.
7. Discuss the spread of cancer in the head and neck region and its relationship to lymph nodes.
8. Correctly complete the review questions and activities for this chapter.
9. Integrate the knowledge about head and neck lymphatics into clinical dental practice.

KEY TERMS

Afferent Vessel (**af**-er-ent) Type of lymphatic vessel in which lymph flows into the lymph node.

Efferent Vessel (**ef**-er-ent) Type of lymphatic vessel in which lymph flows out of the lymph node in the area of the node's hilus.

Hilus (**hi**-lus) Depression on one side of a lymph node where lymph flows out by way of an efferent lymphatic vessel.

Lymph Tissue fluid that drains from the surrounding region and into the lymphatic vessels.

Lymphadenopathy (lim-fad-in-**op**-ah-thee) Process in which there is an increase in the size and a change in the consistency of lymphoid tissue.

Lymphatic Ducts (lim-**fat**-ik) Larger lymphatic vessels that drain smaller vessels and then empty into the venous system.

Lymphatics Portion of the immune system with ducts, nodes, tonsils, and vessels.

Lymphatic Vessels System of channels that drains tissue fluid from the surrounding regions.

Lymph Nodes Organized, bean-shaped lymphoid tissue that filters the lymph by way of lymphocytes to fight disease and is grouped into clusters along the connecting lymphatic vessels.

Metastasis (meh-**tas**-tah-sis) Spread of cancer from the original or primary site to another or secondary site.

Primary Node Lymph node that drains lymph from a particular region.

Secondary Node Lymph node that drains lymph from a primary node.

Tonsillar Tissue (**ton**-sil-lar) Masses of lymphoid tissues located in the oral cavity and pharynx to protect the body against disease processes.

OVERVIEW OF THE LYMPHATIC SYSTEM

The **lymphatics** are part of the immune system. They help fight disease processes and serve other functions in the body. The lymphatic system consists of a network of lymphatic vessels linking lymph nodes throughout most of the body. Tonsillar tissue located in the oral cavity and pharynx is also a portion of the lymphatic system. Although not part of the lymphatic system, the thymus gland also works as a portion of the immune system and is discussed in Chapter 7.

Lymphatic Vessels

The **lymphatic vessels** are a system of channels that mainly parallel the venous blood vessels in location yet are more numerous (Figure 10-1). Tissue fluid drains from the surrounding region into the lymphatic vessels as **lymph.** Not only do the lymphatic vessels drain their region, but they also communicate with each other. Lymphatic vessels are larger and thicker than the vascular system's capillaries. Unlike capillaries, lymphatic vessels have valves similar to many veins. These valves ensure a one-way flow of lymph through the lymphatic vessel. Lymphatic vessels are even found within the tooth's pulp tissue.

Lymph Nodes

The **lymph nodes** are bean-shaped bodies grouped in clusters along the connecting lymphatic vessels (Figure 10-2). Along the lymphatic vessels, the lymph nodes are positioned to filter toxic products from the lymph to prevent their entry into the vascular system. The lymph nodes are composed of organized lymphoid tissue and contain lymphocytes, white blood cells of the immune system that actively remove the toxic products. The removal of the toxic products helps fight disease processes in the body.

The lymph nodes can be superficial in location with the superficial veins or located deep in the tissue with the deep blood vessels. In healthy patients, lymph nodes are usually small, soft, and free or mobile in the surrounding tissue. Therefore lymph nodes normally cannot be visualized or palpable during an extraoral examination of a healthy patient.

DRAINAGE PATTERNS OF LYMPH NODES

The lymph flows into the lymph node by way of **afferent vessels.** On one side of the node is a depression or **hilus,** where the lymph flows out of the node by way of a single **efferent vessel.**

Lymph nodes can be classified as primary or secondary. Lymph from a particular tissue region drains into a **primary node** or regional node. The primary node may also be called a *master node.* Primary nodes, in turn, drain into a **secondary node** or central node.

Tonsillar Tissue

Tonsillar tissue consists of masses of lymphoid tissue located in the oral cavity and pharynx. Tonsils, like lymph nodes, contain lymphocytes that remove toxic products. Tonsillar tissue is located near airway and food passages to protect the body against disease processes from toxic products.

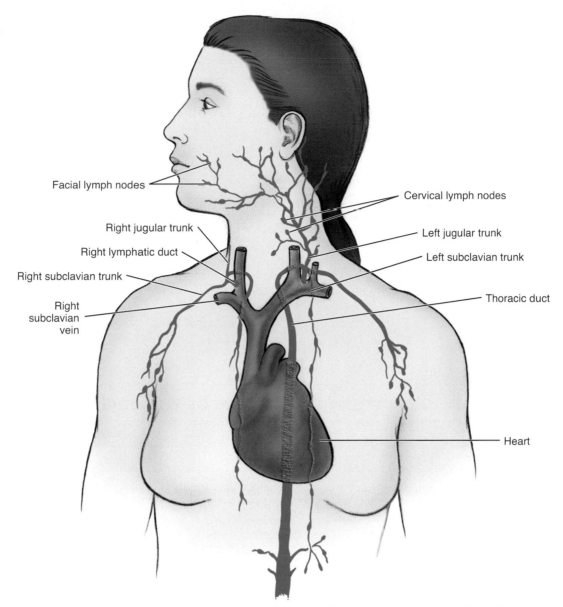

Facial lymph nodes

Right jugular trunk

Right lymphatic duct

Right subclavian trunk

Right subclavian vein

Cervical lymph nodes

Left jugular trunk

Left subclavian trunk

Thoracic duct

Heart

FIGURE 10-1 Lymphatic vessels and lymphatic ducts of the right and left sides of the upper body.

Lymphatic Ducts

Smaller lymphatic vessels containing lymph converge into larger **lymphatic ducts** (see Figure 10-1), which empty into the venous system of the blood in the chest area. The drainage pattern of the lymphatic vessels into the lymphatic ducts depends on which side of the body is involved.

The lymphatics of the right side of the head and neck converge by way of the right **jugular trunk** (jug-you-lar), joining lymphatics from the right arm and thorax to form the right **lymphatic duct,** which drains into the venous system at the junction of the right subclavian and right internal jugular veins.

The lymphatic vessels of the left side of the head and neck converge into the left jugular trunk, actually

a short vessel, and then into the **thoracic duct** (tho-**ras**-ik), which joins the venous system at the junction of the left subclavian and left internal jugular veins. Lymphatics from the left arm and thorax also join the thoracic duct. The thoracic duct is much larger than the right lymphatic duct because it drains the lymph from the entire lower half of the body (both right and left sides).

LYMPH NODES OF THE HEAD AND NECK

A dental professional needs to examine carefully for any palpable lymph nodes of the head and neck during an extraoral examination and record whether any are present (see Appendix B). The lymph nodes

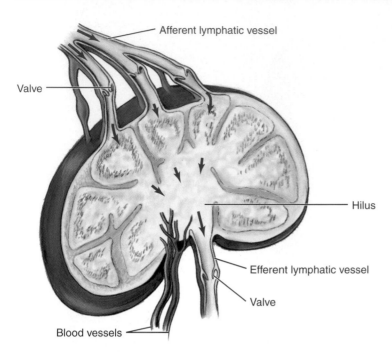

FIGURE 10-2 Lymph node and components.

TABLE 10-1

LYMPH NODE DRAINAGE PATTERN FOR TISSUES OF THE ORAL CAVITY

Tissue	Primary Nodes	Secondary Nodes
Buccal mucosal tissues	Buccal and mandibular	Submandibular
Anterior hard palate	Submandibular and retropharyngeal	Superior deep cervical
Posterior hard palate	Superior deep cervical and retropharyngeal	Inferior deep cervical
Soft palate	Superior deep cervical and retropharyngeal	Inferior deep cervical
Maxillary anterior teeth and associated tissues	Submandibular	Superior deep cervical
Maxillary first and second molars and premolars and associated tissues	Submandibular	Superior deep cervical
Maxillary third molars and associated tissues	Superior deep cervical	Inferior deep cervical
Mandibular incisors and associated tissues	Submental	Submandibular and deep cervical
Mandibular canines, premolars, and molars and associated tissues	Submandibular	Superior deep cervical
Floor of mouth	Submental	Submandibular and deep cervical
Tongue apex	Submental	Submandibular and deep cervical
Tongue body	Submandibular	Superior deep cervical
Tongue base	Superior deep cervical	Inferior deep cervical
Palatine tonsils and lingual tonsil	Superior deep cervical	Inferior deep cervical

that are palpable may help determine where a disease process such as cancer or infection is active (cancer is discussed later). The examination also may help determine whether the disease process has become widespread and involves a larger region and thus more secondary lymph nodes and related tissues.

This documentation and history concerning palpable lymph nodes will assist in the diagnosis, treatment, and outcome of any disease process that may be present in the patient. Therefore a dental professional must understand the relationship between node location and node drainage patterns in the tissues of the oral cavity (Table 10-1), face and scalp (Table 10-2), and neck (Table 10-3).

The dental professional also needs to remember that these lymph nodes drain not only intraoral dental structures such as the teeth but also the eyes, ears, nasal cavity, and deeper areas of the pharynx. Many times a patient needs a referral to a physician when lymph nodes are palpable due to a disease process in these other organs and regions.

Lymph Nodes of the Head

The lymph nodes of the head are located in either a superficial or a deep position relative to the surrounding tissues. All the nodes of the head drain either the right or left tissues in each region, depending on their location.

SUPERFICIAL LYMPH NODES OF THE HEAD

Five groups of superficial lymph nodes are located in the head: the occipital, retroauricular, anterior auricular, superficial parotid, and facial nodes (Figure 10-3; see Figure 10-8).

Occipital Lymph Nodes.

The **occipital lymph nodes** (ok-**sip**-it-al) (one to three in number) are located bilaterally on the posterior base of the head in the occipital region and drain this portion of the scalp. Having the patient lean the head

TABLE 10-2

LYMPH NODE DRAINAGE PATTERNS FOR TISSUES OF THE SCALP AND FACE

Tissues	Primary Nodes	Secondary Nodes
Scalp	Retroauricular, anterior auricular, superficial parotid, occipital, and accessory	Deep cervical and supraclavicular
Lacrimal gland	Superficial parotid	Superior deep cervical
External ear	Retroauricular, anterior auricular, and superficial parotid	Superior deep cervical
Middle ear	Deep parotid	Superior deep cervical
Pharyngeal tonsil and tubal tonsil	Superior deep cervical	Inferior deep cervical
Paranasal sinuses	Retropharyngeal	Superior deep cervical
Infraorbital region and nasal cavity	Malar, nasolabial, retropharyngeal, and superior deep cervical	Submandibular and deep cervical
Cheek	Buccal, malar, mandibular, and submandibular	Superior deep cervical
Parotid gland	Deep parotid	Superior deep cervical
Upper lip	Submandibular	Superior deep cervical
Lower lip	Submental	Submandibular and deep cervical
Chin	Submental	Submandibular and deep cervical
Sublingual gland	Submandibular	Superior deep cervical
Submandibular gland	Submandibular	Superior deep cervical

TABLE 10-3

LYMPH NODE DRAINAGE PATTERNS FOR TISSUES OF THE NECK

Tissues	Primary Nodes	Secondary Nodes
Superficial anterior cervical triangle	Anterior jugular	Inferior deep cervical
Superficial lateral and posterior cervical triangles	External jugular and accessory	Deep cervical and supraclavicular
Deep posterior cervical triangle	Inferior deep cervical	Pass directly into the jugular trunk on the right side or thoracic duct on the left
Pharynx	Retropharyngeal	Superior deep cervical
Thyroid gland	Superior deep cervical	Inferior deep cervical
Larynx	Laryngeal	Inferior deep cervical
Esophagus	Superior deep cervical	Inferior deep cervical
Trachea	Superior deep cervical	Inferior deep cervical

forward allows for effective bilateral palpation at the base of the head for these nodes (Figure 10-4). The occipital nodes empty into the deep cervical nodes of the neck.

Retroauricular, Anterior Auricular, and Superficial Parotid Lymph Nodes.

The nodes known as **retroauricular lymph nodes** (ret-ro-aw-**rik**-you-lar) or mastoid or posterior auricular nodes (one to three in number) are located posterior to each ear, where the sternocleidomastoid muscle inserts on the mastoid process. The **anterior auricular lymph nodes** (aw-**rik**-you-lar) (one to three in number) are located anterior to each ear.

The **superficial parotid lymph nodes** (pah-**rot**-id) or paraparotid nodes (up to 10 in number along with the deep parotid group) are just superficial to each parotid salivary gland. Anatomists sometimes tend to group

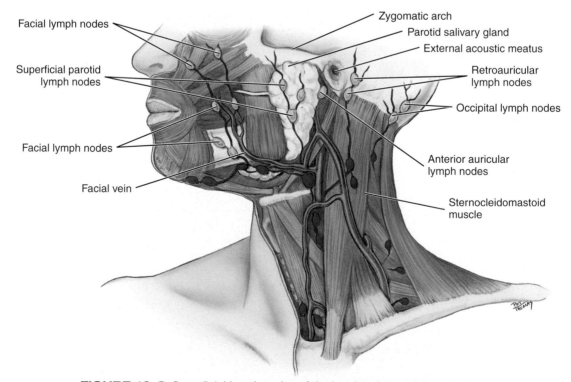

FIGURE 10-3 Superficial lymph nodes of the head and associated structures.

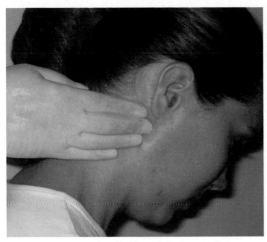

FIGURE 10-4 Palpating the occipital lymph nodes by having the patient's head forward.

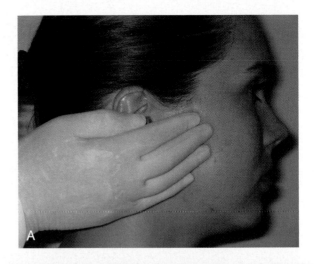

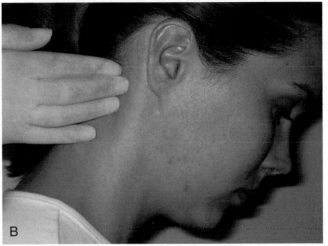

FIGURE 10-5 Palpating the auricular lymph nodes using gentle pressure on the face **(A)** and scalp around each ear **(B)**.

the anterior auricular and superficial parotid nodes together.

The retroauricular, anterior auricular, and superficial parotid nodes drain the external ear, lacrimal gland, and adjacent regions of the scalp and face. All of these nodes empty into the deep cervical lymph nodes. During an extraoral examination, standing near the patient, bilaterally palpate these nodes, as well as the face and scalp anterior to and around each ear (Figure 10-5).

Facial Lymph Nodes.

The final group of superficial nodes of the head is the **facial lymph nodes** (up to 12 in number), which are located along the length of the facial vein. These nodes are typically small and variable in number. The facial nodes are further categorized into four subgroups: malar, nasolabial, buccal, and mandibular nodes.

Nodes in the infraorbital region are the **malar lymph nodes** (**may**-lar) or infraorbital nodes. Nodes located near the nose are the **nasolabial lymph nodes** (nay-zo-**lay**-be-al). Nodes at the labial commissure and just superficial to the buccinator muscle are the **buccal lymph nodes**. Nodes in the tissues over the surface of the mandible, anterior to the masseter muscle, are the **mandibular lymph nodes** (man-**dib**-you-lar).

Each facial node subgroup drains the skin and mucous membranes where the nodes are located. The facial nodes also drain from one to the other, superior to inferior, and then finally drain together into the submandibular nodes. During an extraoral examination, bilaterally palpate these nodes on each side of the space, moving from the infraorbital region to the labial commissure and then to the surface of the mandible (Figure 10-6). Infections from the teeth may spread to one of these nodes, which, when enlarged, can be described as being firm like a dried pea.

DEEP LYMPH NODES OF THE HEAD

Deep lymph nodes in the head region can never be palpated during an extraoral examination due to their depth in the tissues. The deep nodes of the face include the deep parotid and retropharyngeal nodes (Figures 10-7 and 10-8). All of these deep nodes of the head drain into the deep cervical lymph nodes of the neck.

Deep Parotid Lymph Nodes.

The **deep parotid lymph nodes** (up to 10 in number along with the superficial parotid nodes) are located deep in the parotid salivary gland and drain the middle ear, auditory tube, and parotid salivary gland.

Retropharyngeal Lymph Nodes.

Also located near the deep parotid nodes and at the level of the atlas, the first cervical vertebra, are the **retropharyngeal lymph nodes** (ret-ro-far-**rin**-je-al) (up to three in number), which drain the pharynx, palate, paranasal sinuses, and nasal cavity.

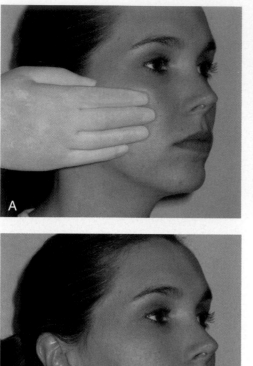

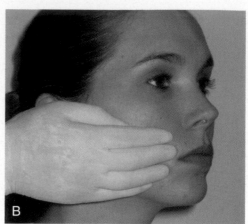

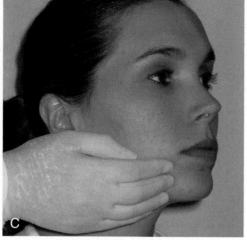

FIGURE 10-6 Palpating the facial nodes from the malar to the nasolabial **(A)**; from the nasolabial to the buccal **(B)**; and then to the mandibular nodes **(C)**.

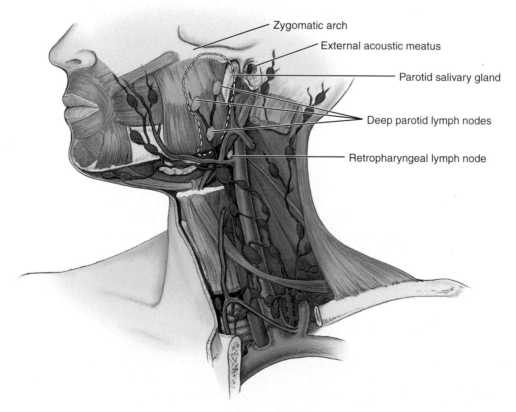

Zygomatic arch

External acoustic meatus

Parotid salivary gland

Deep parotid lymph nodes

Retropharyngeal lymph node

FIGURE 10-7 Deep lymph nodes of the head and associated structures.

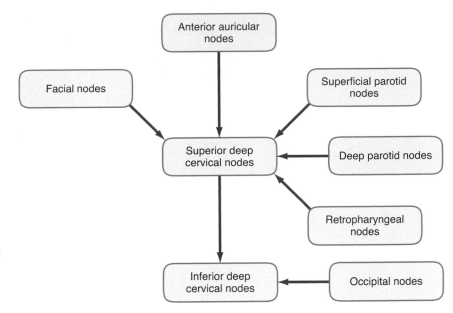

FIGURE 10-8 Flow chart of the lymphatic drainage of the head into the neck (note that the external jugular nodes may be secondary nodes for the occipital, retroauricular, anterior auricular, and superficial parotid nodes).

Cervical Lymph Nodes

Nodes of the neck or cervical lymph nodes can be in either a superficial or deep location in the tissues. All the cervical nodes drain either the right or left portions of the tissues in which they are located, except the midline submental nodes, which drain the tissues in the region bilaterally.

Many clinicians record all the cervical nodes (except those directly inferior to the chin) in relationship to the sternocleidomastoid muscle. Thus the cervical nodes can be discussed as if they were in three overlapping categories: superior or inferior, anterior or lateral/posterior, superficial or deep. This text is more specific but recognizes this other method as workable for clinicians in a dental setting. Older names are included for completeness.

SUPERFICIAL CERVICAL LYMPH NODES

Four groups of superficial cervical lymph nodes exist: the submental, submandibular, external jugular, and anterior jugular nodes (Figures 10-9 and 10-10).

Submental Lymph Nodes.

The **submental lymph nodes** (sub-**men**-tal) (two to three in number) are located inferior to the chin in the submental fascial space. The submental nodes are also just superficial to the mylohyoid muscle, near the midline between the mandible's symphysis and hyoid bone. These nodes drain both sides of the chin and the lower lip, floor of the mouth, apex of the tongue, and mandibular incisors and associated tissues. The submental nodes then empty into the submandibular nodes or directly into the deep cervical nodes.

Submandibular Lymph Nodes.

Submandibular lymph nodes (sub-man-**dib**-you-lar) (three to six in number) are located at the inferior border of the ramus of the mandible, just superficial to the submandibular salivary gland, and within the submandibular fascial space. These nodes drain the cheeks, upper lip, body of the tongue, anterior portion of the hard palate, and associated teeth, except the mandibular incisors and maxillary third molars.

The submandibular nodes may be secondary nodes for the submental nodes and facial regions. Lymphatics from both the sublingual and submandibular salivary glands also drain into these nodes. The submandibular nodes then empty into the deep cervical nodes.

During an extraoral examination of the submental and submandibular nodes directly inferior to the chin, manually palpate the nodes after having the patient lower the chin (Figure 10-10). Then, tissue in the area is pushed over the bony edge of the mandible on each side, where it is grasped and rolled (Figure 10-11). Some dental professionals recommend that the patient put the chin up, with the mouth slightly open and the apex of the tongue on the hard palate, to allow palpation of the nodes directly inferior to the chin.

External Jugular Lymph Nodes.

The **external jugular lymph nodes** or superior superficial lateral cervical nodes are located on each side of the neck along the external jugular vein, superficial to

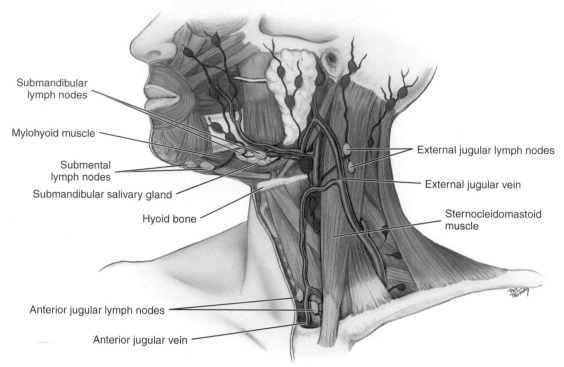

FIGURE 10-9 Superficial cervical lymph nodes and associated structures.

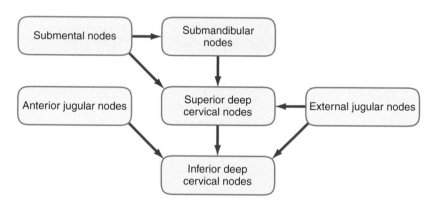

FIGURE 10-10 Superficial lymphatic drainage of the neck.

the sternocleidomastoid muscle. The external jugular nodes may be secondary nodes for the occipital, retroauricular, anterior auricular, and superficial parotid nodes. These nodes then empty into the deep cervical nodes.

Anterior Jugular Lymph Nodes.

The **anterior jugular lymph nodes** or anterior superficial cervical nodes are located on each side of the neck along the length of the anterior jugular vein, anterior to the sternocleidomastoid muscle, to drain the infrahyoid region of the neck. The anterior jugular nodes then empty into the deep cervical nodes.

During an extraoral examination of the external and anterior jugular nodes in the midportion of the neck,

having the patient turn the head to the opposite side makes the important landmark of the sternocleidomastoid muscle more prominent (Figure 10-13). Palpation of these nodes should start inferior to the ear and continue the whole length of the muscle's surface to the clavicles.

DEEP CERVICAL LYMPH NODES

The **deep cervical lymph nodes** (15 to 30 in number) are located along the length of the internal jugular vein on each side of the neck, deep to the sternocleidomastoid muscle (Figures 10-14 and 10-15). The deep cervical nodes extend from the base of the skull to the root of the neck, adjacent to the pharynx, esophagus, and trachea.

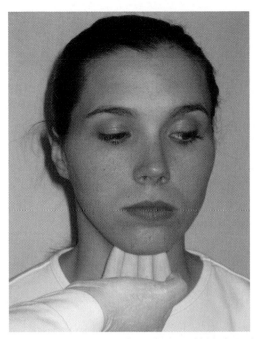

FIGURE 10-11 Palpating the submental lymph nodes.

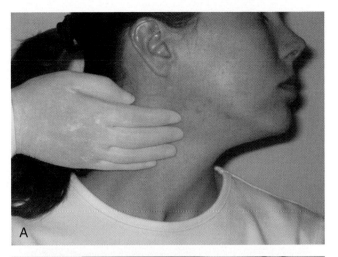

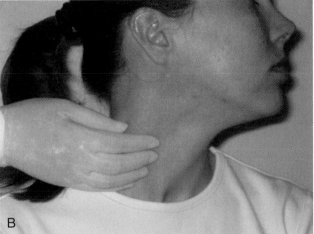

FIGURE 10-13 Palpating the external and anterior jugular lymph nodes using a prominent sternocleidomastoid muscle, starting at the ear **(A)** and continuing down the length of the muscle **(B).**

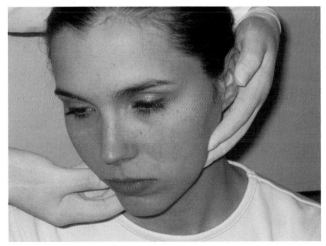

FIGURE 10-12 Palpating the submandibular lymph nodes inferior to the chin by having the patient's chin lowered.

Unlike the deep nodes of the head, the deep cervical nodes of the neck can be palpated. Again, during an extraoral examination, having the patient turn the head to the opposite side makes the important landmark of the sternocleidomastoid muscle more prominent and increases accessibility for effective palpation of these nodes (Figure 10-16). Palpation of the deep cervical nodes is performed on the underside of the anterior and posterior aspects of the muscle in contrast to the superficial cervical nodes that are on the muscle's surface. Again, palpation should start inferior to the ear and continue down the length of the muscle to the clavicles.

For those nodes in the most inferior portion of the neck in the area of the clavicles, having the patient raise the shoulders up and forward allows for effective palpation during an extraoral examination (Figure 10-17).

The deep cervical nodes can be divided into two groups, the superior and inferior deep cervical nodes. This division is based on whether the nodes are superior or inferior to the point where the omohyoid muscle crosses the internal jugular vein. However, the specificity of this division is not as important in the overall drainage of the head and neck to dental professionals as it is to medical professionals.

Superior Deep Cervical Lymph Nodes.
The superior deep (lateral) cervical lymph nodes or internal jugular nodes are located deep beneath the sternocleidomastoid muscle, superior to where the omohyoid muscle crosses the internal jugular vein. The superior deep cervical nodes are primary nodes

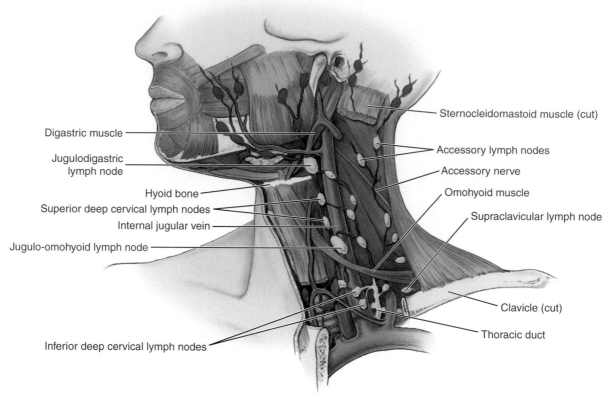

FIGURE 10-14 Deep cervical lymph nodes and associated structures.

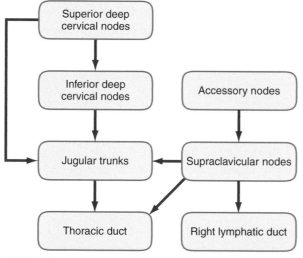

FIGURE 10-15 Deep lymphatic drainage of the neck.

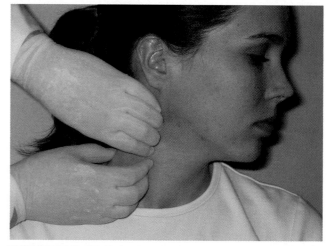

FIGURE 10-16 Palpating the deep cervical lymph nodes by having the patient's head turned.

for and drain the posterior nasal cavity, posterior portion of the hard palate, soft palate, base of the tongue, maxillary third molars and associated tissues, esophagus, trachea, and thyroid gland. Remembering that the lymphatic drainage of the base of the tongue is bilateral posteriorly and that the contralateral node may therefore be affected is important.

The superior deep cervical nodes may be secondary nodes for all other nodes of the head and neck, except

inferior deep cervical nodes. The superior deep cervical nodes empty into the inferior deep cervical nodes or directly into the jugular trunk.

One node of the superior deep cervical nodes, the **jugulodigastric lymph node** (jug-you-lo-di-**gas**-tric) or tonsillar node, easily becomes palpable when the palatine tonsils or pharynx is inflamed. The jugulodigastric node is located inferior to the posterior belly of the digastric muscle.

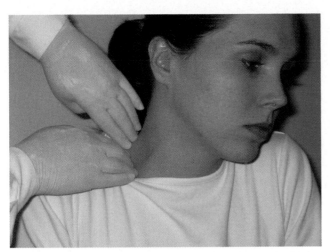

FIGURE 10-17 Palpating the most inferior deep cervical lymph nodes by having the patient's shoulders raised up and forward.

Inferior Deep Cervical Lymph Nodes.

The inferior deep (lateral) cervical lymph nodes are a continuation of the superior deep cervical group. The inferior deep cervical nodes are located deep to the sternocleidomastoid muscle, inferior to where the omohyoid muscle crosses the internal jugular vein, extending into the supraclavicular fossa, superior to each clavicle. The inferior deep cervical nodes are primary nodes for and drain the posterior portion of the scalp and neck, the superficial pectoral region, and a portion of the arm.

A sometimes prominent node of the inferior deep cervical nodes, the **jugulo-omohyoid lymph node** (jug-you-lo-o-mo-**hi**-oid), is located at the actual crossing of the omohyoid muscle and internal jugular vein. The jugulo-omohyoid node drains the tongue and submental region.

The inferior deep cervical nodes may be secondary nodes for the superficial lymph nodes of the head and superior deep cervical nodes. Their efferent vessels form the jugular trunk, which is one of the tributaries of the right lymphatic duct (on the right side) and the thoracic duct (on the left). The inferior deep cervical nodes also communicate with the axillary lymph nodes that drain the breast region. These nodes in the area of the armpit may be involved when the patient has breast cancer (adenocarcinoma), which is discussed later.

ACCESSORY AND SUPRACLAVICULAR LYMPH NODES

In addition to the deep cervical lymph nodes are the accessory and supraclavicular node groups in the most inferior portion of the neck. The (spinal) **accessory lymph nodes** (ak-**ses**-o-ree) (two to six in number) or posterior lateral superficial cervical nodes are located along the eleventh cranial or accessory nerve. They drain the scalp and neck regions and then drain into the supraclavicular nodes. The **supraclavicular lymph nodes** (soo-prah-klah-**vik**-you-ler) or transverse cervical chain of nodes (1 to 10 in number) are located along the clavicle and drain the lateral cervical triangles. The supraclavicular nodes may empty into one of the jugular trunks or directly into the right lymphatic duct or thoracic duct. These nodes are located in the final common pathway of lymphatic drainage from the entire body. For instance, cancer arising from the lungs, esophagus, and stomach may present in these nodes. Therefore inspection of these nodes is important in any comprehensive assessment.

TONSILS

The **tonsils** (**ton**-sils) are masses of lymphoid tissue located in the oral cavity and pharynx. Unlike lymph nodes, tonsils are not located along lymphatic vessels. All the tonsillar tissue drains into the superior deep cervical lymph nodes, particularly the jugulodigastric lymph node (see Tables 10-1 and 10-2).

Palatine and Lingual Tonsils

The **palatine tonsils** (**pal**-ah-tine) are two rounded masses of variable size located in the oral cavity between the anterior and posterior faucial pillars (Figure 10-18; see Chapters 2 and 4).

The **lingual tonsil** is an indistinct layer of lymphoid tissue located intraorally on the base of the dorsal surface of the tongue (Figure 10-19).

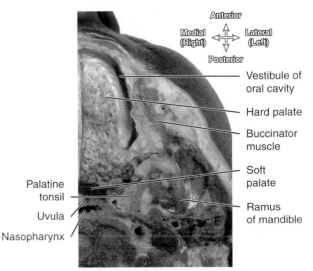

FIGURE 10-18 Palatine tonsils in a transverse section of the palate and oral cavity. (From Logan BM, Reynold PA, Hutching RT: *McMinn's color atlas of head and neck anatomy*, ed 3, London, 2004, Mosby Ltd.)

Pharyngeal and Tubal Tonsils

The **pharyngeal tonsil** (fah-**rin**-je-il) is located on the posterior wall of the nasopharynx (Figure 10-20). This tonsil is also called the **adenoids** (**ad**-in-oidz) and is normally enlarged in children. The **tubal tonsil** (**tube**-al) is also located in the nasopharynx, posterior to the openings of the eustachian or auditory tube (see Figure 10-20).

LYMPHADENOPATHY

When a patient has a disease process such as cancer or infection active in a region, the region's lymph nodes respond. The resultant increase in size and change in consistency of the lymphoid tissue is termed **lymphadenopathy** (Figure 10-21). Lymphadenopathy results from an increase in both the size of each individual lymphocyte and the overall cell count in the lymphoid tissue. With more and larger lymphocytes, the lymphoid tissue can better fight the disease process.

The lymph nodes can also be involved in the spread of infection such as dental infection from the teeth, which is discussed in Chapter 12. This spread of infection occurs along the connecting lymphatic vessels of the involved nodes.

This lymphadenopathy may allow the lymph node to be visualized during an extraoral examination. More important, changes in consistency allow the node to be palpated during the extraoral examination along the even firmer backdrop of underlying bones and muscles or the clinician's hands.

This change in lymph node consistency can range from firm to bony hard. Nodes can remain mobile or free from the surrounding tissue during a disease. However, they can also become attached or fixed to the surrounding tissues such as skin, bone, or muscle, as the disease process progresses to involve the

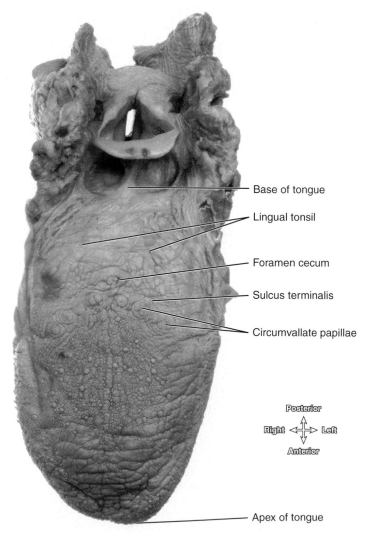

- Base of tongue
- Lingual tonsil
- Foramen cecum
- Sulcus terminalis
- Circumvallate papillae

Posterior
Right ⟷ Left
Anterior

- Apex of tongue

FIGURE 10-19 Gross specimen of the dorsal surface of the tongue noting the lingual tonsil. (From Logan BM, Reynold PA, Hutching RT: *McMinn's color atlas of head and neck anatomy,* ed 3, London, 2004, Mosby Ltd.)

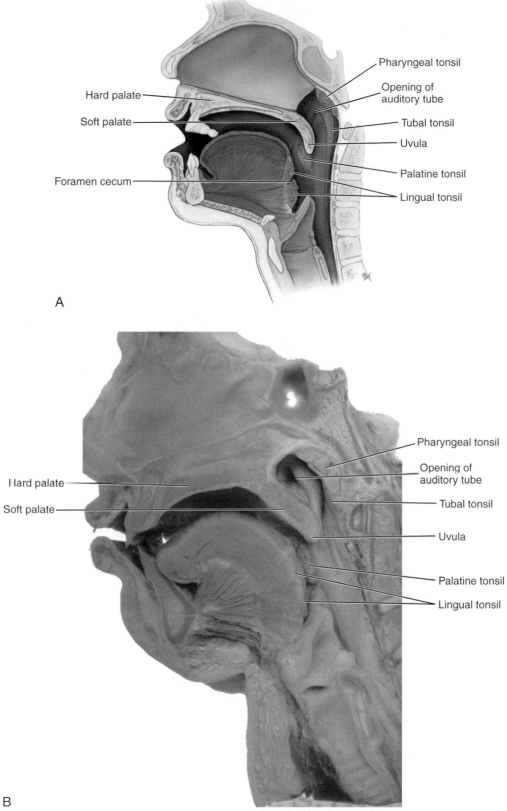

A

B

FIGURE 10-20 Pharyngeal tonsil and tubal tonsil on diagram **(A)** and in a sagittal section of the nasal, oral, and pharyngeal regions **(B)**. (**B,** From Reynolds PA, Abrahams PH: *McMinn's interactive clinical anatomy: head and neck,* ed 2, London, 2001, Mosby Ltd.)

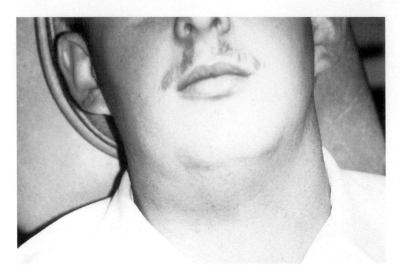

FIGURE 10-21 Excessive unilateral lymphadenopathy of the submandibular lymph nodes causing enlargement and loss of cervical symmetry of the neck.

regional tissues. When the nodes are involved with lymphadenopathy, the node can also feel tender to the patient when palpated. This tenderness is due to pressure on the area nerves resulting from the nodes' enlargement.

Again, any palpable lymph nodes found in a patient need to be recorded, and any appropriate physician referrals made by the dental professional. The changes in a node when it is involved with infection are discussed in Chapter 12.

Lymphadenopathy can also occur to the tonsils, causing tissue enlargement (Figure 10-22). In most cases this enlargement of the tonsils, with the exception of the tonsils located in the tissues of the pharynx, can be visualized during an intraoral examination of the patient (compare Figures 10-22 and 10-18). The intraoral tonsils may also be tender when palpated. Lymphadenopathy of the tonsils in both the oral cavity and pharynx may cause airway obstruction with its complications and lead to infection of the tonsillar tissue. A dental professional may need to refer the patient to a physician if lymphadenopathy and infection of intraoral tonsillar tissue are noted.

METASTASIS AND CANCER

Even though the lymph nodes usually assist in fighting the disease process, the nodes can become involved in the spread of certain cancers, called *carcinomas,* from epithelial tissues in the region they filter.

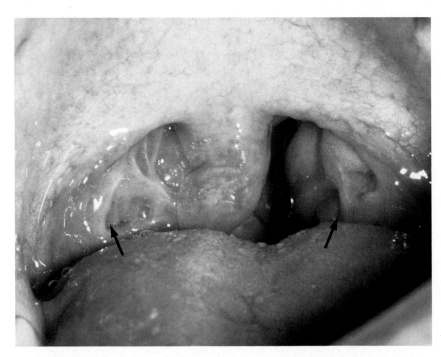

FIGURE 10-22 Enlarged palatine tonsils undergoing lymphadenopathy *(arrows).*

The spread of a cancer from the original or primary site of the tumor to another or secondary site is called **metastasis.** Primary nodes are the initial secondary site in which the cancer will metastasize from the tumor.

Often if the cancer is caught early enough at the primary tumor site or even at the initial secondary site of the primary lymph nodes, surgery to remove the tumor as well as the primary nodes may successfully stop metastasis. If the cancer is not caught early or stopped by the primary nodes, it will spread to secondary nodes and metastasis will continue to progress. Cancerous cells can slowly travel, unchecked in the lymph from node to node, if they are not stopped by any of the nodes along the lymphatic vessels.

If the cancer metastasizes past all the lymph nodes, the cancer cells of a carcinoma can enter the vascular system by way of the lymphatic ducts. The spread of cancer or metastasis by way of the blood vessels is quicker than by way of the nodes, so the cancer can quickly metastasize to the rest of the body, causing possibly fatal systemic involvement with the cancer. Thus an increase in the number of nodes involved with the cancer before involving the lymphatic duct and associated blood vessels may mean a better outcome for the patient.

When they are involved with cancer, the lymph nodes can become bony, hard, and possibly fixed to surrounding tissues and structures, thus making them nonmobile as the cancer grows and spreads. The cancerous nodes are usually not tender. In comparison, those nodes involved with acute infection are only firm, mobile, and tender (see Chapter 12).

Identification Exercises

Identify the structures on the following diagrams by filling in each blank with the correct anatomical term. You can check your answers by looking back at the figure indicated in parentheses for each identification diagram.

1. (Figure 10-1)

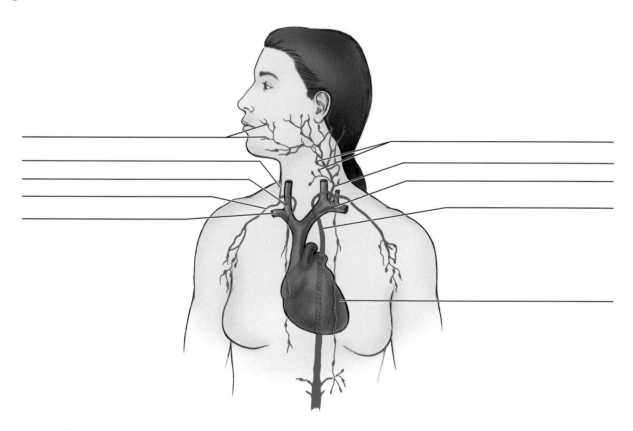

2. (Figure 10-2)

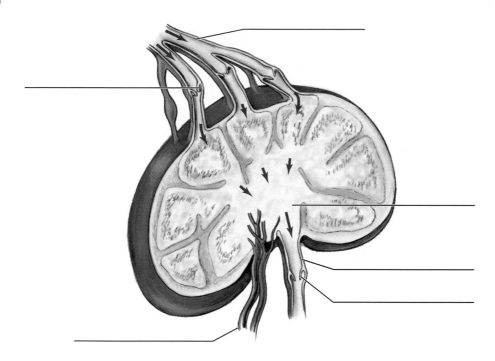

3. (Figure 10-3)

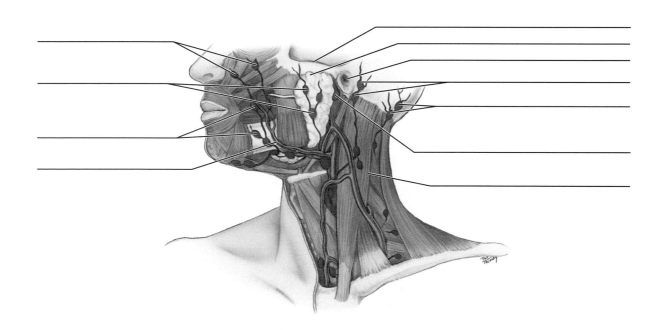

4. (Figure 10-7)

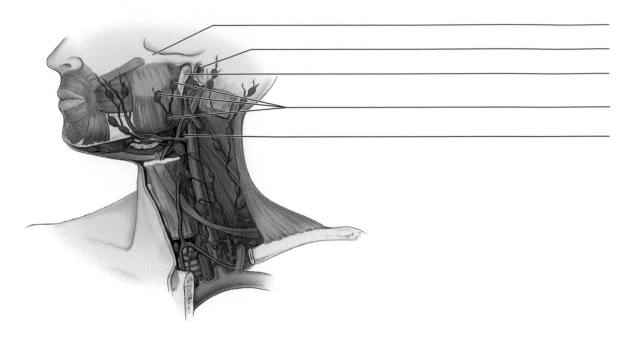

5. (Figure 10-9)

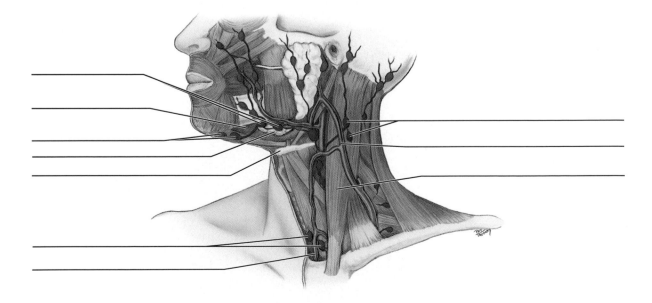

6. (Figure 10-14)

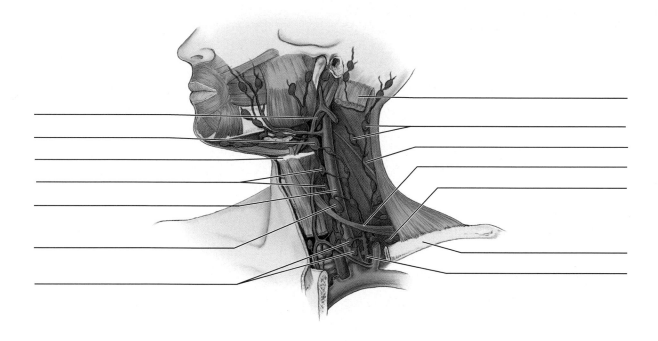

7. (Figure 10-20, *A*)

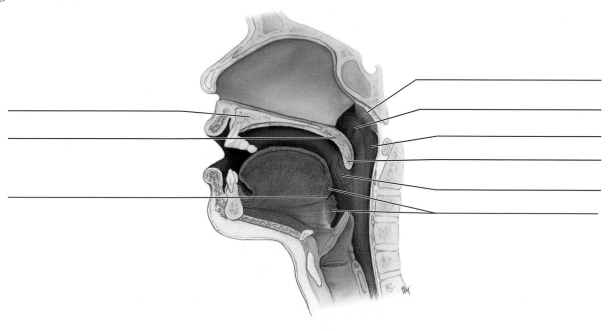

■ REVIEW QUESTIONS

1. Which of the following lymph node groups have both superficial and deep nodes within the group?
   A. Facial nodes
   B. Buccal nodes
   C. Parotid nodes
   D. Occipital nodes
   E. Submandibular nodes

2. Which of the following structures leave each individual lymph node at the hilus?
   A. Lymphatic ducts
   B. Tonsillar tissue
   C. Efferent lymphatic vessels
   D. Afferent lymphatic vessels

3. Which of the following lymph nodes are considered within the facial lymph node group?
   A. Sublingual, submandibular, zygomatic, and buccal nodes
   B. Infraorbital, nasal, buccal, and submental nodes
   C. Mandibular, lingual, malar, and zygomatic nodes
   D. Malar, buccal, nasolabial, and mandibular nodes
   E. Zygomatic, nasolabial, masseteric, and submental nodes

4. Which of the following components of the lymphatic system have one-way valves?
   A. Arteries
   B. Veins
   C. Vessels
   D. Nodes
   E. Ducts

5. Which of the following nodes drain lymph from a local region before the lymph flows to a more distant region?
   A. Primary
   B. Secondary
   C. Central
   D. Tertiary

6. The buccal lymph nodes are located superficial to which of the following?
   A. Sublingual gland
   B. Buccinator muscle
   C. Sternocleidomastoid muscle
   D. Parotid gland
   E. Submandibular gland

7. Which of the following lymph node groups extend from the base of the skull to the root of the neck?
   A. Facial nodes
   B. Deep cervical nodes
   C. Occipital nodes
   D. Jugulodigastric nodes
   E. Anterior jugular nodes

8. Where are the external jugular lymph nodes located?
   A. Anterior to the hyoid bone
   B. Along the external jugular vein
   C. Deep to the sternocleidomastoid muscle
   D. Close to the symphysis of the mandible

9. Into which area does the thoracic duct empty?
   A. Aortic arch of the body
   B. Superior vena cava of the body
   C. Junction of the right and left brachiocephalic veins
   D. Junction of the left internal jugular and subclavian veins

10. Which of the following are the primary lymph nodes that drain the skin and mucous membranes of the lower face?
    A. Occipital nodes
    B. Malar nodes
    C. Submandibular nodes
    D. Superficial parotid nodes
    E. Deep parotid nodes

11. Which of the following are secondary lymph nodes for the occipital nodes?
    A. Buccal nodes
    B. Submental nodes
    C. Submandibular nodes
    D. Deep cervical nodes
    E. Supraclavicular nodes

12. Which of the following pairs of lymph nodes are both considered portions of the superficial cervical lymph node group?
    A. External and anterior jugular nodes
    B. Superficial and deep jugular nodes
    C. Medial and lateral jugular nodes
    D. Internal and external jugular nodes

13. Which of the following statements concerning the submental lymph nodes is correct?
    A. They are located deep to the mylohyoid muscle.
    B. They are located between the mandible's symphysis and hyoid bone.
    C. They drain the labial commissure and base of tongue.
    D. They are secondary nodes for deep cervical nodes.

14. Which muscle needs to be made more prominent on a patient to achieve effective palpation of the region where the superior deep cervical lymph nodes are located?
    A. Masseter muscle
    B. Trapezius muscle
    C. Sternocleidomastoid muscle
    D. Epicranial muscle

15. Where is the lingual tonsil located?
    A. Posterior to the auditory tube's opening
    B. On the superior posterior wall of the nasopharynx
    C. At the base of the tongue
    D. Between the anterior and posterior faucial pillars

16. Which of the following nodes often become easily palpable when the palatine tonsils are inflamed?
    A. Jugulo-omohyoid node
    B. Jugulodigastric node
    C. Submental nodes
    D. Facial nodes

17. Which of the following are primary nodes for the maxillary third molar if it becomes infected?
    A. Submental nodes
    B. Submandibular nodes
    C. Superior deep cervical nodes
    D. Inferior deep cervical nodes

18. If a patient with breast cancer has involvement with the axillary nodes, which lymph nodes in the neck area primarily communicate with these nodes?
    A. Superior deep cervical nodes
    B. Inferior deep cervical nodes
    C. Submental nodes
    D. Submandibular nodes

19. At which intraoral site are the palatine tonsils located?
    A. Dorsal surface of tongue
    B. Submandibular fossa
    C. Between anterior and posterior faucial pillars
    D. Surrounding the faucial arch

20. When lymph nodes are involved in the metastasis of cancer, what characterizes them?
    A. Always tender
    B. Usually bony hard
    C. Always mobile
    D. Usually decreased in size

21. Where is the last stop for the lymph before reentering the systemic circulation?
    A. Several deep lymph nodes
    B. Entry into the lymphatic vessels through the walls
    C. The thoracic duct
    D. The thymus gland

22. Enlargement of the lymph nodes occurs because of which of the following?
    A. The amount of intergland lymph is large.
    B. Accumulation of bacteria and viruses causes the node to expand.
    C. More protein is lost from the circulatory system and winds up in the nodes.
    D. White blood cells in the node multiply to fight an infection.

23. Which of the following nodes are prominent nodes that drain the tongue and submental region?
    A. Jugulo-omohyoid nodes
    B. Jugulodigastric nodes
    C. Mandibular nodes
    D. Accessory nodes

24. Which tonsil is also called the *adenoids* and is normally enlarged in children?
    A. Palatine tonsil
    B. Pharyngeal tonsil
    C. Tubal tonsil
    D. Lingual tonsil

25. Which nodes drain the infrahyoid region of the neck?
    A. Malar nodes
    B. External jugular nodes
    C. Anterior jugular nodes
    D. Accessory nodes

Fascia and Spaces

LEARNING OBJECTIVES

After studying this chapter, the reader should be able to do the following:

1. Define and pronounce all the key terms and anatomical terms in this chapter.
2. Locate and identify the fasciae of the head and neck on a diagram, skull, and patient.
3. Locate and identify the major spaces of the head and neck on a diagram, skull, and patient.
4. Discuss the communication between the major spaces of the head and neck.
5. Correctly complete the review questions and activities for this chapter.
6. Integrate the knowledge of head and neck fasciae and spaces into the clinical dental practice.

KEY TERMS

Fascia, Fasciae (fash-e-ah, **fash**-e-ay) Layers of fibrous connective tissue that underlie the skin and surround the muscles, bones, vessels, nerves, organs, and other structures of the body.

Fascial Spaces (fash-e-al) Potential spaces between the layers of fascia in the body.

This chapter first discusses the fascia of the head and neck that surrounds all these structures. Later, the chapter discusses the potential spaces that are created between the layers of fascia of the body. In this chapter, the dental professional also has an opportunity to view the head and neck systems and their structures on the basis of their regional location in a three-dimensional mode, allowing completeness in their studies.

OVERVIEW OF THE FASCIA

Fascia (plural, **fasciae**) consists of layers of fibrous connective tissue. The fascia lies underneath the skin and surrounds the muscles, bones, vessels, nerves, organs, and other structures. The fasciae can be divided into superficial fascia and deep fascia.

Superficial Fascia

In all areas of the body the superficial fascia is found just deep to and attached to the skin. The superficial fascia generally separates the skin from the deeper structures, allowing the skin to move independently of these deeper structures. The superficial fascia varies in thickness in different portions of the body. The superficial fascia is composed of fat as well as irregularly arranged connective tissue. The vessels and nerves of the skin travel in the superficial fascia.

SUPERFICIAL FASCIA OF THE HEAD AND NECK

The superficial fascia of the body does not usually enclose muscles, except in the superficial fascia of the head and neck (Figure 11-1). The superficial facial fascia encloses the muscles of facial expression. The superficial cervical fascia of the neck contains the platysma muscle, which covers most of the anterior cervical triangle.

Deep Fascia

The deep fascia covers the deeper structures of the body such as the bones, muscles, vessels, and nerves. This fascia consists of a dense and inelastic fibrous tissue forming sheaths around these deeper structures.

DEEP FASCIA OF THE FACE AND JAWS

The deep fascia of the face and jaws is divided into fascial layers that are continuous with each other and with the deep cervical fascia (see Figure 11-1). This fascia includes the temporal, masseteric-parotid, and pterygoid fasciae.

The **temporal fascia** (**tem**-poh-ral) covers the temporalis muscle down to the zygomatic arch. The **masseteric-parotid fascia** (mass-et-**tehr**-ik-pah-**rot**-id) is located inferior to the zygomatic arch and over the masseter muscle and surrounds the parotid salivary gland. The **pterygoid fascia** (**teh**-ri-goid) is located on the medial surface of the medial pterygoid muscle. These fasciae are all continuous with the investing layer of the deep cervical fascia.

DEEP CERVICAL FASCIA

The deep cervical fascia is composed of layers that include the investing fascia, carotid sheath, visceral fascia, and vertebral fascia (Figures 11-2 and 11-3; see Chapter 3). Again, it is important to note that the layers of this fascia are continuous with each other and with the deep fascia of the face and jaws.

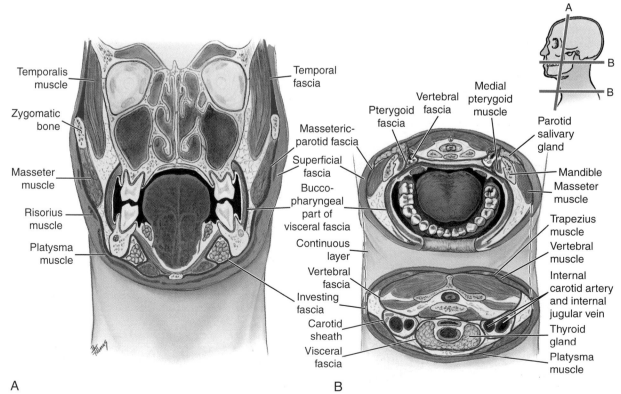

A   B

FIGURE 11-1 Frontal section **(A)** of the head highlighting the fasciae of the face. Transverse sections **(B)** at the oral cavity and neck highlighting the continuous nature of the investing fascia.

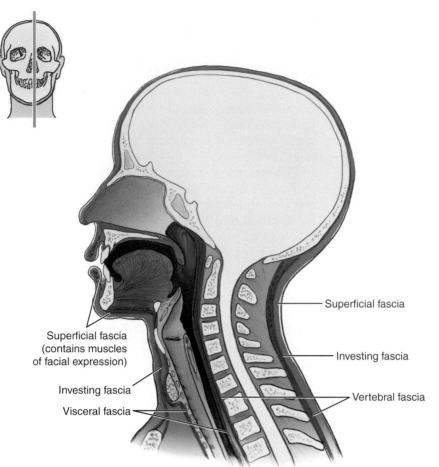

Superficial fascia

Superficial fascia
(contains muscles
of facial expression)

Investing fascia

Investing fascia

Visceral fascia

Vertebral fascia

FIGURE 11-2 Midsagittal section of the
head and neck highlighting the deep
cervical fasciae.

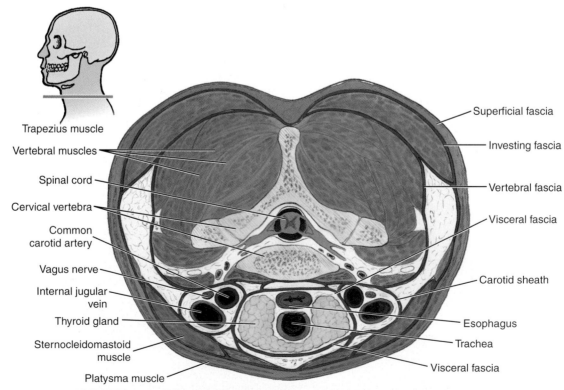

Trapezius muscle

Vertebral muscles

Spinal cord

Cervical vertebra

Common
carotid artery

Vagus nerve

Internal jugular
vein

Thyroid gland

Sternocleidomastoid
muscle

Platysma muscle

Superficial fascia

Investing fascia

Vertebral fascia

Visceral fascia

Carotid sheath

Esophagus

Trachea

Visceral fascia

FIGURE 11-3 Transverse section of the neck highlighting the deep cervical fasciae.

Investing Fascia.

The **investing fascia** is the most external layer of deep cervical fascia. This fascia surrounds the neck, continuing onto the masseteric-parotid fascia. This fascia also splits around two salivary glands (submandibular and parotid) and two muscles (sternocleidomastoid and trapezius), enclosing them completely. Branching laminae from this fascia also provide the deep fasciae that surround the infrahyoid muscles, from the hyoid bone inferiorly to the sternum.

Carotid Sheath and Visceral Fascia.

The **carotid sheath** (kah-**rot**-id) is a tube of deep cervical fascia deep to the investing fascia and sternocleidomastoid muscle, running inferiorly along each side of the neck from the base of the skull to the thorax. This sheath houses the internal carotid and common carotid arteries and the internal jugular vein, as well as the tenth cranial or vagus nerve. All these structures travel between the braincase and thorax.

Deep to the carotid sheath is the **visceral fascia** (**vis**-er-al) or pretracheal fascia, which is a single, midline tube of deep cervical fascia running inferiorly along the neck. This fascia surrounds the air and food passageway including the trachea, esophagus, and thyroid gland.

Nearer to the skull, the visceral fascia located posterior and lateral to the pharynx is known as the **buccopharyngeal fascia** (buk-o-fah-**rin**-je-al). This deep cervical fascial layer encloses the entire superior portion of the alimentary canal and is continuous with the fascia on the surface of the buccinator muscle, where that muscle and the superior pharyngeal constrictor muscle come together at the pterygomandibular raphe (see Chapter 4).

Vertebral Fascia.

The deepest layer of the deep cervical fascia, the **vertebral fascia** (**ver**-teh-brahl) or prevertebral fascia, covers the vertebrae, spinal column, and associated muscles. Some clinicians distinguish a branch of the vertebral fascia, called the *alar fascia*, which is said to run from the base of the skull to connect with the visceral fascia inferiorly in the neck.

FASCIAL SPACES

Potential spaces are created between the layers of fascia of the body because of the sheetlike nature of the fasciae. These potential spaces are termed **fascial spaces** or planes. Importantly, these fascial spaces are not actually empty spaces in healthy patients because they contain loose connective tissue. Other spaces are present in the head and neck but not created necessarily by the fascia.

Fascial Spaces of the Head and Neck

A dental professional must have knowledge of the anatomical aspects of the fascial spaces of the head and neck when examining a patient. These spaces are important because they can be involved in infections arising in dental tissues. These spaces also communicate with each other directly, as well as through their blood and lymph vessels. This communication may allow the spread of dental infection from an initial superficial area to more vital deeper structures. The spread of infection by way of these spaces may result in serious consequences. The role of spaces in the spread of dental infection is discussed further in Chapter 12. Again, the study of these spaces allows the clinician to also form a three-dimensional view of head and neck anatomy.

SPACES OF THE FACE AND JAWS

The major spaces of the face and jaws include the vestibular spaces of the maxilla and mandible; the canine, parotid, buccal, and masticatory spaces; the space of the body of the mandible; and the submental, submandibular, and sublingual spaces (Table 11-1). Importantly, these spaces can communicate with each other and with the cervical fascial spaces. Unlike the neck, the spaces of the face and jaws are often defined by the arrangement of muscles and bones, in addition to the fasciae. Thus many of the spaces are not considered fascial spaces.

Vestibular Space of the Maxilla.

The space of the upper jaw, the **vestibular space of the maxilla** (mak-**sil**-ah), is located medial to the buccinator muscle and inferior to the attachment of this muscle along the alveolar process of the maxilla (Figure 11-4). Its lateral wall is the oral mucosa. This space communicates with the maxillary molar teeth and periodontium and thus can become involved with infections of these tissues.

Vestibular Space of the Mandible.

The **vestibular space of the mandible** (**man**-di-bl) is located between the buccinator muscle and overlying oral mucosa (see Figure 11-4). This space is bordered by the attachment of the buccinator muscle onto the mandible. This important space of the lower jaw communicates with the mandibular teeth and periodontium, as well as the space of the body of the mandible.

Canine Space.

The **canine space** (**kay**-nine) is located superior to the upper lip and lateral to the apex of the maxillary canine (Figure 11-5). This space is deep to the overlying skin and muscles of facial expression that elevate the upper lip (levator labii superioris and zygomaticus

TABLE 11-1

MAJOR SPACES OF THE FACE AND JAWS WITH THEIR LOCATIONS, CONTENTS, AND COMMUNICATION PATTERNS

Space	Location	Contents	Communication Patterns
Maxillary vestibular space	Between buccinator muscle and oral mucosa		Maxillary teeth and periodontium
Mandibular vestibular space	Between buccinator muscle and oral mucosa		Mandibular teeth and periodontium, body of mandible
Canine	Within superficial fascia covering canine fossa		Buccal
Buccal	Lateral to buccinator muscle	Buccal fat pad	Canine, pterygomandibular, and body of mandible
Parotid	Within parotid gland	Parotid gland, facial nerve, external carotid artery, and retromandibular vein	
Masticator	Area of mandible and muscles of mastication	Temporal, submasseteric, and infratemporal spaces	All portions communicate with each other and submandibular and parapharyngeal
Temporal	Portion of masticator space between temporal fascia and temporalis muscle	Fat	Infratemporal and submasseteric
Infratemporal	Portion of masticator space between lateral pterygoid plate, maxillary tuberosity, and ramus	Maxillary artery and branches, mandibular nerve and branches, and pterygoid plexus	Temporal, submasseteric, submandibular, and parapharyngeal
Pterygomandibular	Portion of infratemporal space between medial pterygoid muscle and ramus	Inferior alveolar nerve and vessels	Submandibular and parapharyngeal
Submasseteric	Portion of masticator space between masseter muscle and external surface of ramus	Temporal and infratemporal	
Body of mandible	Periosteum covering mandible	Mandible and inferior alveolar nerve, artery, and vein	Vestibular space of mandible, buccal, submental, submandibular, and sublingual
Submental	Midline between symphysis and hyoid bone	Submental nodes and anterior jugular vein	Body of mandible, submandibular, and sublingual
Submandibular	Medial to mandible and inferior to mylohyoid muscle	Submandibular nodes and gland and facial artery	Infratemporal, body of mandible, submental, sublingual and parapharyngeal
Sublingual	Medial to mandible and superior to mylohyoid muscle	Sublingual gland and ducts, submandibular duct, lingual nerve and artery, and hypoglossal nerve	Body of mandible, submental, and submandibular

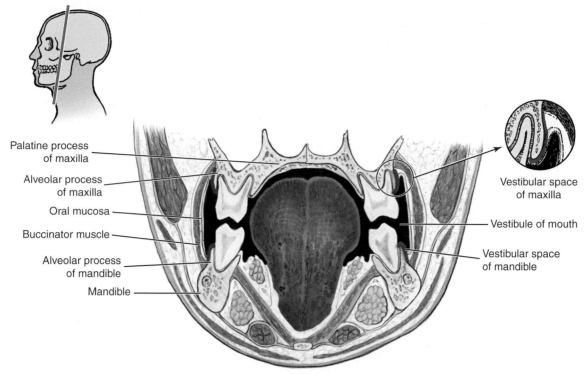

Palatine process of maxilla

Alveolar process of maxilla

Oral mucosa

Buccinator muscle

Alveolar process of mandible

Mandible

Vestibular space of maxilla

Vestibule of mouth

Vestibular space of mandible

FIGURE 11-4 Frontal section of the head highlighting the maxillary vestibular space and mandibular vestibular space.

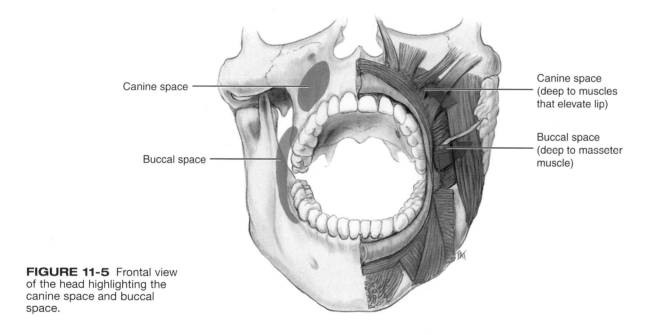

Canine space

Buccal space

Canine space (deep to muscles that elevate lip)

Buccal space (deep to masseter muscle)

FIGURE 11-5 Frontal view of the head highlighting the canine space and buccal space.

minor). The floor of the space is the canine fossa, which is covered by periosteum. This space is bordered anteriorly by the orbicularis oris muscle and posteriorly by the levator anguli oris muscle. The canine space communicates with the buccal space.

Buccal Space.

The **buccal space** is the fascial space formed between the buccinator muscle (actually the buccopharyngeal fascia) and masseter muscle (see Figure 11-5). Therefore the buccal space is inferior to the zygomatic arch, superior to the mandible, lateral to the buccinator muscle, and medial and anterior to the masseter muscle.

This bilateral space is partially covered by the platysma muscle, as well as by an extension of fascia from the parotid salivary gland capsule. The space contains the buccal fat pad. The buccal space communicates with the canine space, pterygomandibular space, and space of the body of the mandible.

Parotid Space.

The **parotid space** (pah-**rot**-id) is a fascial space created inside the investing fascial layer of the deep cervical fascia as it envelops the parotid salivary gland (Figure 11-6). The space contains not only the entire parotid gland but also much of the seventh cranial or facial nerve and a portion of the external carotid artery and retromandibular vein. The fascial boundaries of this space help to keep infections of the parotid salivary gland from spreading to other sites.

Masticator Space.

The **masticator space** (mass-ti-**kay**-tor) is a general term used to include the entire area of the mandible and muscles of mastication. Thus it includes the temporal, infratemporal, and submasseteric spaces, as well as the masseter muscle and ramus and body of the mandible. All portions of the space communicate with each other, as well as with the submandibular space and a cervical fascial space, the parapharyngeal space (discussed later).

A portion of the masticator space is the **temporal space** (**tem**-poh-ral), which is formed by the temporal fascia covering the temporalis muscle (Figure 11-7). This space is between the fascia and muscle and therefore extends from the superior temporal line inferiorly to the zygomatic arch and infratemporal crest. The space contains fat tissue and communicates with the infratemporal and submasseteric spaces.

The **infratemporal space** (in-frah-**tem**-poh-ral) occupies the infratemporal fossa, an area adjacent to the lateral pterygoid plate and maxillary tuberosity (Figure 11-8, *A*; see Figure 11-7). The space is bordered laterally by the medial surface of the mandible and the temporalis muscle. Its roof is formed by the infratemporal surface of the greater wing of the sphenoid bone. Medially, the space is bordered by the lateral pterygoid plate anteriorly and by the pharynx with its visceral layer of deep fascia posteriorly. There is no boundary inferiorly and posteriorly, where the infratemporal space is continuous with the cervical fascial space, the parapharyngeal space (discussed later).

The infratemporal space contains a portion of the maxillary artery as it branches, the mandibular nerve and its branches, and the pterygoid plexus of veins. It also houses the medial and lateral pterygoid muscles. This space communicates with the temporal and submasseteric spaces, as well as with the submandibular and parapharyngeal spaces.

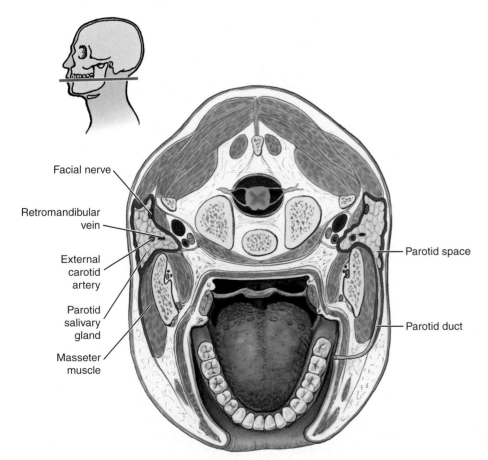

Facial nerve

Retromandibular vein

External carotid artery

Parotid salivary gland

Masseter muscle

Parotid space

Parotid duct

FIGURE 11-6 Transverse section of the head highlighting the parotid space.

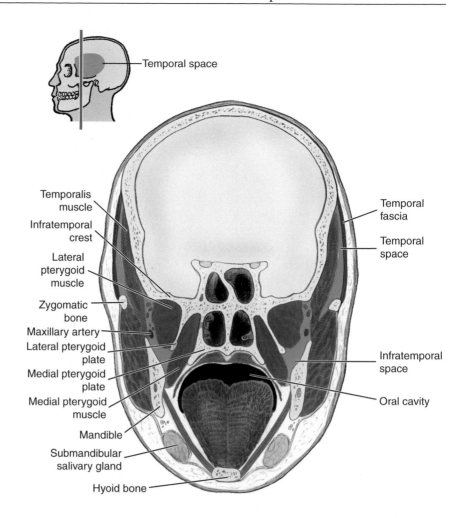

FIGURE 11-7 Frontal section of the head highlighting the temporal space and infratemporal space.

The **pterygomandibular space** (teh-ri-go-man-**dib**-you-lar) is a portion of the infratemporal space, formed by the lateral pterygoid muscle (roof), medial pterygoid muscle (medial wall), and mandibular ramus (lateral wall) (see Figure 11-8).

The pterygomandibular space is important because it contains the inferior alveolar nerve and vessels and is the injection site for the inferior alveolar local anesthetic block (see Chapter 9). This space communicates with the submandibular space and the parapharyngeal space of the neck (discussed later).

Another portion of the masticator space, the **submasseteric space** (sub-mas-et-**tehr**-ik), is located between the masseter muscle and external surface of the vertical ramus (Figure 11-9). This space communicates with the temporal and infratemporal spaces.

Space of the Body of the Mandible.
The **space of the body of the mandible** is formed by the periosteum, covering the body of the mandible from its symphysis to the anterior borders of the masseter and medial pterygoid muscles (Figure 11-10).

This potential space contains the mandible; a portion of the inferior alveolar nerve, artery, and vein; and the dental and alveolar branches of these vessels,

as well as the mental and incisive branches. The space of the mandible communicates with the vestibular space of the mandible, as well as with the buccal, submental, submandibular, and sublingual spaces.

Submental Space.
The **submental space** (sub-**men**-tal) is located in the midline between the mandibular symphysis and hyoid bone (Figure 11-11). The floor of this space is the superficial cervical fascia covering the suprahyoid muscles. The roof is the mylohyoid muscle, covered by the investing fascia. Forming the lateral boundaries of this space are the diverging anterior bellies of the digastric muscles.

The submental space contains the submental lymph nodes and the origin of the anterior jugular vein. The space communicates with the space of the body of the mandible and the submandibular and sublingual spaces.

Submandibular Space.
The **submandibular space** (sub-man-**dib**-you-lar) is located lateral and posterior to the submental space on each side of the jaws (Figure 11-12; see Figure 11-11). The cross-sectional shape of this bilateral potential

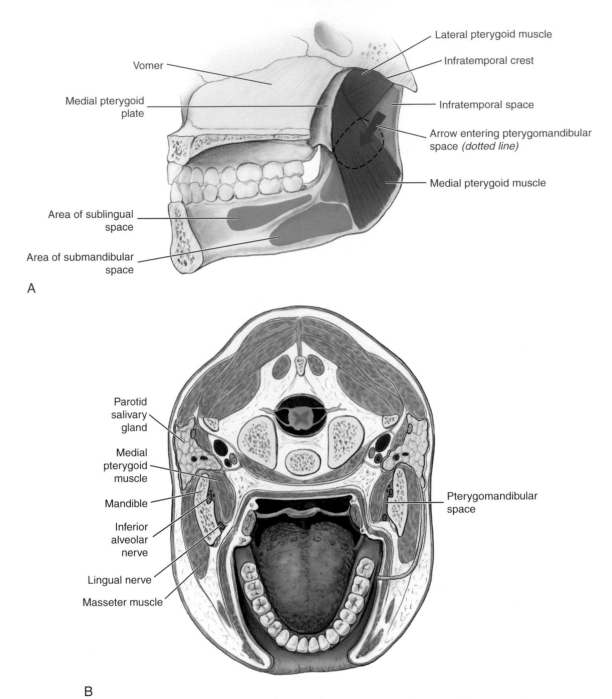

FIGURE 11-8 A, Median section of the skull highlighting the infratemporal space and pterygomandibular space. **B,** Transverse section of the head highlighting the pterygomandibular space.

space is triangular, with the mylohyoid line of the mandible being its superior boundary. The mylohyoid muscle forms the medial, as well as the superior, boundary of the space, and the hyoid bone creates its medial apex.

The submandibular space contains the submandibular lymph nodes, most of the submandibular salivary gland, and portions of the facial artery. This space communicates with the infratemporal, submental, and sublingual spaces and the parapharyngeal space of the

neck (discussed later). This space is usually involved if there is a spread of dental infection.

Sublingual Space.

The **sublingual space** (sub-**ling**-gwal) is located deep to the oral mucosa, thus making this tissue its roof (see Figure 11-12). The floor of this space is the mylohyoid muscle. Thus this muscle creates the division between the submandibular and sublingual spaces. The tongue and its intrinsic muscles form the medial boundary

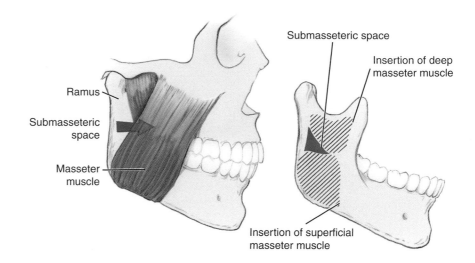

FIGURE 11-9 Lateral views of the face and mandible highlighting the submasseteric space.

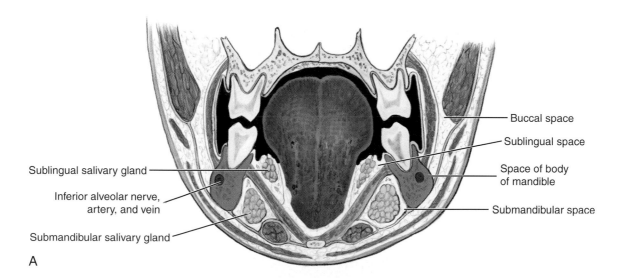

A

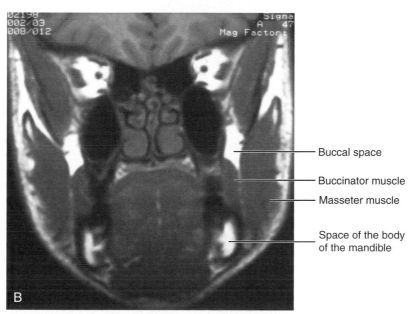

B

FIGURE 11-10 Frontal section of the head highlighting the space of the body of the mandible **(A, B).** (From Reynolds PA, Abrahams PH: McMinn's interactve clinical anatomy: head and neck, ed 2, London, 2001, Mosby Ltd.)

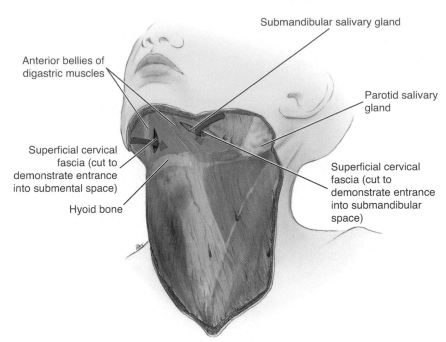

FIGURE 11-11 Anterolateral view of the neck. The skin has been removed, leaving the superficial cervical fascia in place *(platysma has been omitted)*. The location of the submental space at the midline and the two lateral submandibular spaces are indicated.

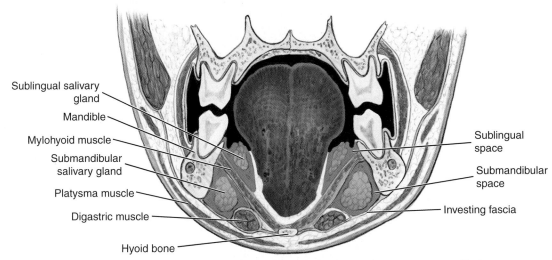

FIGURE 11-12 Frontal section of the head and neck highlighting the submandibular space and sublingual space.

of the sublingual space, and the mandible forms its lateral wall.

The sublingual space contains the sublingual salivary gland and ducts, the duct of the submandibular salivary gland, a portion of the lingual nerve and artery, and the twelfth cranial or hypoglossal nerve. The space communicates with the submental and submandibular spaces and the space of the body of the mandible.

CERVICAL FASCIAL SPACES

The major cervical fascial spaces include the parapharyngeal, retropharyngeal, and previsceral spaces (Figures 11-13 and 11-14; Table 11-2). These fascial spaces of the neck can communicate with the spaces of the face and jaws, as well as with each other. Most importantly, these spaces connect the spaces of the head and neck with those of the thorax, allowing dental infections to spread to vital organs such as the heart and lungs.

Parapharyngeal Space.

The **parapharyngeal space** (pare-ah-fah-**rin**-je-al) is a fascial space lateral to the pharynx and medial to the medial pterygoid muscle, paralleling the carotid sheath. The parapharyngeal space in its posterior portion is adjacent to the carotid sheath, which contains the internal and common carotid arteries and the inter-

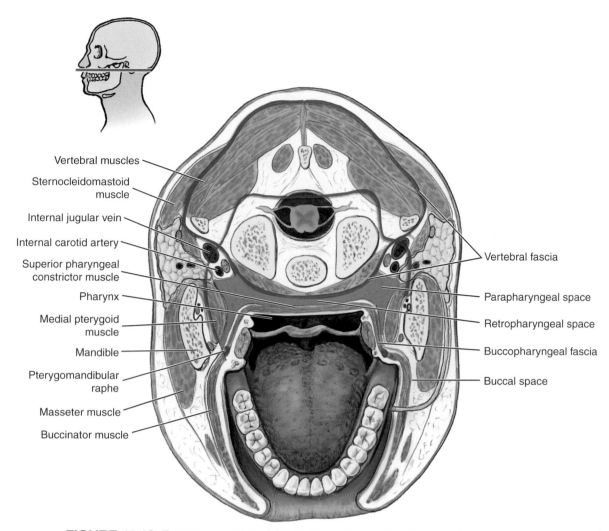

Vertebral muscles

Sternocleidomastoid muscle

Internal jugular vein

Internal carotid artery

Superior pharyngeal constrictor muscle

Pharynx

Medial pterygoid muscle

Mandible

Pterygomandibular raphe

Masseter muscle

Buccinator muscle

Vertebral fascia

Parapharyngeal space

Retropharyngeal space

Buccopharyngeal fascia

Buccal space

FIGURE 11-13 Transverse section of the oral cavity highlighting the retropharyngeal space and parapharyngeal space.

nal jugular vein, as well as the tenth cranial or vagus nerve. It is also adjacent to the ninth, eleventh, and twelfth cranial nerves as they exit the cranial cavity.

Anteriorly, the parapharyngeal space extends to the pterygomandibular raphe, where it is continuous with the infratemporal and buccal spaces. The parapharyngeal space anteriorly contains a few lymph nodes. Posteriorly, the space extends around the pharynx, where it is continuous with another cervical fascial space, the retropharyngeal space. Dental

MAJOR CERVICAL FASCIAL SPACES WITH THEIR LOCATIONS, CONTENTS, AND COMMUNICATION PATTERNS

Fascial Space	Location	Contents	Communication Patterns
Parapharyngeal	Lateral to the visceral fascia around pharynx	Nodes	Masticator, submandibular, retropharyngeal, previsceral, and adjacent to carotid sheath
Retropharyngeal	Between vertebral and visceral fasciae		Parapharyngeal
Previsceral	Between visceral and investing fasciae	Nodes and cervical vessels	Parapharyngeal

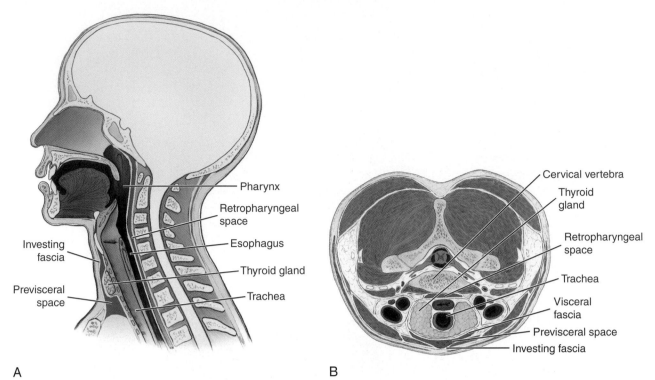

A   B

FIGURE 11-14 A, Midsagittal section of the head and neck highlighting the retropharyngeal space and previsceral space. **B,** Transverse section of the neck highlighting the retropharyngeal space and previsceral space.

infections can become dangerous when they reach the parapharyngeal space because of its connection to the retropharyngeal space.

Retropharyngeal Space.

The **retropharyngeal space** (re-troh-fah-**rin**-je-al) is a fascial space located immediately posterior to the pharynx, between the vertebral and visceral fasciae. The retropharyngeal space extends from the base of the skull, where it is posterior to the superior pharyngeal constrictor muscle, inferiorly to the thorax.

Because of the rapidity with which dental infections can travel inferiorly along the retropharyngeal space, it is also known as the "danger space." This space communicates with the parapharyngeal spaces.

Previsceral Space.

The **previsceral space** (pre-**vis**-er-al) is located between the visceral and investing fasciae, anterior to the trachea. The previsceral space communicates with the parapharyngeal spaces.

Identification Exercises

Identify the structures on the following diagrams by filling in each blank with the correct anatomical term. You can check your answers by looking back at the figure indicated in parentheses for each identification diagram.

1. (Figure 11-1, *A*)

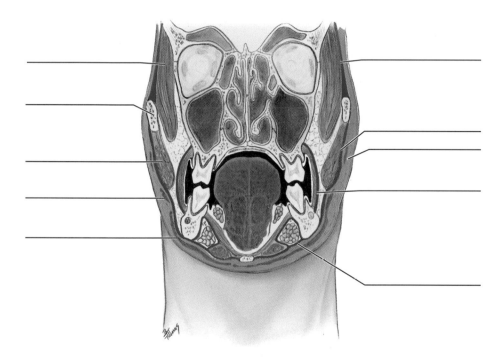

2. (Figure 11-1, *B*)

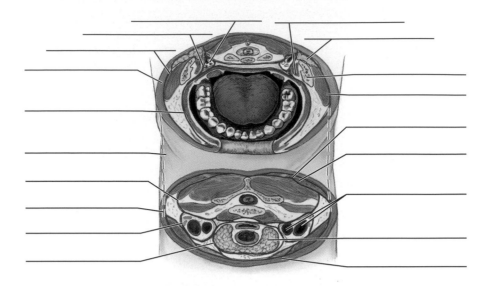

3. (Figure 11-2)

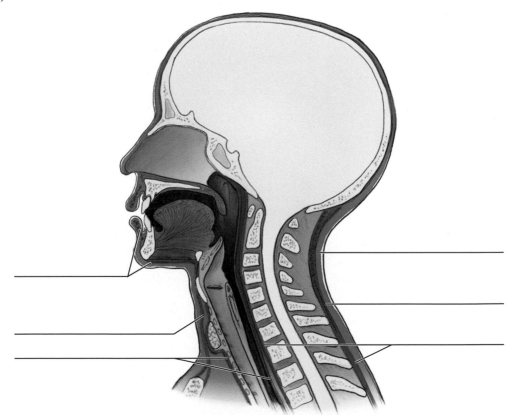

4. (Figure 11-3)

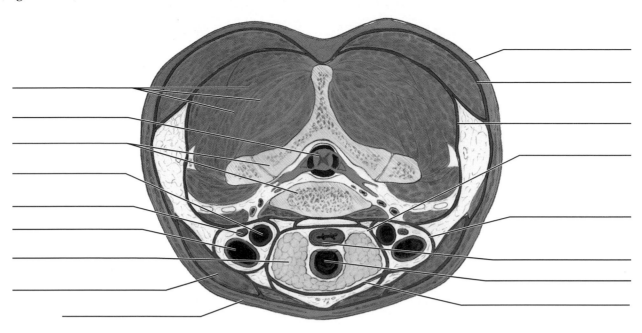

5. (Figure 11-4)

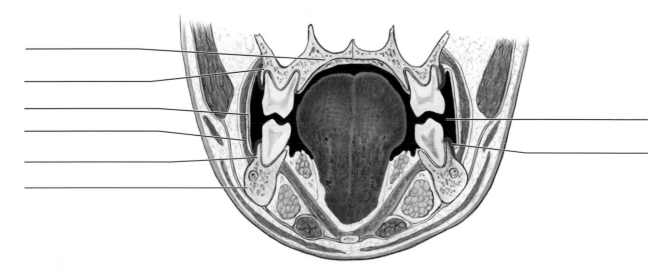

6. (Figure 11-5)

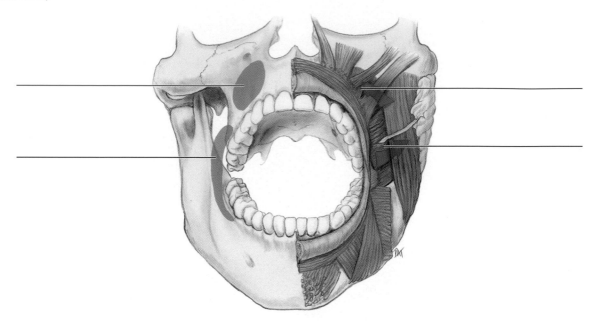

7. (Figure 11-6)

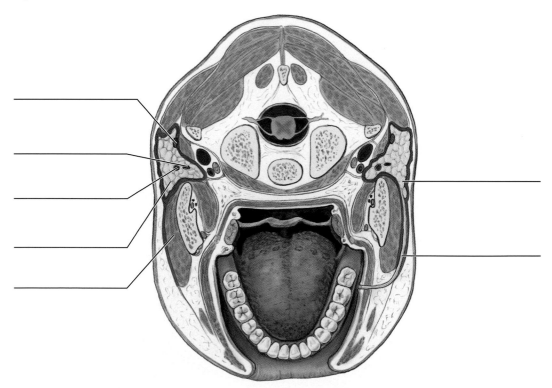

8. (Figure 11-7)

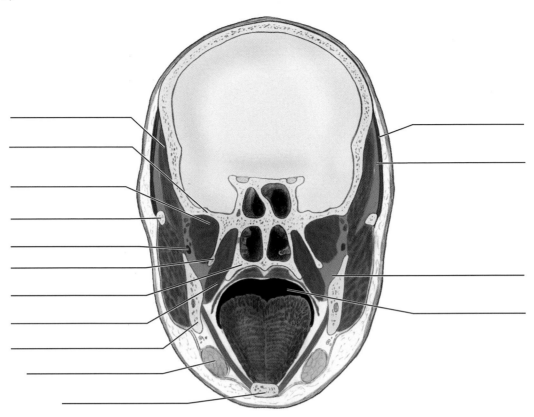

9. (Figure 11-8, *A*)

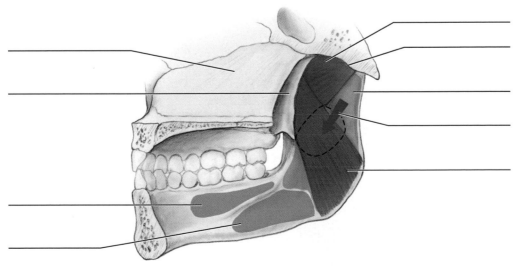

10. (Figure 11-8, *B*)

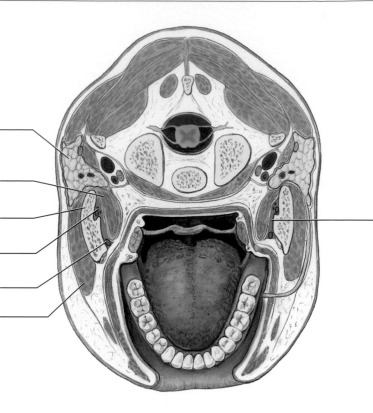

11. (Figure 11-9)

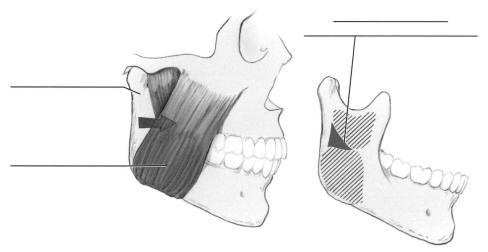

12. (Figure 11-10, *A*)

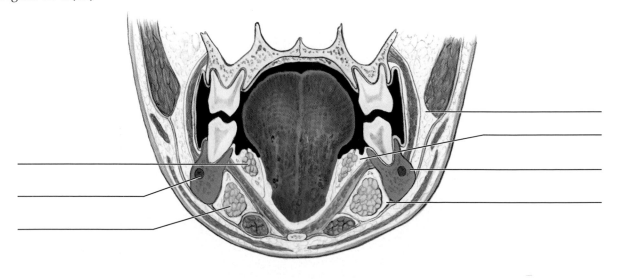

13. (Figure 11-11)

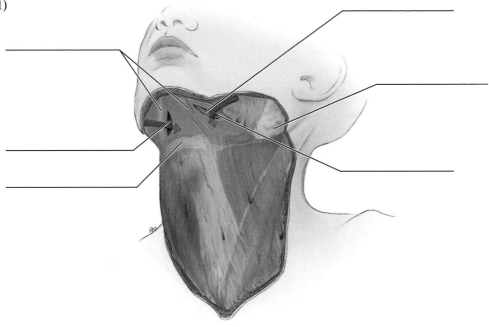

14. (Figure 11-12)

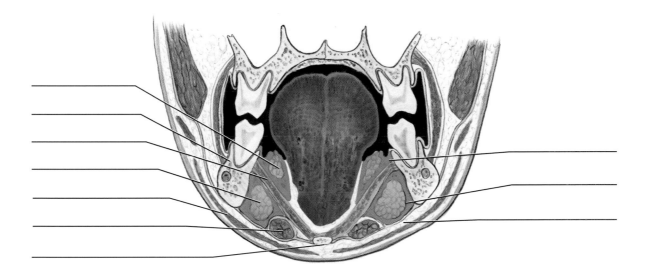

15. (Figure 11-13)

16. (Figure 11-14, *A*)

17. (Figure 11-14, *B*)

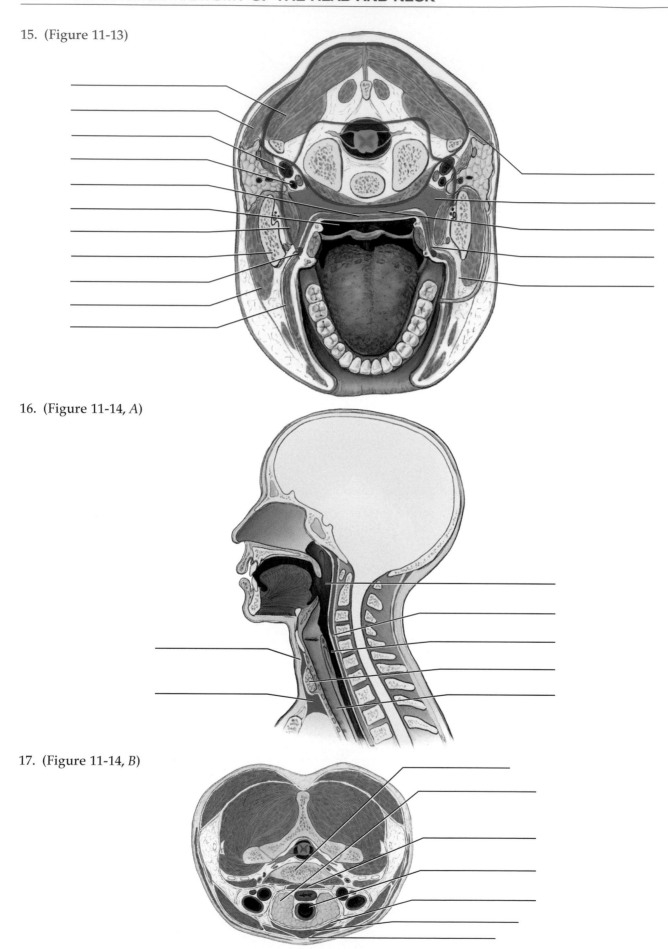

■ REVIEW QUESTIONS

1. Which of the following describes deep fascia?
   A. Dense and inelastic tissue forming sheaths around deep structures
   B. Fatty and elastic fibrous tissue found just deep to the skin
   C. Potential spaces containing loose connective tissue
   D. Fatty and elastic fibrous tissue forming spaces under the skin
   E. Dense and inelastic deep structures of the vascular system

2. Which of the following is covered by the carotid sheath?
   A. Internal and common carotid arteries and tenth cranial nerve
   B. External and common carotid arteries and fifth cranial nerve
   C. External jugular vein and tenth cranial nerve
   D. Internal jugular vein and fifth cranial nerve

3. In which of the following spaces is the pterygoid plexus of veins located?
   A. Parotid space
   B. Temporal space
   C. Infratemporal space
   D. Buccal space
   E. Parapharyngeal space

4. The masticator space includes the submasseteric space and which of the following?
   A. Submental space
   B. Submandibular space
   C. Sublingual space
   D. Pterygomandibular space
   E. Retropharyngeal space

5. Which of the following tissues surrounds the space of the body of the mandible?
   A. Fatty tissue
   B. Loose connective tissue
   C. Periosteum
   D. Elastic tissue

6. The submandibular space communicates most directly with this space:
   A. Temporal
   B. Parotid
   C. Buccal
   D. Sublingual
   E. Canine

7. The parapharyngeal space is located between the superior pharyngeal constrictor muscle and this muscle:
   A. Lateral pterygoid
   B. Medial pterygoid
   C. Mylohyoid
   D. Masseter
   E. Buccinator

8. Which space is located in the midline between the mandibular symphysis and the hyoid bone?
   A. Retropharyngeal space
   B. Sublingual space
   C. Submandibular space
   D. Submental space
   E. Submasseteric space

9. Which of the following nerves is located in the pterygomandibular space?
   A. Infraorbital nerve
   B. Posterior superior alveolar nerve
   C. Inferior alveolar nerve
   D. Anterior superior alveolar nerve

10. Which of the following areas directly communicates with the retropharyngeal space?
    A. Masticator space
    B. Submandibular space
    C. Previsceral space
    D. Parapharyngeal space

11. Which of the following muscles forms the roof of the pterygomandibular space?
    A. Lateral pterygoid muscle
    B. Medial pterygoid muscle
    C. Temporalis muscle
    D. Sternocleidomastoid muscle

12. Which of the following blood vessels is located in the sublingual space?
    A. Facial artery
    B. Anterior jugular vein
    C. Lingual artery
    D. Inferior alveolar vein

13. Which of the following spaces is also known as the "danger space"?
    A. Parapharyngeal space
    B. Body of the mandible
    C. Submandibular space
    D. Retropharyngeal space

14. Which of the following fascial structures are considered deep fascia of the face?
A. Masseteric-parotid fascia
B. Investing fascia
C. Visceral fascia
D. Carotid sheath

15. Which of the following structures are located in the superficial fascia of the head and neck?
A. Temporalis muscle
B. Muscles of facial expression
C. Parotid salivary gland
D. Thyroid gland

Spread of Dental Infection

LEARNING OBJECTIVES

After studying this chapter, the reader should be able to do the following:

1. Define and pronounce all the key terms and anatomical terms in this chapter.
2. Discuss the spread of infection to the sinuses and by the vascular system, lymphatics, and spaces to other areas in the head and neck region.
3. Trace the routes of the spread of dental infection in the head and neck region on a diagram, skull, and patient.
4. Discuss the lesions and complications that can occur with the spread of dental infection in the head and neck region.
5. Discuss the prevention of the spread of dental infection during patient care.
6. Correctly complete the review questions and activities for this chapter.
7. Integrate the knowledge of the spread of dental infection into clinical dental practice.

KEY TERMS

Abducens Nerve Paralysis (ab-**doo**-senz pah-**ral**-i-sis) Loss of function of the sixth cranial nerve.

Abscess (**ab**-ses) Infection with suppuration resulting from the entrapment of pathogens in a contained space.

Bacteremia (bak-ter-**ee**-me-ah) Bacteria traveling within the vascular system.

Cavernous Sinus Thrombosis (**kav**-er-nus **sy**-nus throm-**bo**-sus) Infection of the cavernous venous sinus.

(Continued)

KEY TERMS (continued)

Cellulitis (sel-you-**lie**-tis) Diffuse inflammation of soft tissue spaces.

Embolus, Emboli (**em**-bol-us, **em**-bol-eye) Foreign material or thrombus traveling in the blood that can block the vessel.

Fistula, Fistulae (**fis**-chool-ah, **fis**-chool-ay) Passageway in the skin, mucosa, or even bone allowing drainage of an abscess at the surface.

Ludwig's Angina (**lood**-vigz an-**ji**-nah) Serious infection of the submandibular space, with a risk of spread to the neck and chest.

Lymphadenopathy (lim-fad-in-**op**-ah-thee) Process in which there is an increase in the size and a change in the consistency of lymphoid tissue.

Maxillary Sinusitis (**sy**-nu-**si**-tis) Infection of the maxillary sinus.

Meningitis (men-in-**jite**-is) Inflammation of the meninges of the brain or spinal cord.

Normal Flora (**flor**-ah) Resident microorganisms that usually do not cause infections.

Odontogenic Infections (o-**dont**-o-jen-ic) Dental infections involving the teeth or associated tissues.

Opportunistic Infections (op-or-tu-**nis**-tik) Normal flora creating an infectious process because the body's defenses are compromised.

Osteomyelitis (os-tee-o-my-il-**ite**-is) Inflammation of bone marrow.

Paresthesia (par-es-**the**-ze-ah) Abnormal sensation from an area such as burning or prickling.

Pathogens (**path**-ah-jens) Flora that are not normal body residents and can cause an infection.

Perforation (per-fo-**ray**-shun) Abnormal hole in a hollow organ such as in the wall of a sinus.

Primary Node Lymph node that drains lymph from a particular region.

Pustule (**pus**-tule) Small, elevated, circumscribed suppuration-containing lesion of either the skin or the oral mucosa.

Secondary Node Lymph node that drains lymph from a primary node.

Stoma (**stow**-mah) Opening, such as that which occurs with a fistula.

Suppuration (sup-u-**ray**-shun) Pus containing pathogenic bacteria, white blood cells, tissue fluid, and debris.

Thrombus, Thrombi (**throm**-bus, **throm**-by) Clot that forms on the inner blood vessel wall.

INFECTIOUS PROCESS

A dental professional should understand the infectious process that allows a microorganism to create disease. The healthy body usually lives in balance with a number of resident **normal flora.** However, certain nonresident microorganisms called **pathogens** can invade and initiate an infection. Pathogens contain certain factors that help further the infection process such as capsules, spores, and toxins.

DENTAL INFECTIONS

Dental infections or **odontogenic infections** involving the teeth or associated tissues are caused by oral pathogens that are predominantly anaerobic and usually of more than one species. These organisms inhabit the surface of the teeth and oral mucous membranes and are also found in the gingival crevice and saliva. These infections can be of dental origin or can arise from a nonodontogenic source. Infections of dental origin usually originate from progressive dental caries or extensive periodontal disease, even with implant placement (periimplantitis). Most odontogenic infections result initially from the formation of dental plaque. Pathogens can also be introduced deeper into the oral tissues by the trauma caused by dental procedures such as the contamination of dental surgical sites (e.g., tooth extraction) and needle tracks made during local anesthetic administration. Treatment consists of removal of the source of infection, systemic antibiotics, and area drainage.

Some dental infections are secondary infections incited by an infection from the tissues surrounding the oral cavity such as the skin, tonsils, ears, or sinuses. These nonodontogenic sources of infections must be diagnosed and treated early. Prompt referral to the patient's physician will prevent further spread and potential complications.

Dental Infection Lesions

Dental infections can result in various types of lesions, depending on the location of the infection and thus the type of tissue involved. Dental infections can result in an abscess, cellulitis, or osteomyelitis in the head and neck region.

ABSCESS

An oral **abscess** occurs when there is localized entrapment of pathogens from a dental infection in a closed tissue space such as that created by the oral mucosa (Figures 12-1 to 12-5). The abscess is filled with **suppuration.** Suppuration is pus that contains pathogenic bacteria, white blood cells, tissue fluid, and debris. Periapical abscess formation can occur with progressive caries, when pathogens invade the usually sterile pulp and the infection spreads apically. Pathogens can also become entrapped in deep pockets in cases of severe periodontal disease and cause a periodontal abscess. An erupting third molar can cause a pericoronal abscess (pericoronitis).

Abscess formation may not be detectable radiographically during the early stages. In the later stages

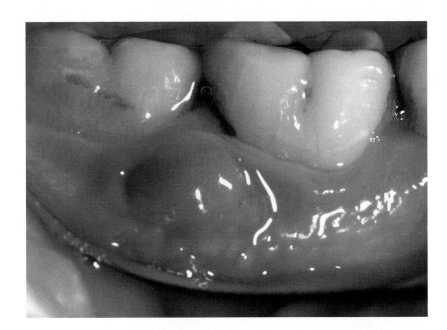

FIGURE 12-1 Intact periodontal abscess formation noted between the apices of the permanent mandibular first and second molars.

of infection, abscess formation can lead to the formation of a passageway or **fistula** (plural, **fistulae**) in the skin, oral mucosa, or even bone that allows drainage of the infection and creates suppuration on a surface (see Figures 12-2 and 12-3). The infectious process causes the overlying tissue to undergo necrosis, which allows this tract or canal to form in the tissue. The opening of the fistula is called a **stoma.** If the dental infection is surrounded by the alveolar bone, it will break down the bone in its thinnest portion (either the facial or lingual cortical plate), following the path of least resistance, and thus will be noted

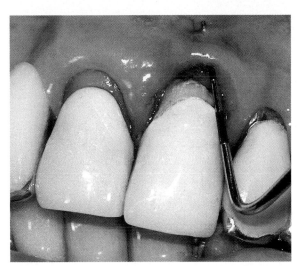

FIGURE 12-3 Periodontal abscess of the permanent maxillary central incisor with fistula and stoma formation (probe inserted) in the maxillary vestibule.

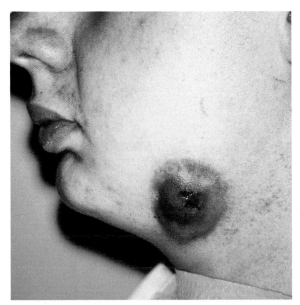

FIGURE 12-2 Extraoral abscess on the buccal skin surface resulting from the formation of a fistula and stoma caused by periapical involvement of the permanent mandibular second molar. (Courtesy Dr. Mark Gabrielson.)

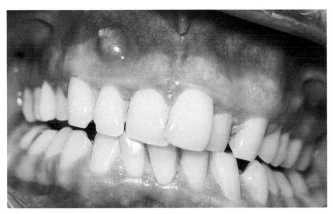

FIGURE 12-4 Periapical abscess of the permanent maxillary lateral incisor with pustule formation.

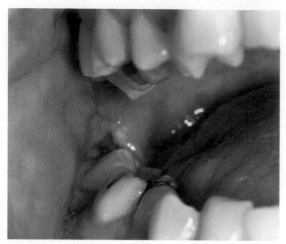

FIGURE 12-5 Pericoronal abscess of the permanent mandibular third molar with abscess formation (pericoronitis).

radiographically. The abscess can be either acute or chronic in nature.

The soft tissue over a fistula in the alveolar bone may also have an extraoral or intraoral **pustule.** A pustule is a small, elevated, circumscribed lesion of either the skin or oral mucosa that contains suppuration (see Figure 12-4). The position of the pustule is determined largely by the relationship between the fistula and the overlying muscle attachments. Again, the infection will follow the path of least resistance (Table 12-1). Importantly, muscle attachments to the bones, unlike the other facial soft tissues, serve as barriers to the spread of infection.

CELLULITIS

Cellulitis of the face and neck can also occur with dental infections, resulting in the diffuse inflammation

TABLE 12-1

TEETH AND ASSOCIATED PERIODONTIUM MOST COMMONLY INVOLVED IN CLINICAL PRESENTATIONS OF ABSCESSES AND FISTULAE*

Clinical Presentation of Lesion	Teeth and Associated Periodontium Most Commonly Involved
Maxillary vestibule	Maxillary central or lateral incisor, all surfaces and root Maxillary canine, all surfaces and root (short root inferior to levator anguli oris) Maxillary premolars, buccal surfaces and roots Maxillary molars, buccal surfaces or buccal roots (short roots inferior to buccinator)
Penetration of nasal floor	Maxillary central incisor, root
Nasolabial skin region	Maxillary canine, all surfaces and root (long root superior to levator anguli oris)
Palate	Maxillary lateral incisor, lingual surface and root Maxillary premolars, lingual surfaces and roots Maxillary molars, lingual surfaces or palatal roots
Perforation into maxillary sinus	Maxillary molars, buccal surface and buccal roots (long roots)
Buccal skin surface	Maxillary molars, buccal surfaces and buccal roots (long roots superior to buccinator) Mandibular first and second molars, buccal surfaces and buccal roots (long roots inferior to buccinator)
Mandibular vestibule	Mandibular incisors, all surfaces and roots (short roots superior to mentalis) Mandibular canine and premolars, all surfaces and roots (all roots superior to depressors) Mandibular first and second molars, buccal surfaces and roots (short roots superior to buccinator)
Submental skin region	Mandibular incisors, root (long roots inferior to mentalis)
Sublingual region	Mandibular first molar, lingual surface and roots (all roots superior to mylohyoid) Mandibular second molar, lingual surface and roots (short roots superior to mylohyoid)
Submandibular skin region	Mandibular second molar, lingual surface and roots (long roots inferior to mylohyoid) Mandibular third molars, all surfaces and roots (all roots inferior to mylohyoid)

*Only permanent teeth are considered in this table.

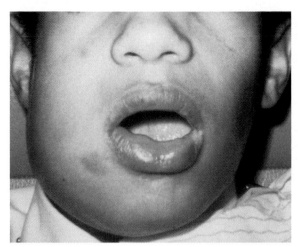

FIGURE 12-6 Cellulitis involving the buccal space resulting from an abscess of the permanent mandibular first molar with swelling noted. (Courtesy Dr. Mark Gabrielson.)

of soft tissue spaces (Figure 12-6; see Chapter 11). The clinical signs and symptoms are pain, tenderness, redness, and diffuse edema of the involved soft tissue space, causing a massive and firm swelling (Table 12-2). Difficulty swallowing (dysphagia) or restricted eye opening (ptosis) may also happen if the cellulitis occurs within the pharynx or orbital regions, respectively. Usually the infection remains localized and a facial abscess tends to form; if not initially treated, it may discharge on the facial surface. Without treatment, cellulitis can possibly spread due to perforation of the surrounding bone, causing serious complications such as Ludwig's angina (discussed later).

Cellulitis is treated by administration of antibiotics and removal of the cause of the infection.

OSTEOMYELITIS

Another type of lesion that can be related to dental infections is **osteomyelitis,** an inflammation of the bone marrow. Osteomyelitis can locally involve any bone in the body or can be generalized. This inflammation develops from the invasion of the tissue of a long bone by pathogens, usually from a skin or pharyngeal infection. In osteomyelitis involving the jawbones, the pathogens are most likely to derive from a periapical abscess, from an extension of cellulitis, or from contamination of a surgical site (Figure 12-7).

Osteomyelitis most commonly occurs in the mandible; it occurs only rarely in the maxilla because of the mandible's thicker cortical plates and reduced vascularization. Continuation of osteomyelitis leads to bone resorption and formation of sequestra, pieces of dead bone separated from the sound bone within the area. This bone damage can be detected by radiographic evaluation (see Figure 12-7).

Paresthesia, evidenced by burning or prickling, may develop in the mandible if the infection involves the mandibular canal carrying the inferior alveolar nerve. Many patients say it feels like "pins and needles." Localized paresthesia of the lower lip may occur if the infection is distal to the mental foramen where the mental nerve exits. Treatment consists of drainage, surgical removal of any sequestra, and antibiotic administration; in some patients the additional use of hyperbaric oxygen may be necessary.

TABLE 12-2

SPACES, TEETH, AND PERIODONTIUM POSSIBLY INVOLVED WITH A CLINICAL PRESENTATION OF CELLULITIS RESULTING FROM THE SPREAD OF DENTAL INFECTION*

Clinical Presentation of Lesion	Space Involved	Teeth and Associated Periodontium Most Commonly Involved in Infection
Infraorbital, zygomatic, and buccal regions	Buccal space	Maxillary premolars and maxillary and mandibular molars
Posterior border of mandible	Parotid space	Not generally of odontogenic origin
Submental region	Submental space	Mandibular anterior teeth
Unilateral submandibular region	Submandibular space	Mandibular posterior teeth
Bilateral submandibular region	Submental, sublingual, and submandibular spaces with Ludwig's angina	Spread of mandibular dental infection
Lateral cervical region	Parapharyngeal space	Spread of mandibular dental infection

*Only permanent teeth are considered in this table.

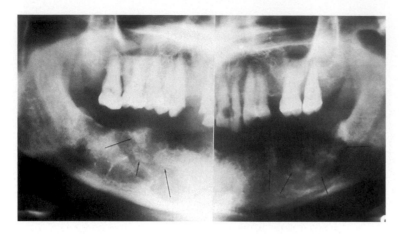

FIGURE 12-7 Panoramic radiograph of osteomyelitis, with bone resorption and formation of sequestra *(arrows)*.

Today, osteomyelitis of the jaw is uncommon because dental care and antibiotics are readily available.

Medically Compromised Patients

Normal flora usually do not create an infectious process. If, however, the body's natural defenses are compromised, then they can create **opportunistic infections.** Medically compromised individuals include those with AIDS, diabetes, or cancer and those undergoing cancer or transplant therapy (Figure 12-8). Some patients have a higher risk of complications resulting from dental infections because of their medical histories. Patients in this category include those at risk for infective endocarditis or infection with their implanted prosthetic joints.

INFECTION RESISTANCE FACTORS

More than half of the gram-negative anaerobic bacteria are capable of producing the beta-lactamase enzyme, which is responsible for the initial etiology of head and neck infections, as well as many treatment failures in dental infections. This enzyme may not only survive penicillin therapy but also may shield penicillin-susceptible co-pathogens from the activity of penicillin by releasing the free enzyme into their environment. Careful use of antimicrobials in the future may reduce and control the emergence of penicillin-resistant organisms.

SPREAD OF DENTAL INFECTIONS

Many odontogenic infections that start in the teeth and associated oral tissues can have significant consequences if they spread to vital tissues or organs. Usually a localized abscess establishes a fistula in the skin, oral mucosa, or associated bone, allowing natural drainage of the infection and diminishing the risk of spread of the infection. However, fistula formation or even establishment of drainage does not always occur. Occasionally, a dental infection can spread to the paranasal sinuses or can be spread by the vascular system, lymphatics, or spaces in the head and neck. Reviewing the communication patterns that are possible in these various tissues is important so as to understand the possible routes of infection that may occur (see Chapters 3, 6, 10, and 11).

Spread to the Paranasal Sinuses

The paranasal sinuses of the skull can become infected as a result of the direct spread of infection from the teeth and associated oral tissues, resulting in a **secondary sinusitis.** A **perforation,** an abnormal hole in the wall of the sinus, can also be caused by an infection.

MAXILLARY SINUSITIS

Secondary sinusitis of dental origin occurs mainly in the maxillary sinuses because the maxillary posterior teeth and associated tissues are in close proximity to these sinuses. Thus **maxillary sinusitis** can result from

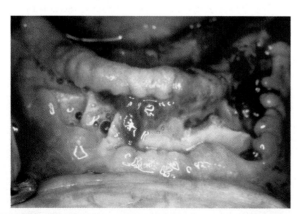

FIGURE 12-8 Osteoradionecrosis of the mandible with loss of bone vitality and inflammation noted after radiation therapy for oral cancer. This therapy and its result increases the risk of dental infections due to the medically compromised situation.

the spread of infection from a periapical abscess initiated by a maxillary posterior tooth that perforates the sinus floor to involve the sinus mucosa. In addition, a contaminated tooth or root fragments can be displaced into the maxillary sinus during an extraction, creating an infection.

However, most infections of the maxillary sinuses are not of dental origin but are caused by an upper respiratory infection, an infection in the nasal region that spreads to the sinuses. An infection in one sinus can travel through the nasal cavity to other sinuses and lead to serious complications for the patient such as infection of the cranial cavity and brain. Thus it is important that any sinusitis be treated aggressively by the patient's physician to eliminate the initial infection.

The symptoms of sinusitis are headache, usually near the involved sinus, and foul-smelling nasal or pharyngeal discharge, possibly with fever and weakness. The skin over the involved sinus can be tender, hot, and red due to the inflammation in the area. Difficulty in breathing (dyspnea) occurs, as well as pain, when the nasal passages become blocked by the effects of tissue inflammation. Early radiographic evidence of sinusitis is the thickening of the sinus walls, with subsequent radiographic evaluation showing increased opacity and possibly perforation. A panoramic radiographic view of the skull is helpful because bilateral comparisons can be made. Even magnetic resonance imaging (MRI) may be indicated.

Acute sinusitis usually responds to antibiotic therapy, while drainage is aided by the use of decongestants. Surgery may be necessary in cases of chronic maxillary sinusitis to enlarge the ostia of the lateral walls in the nasal cavity so that adequate drainage can diminish the effects of the infection. The surgical approach to the maxillary sinus is through the thin bone of the canine fossa. Recent studies show that removal of the toxic mucus with its inflammatory products is of prime importance in chronic sinusitis.

Spread by Vascular System

The vascular system of the head and neck can allow the spread of infection from the teeth and associated oral tissues because pathogens can travel in the veins and drain the infected oral site into other tissues or organs. The spread of dental infection by way of the vascular system can occur because of bacteremia or an infected thrombus.

BACTEREMIA

Bacteria traveling in the vascular system can cause transient **bacteremia**, which can occur during dental treatment. In an individual with a high risk for infective endocarditis, these bacteria may lodge in the compromised tissues and set up serious infection deep in the heart, which can result in massive and fatal heart damage. Such a patient may need antibiotic premedication to prevent bacteremia from occurring during invasive dental treatment. Bacteremia may also be implicated in patients at risk for deep tissue infection surrounding a newly placed prosthesis device or those placed in medically compromised patients. These patients may also need antibiotic premedication to prevent bacteremia from occurring during invasive dental treatment.

CAVERNOUS SINUS THROMBOSIS

An infected intravascular clot or **thrombus** (plural, **thrombi**) can dislodge from the inner blood vessel wall and travel as an **embolus** (plural, **emboli**). Emboli can travel in the veins, draining the oral cavity into areas such as the dural venous sinuses within the cranial cavity. These dural sinuses are channels by which blood is conveyed from the cerebral veins into the veins of the head and neck, particularly the internal jugular vein. However, because these veins lack functional valves, venous blood can flow both into and out of the cranial cavity.

The cavernous sinus is most likely to be involved in the possible fatal spread of dental infection. An infection of this venous sinus is called **cavernous sinus thrombosis**. The cavernous sinus is located on the side of the body of the sphenoid bone. Each cavernous venous sinus communicates with the one on the opposite side and also with the pterygoid plexus of veins and the superior ophthalmic vein, which anastomoses with the facial vein. These major veins drain teeth through the posterior superior and inferior alveolar veins and the lips through the superior and inferior labial veins.

None of these major veins that communicate with the cavernous sinus have valves to prevent the retrograde flow of blood back into the cavernous sinus. Therefore dental infections that drain into these major veins may initiate an inflammatory response resulting in an increase in blood stasis, thrombus formation, and increasing extravascular fluid pressure. Increased pressure can reverse the direction of venous blood flow, enabling the transport of the infected thrombus into this venous sinus and thus causing cavernous sinus thrombosis.

Needle track contamination can also result in a spread of infection to the pterygoid plexus if a posterior superior alveolar anesthetic block is incorrectly administered. Nonodontogenic infections of the area considered by physicians to be the "dangerous triangle of the face," the orbital region, nasal region, and paranasal sinuses, also may result in the spread of infection to the cavernous venous sinus.

The signs and symptoms of cavernous sinus thrombosis include fever, drowsiness, and rapid pulse. In addition, there is loss of function of the sixth cranial nerve or abducens because it runs through the cavernous venous sinus, resulting in **abducens nerve paralysis.** Because the muscle supplied by the nerve moves the eyeball laterally, inability to perform this movement suggests nerve damage. Additionally, the patient usually has double vision (diplopia) because of the restricted movement of the one eye, as well as edema of the eyelids and conjunctivae, tearing (lacrimation), and extruded eyeballs (exophthalmus), depending on the course of the infection (Figure 12-9).

With cavernous sinus thrombosis there may also be damage to the other cranial nerves such as the oculomotor nerve (third) and trochlear nerve (fourth), as well as to the ophthalmic and maxillary divisions of the trigeminal nerve (fifth) and changes in the tissues they innervate because all these nerves travel in the cavernous sinus wall. Finally, this infection can be fatal because it may lead to **meningitis,** inflammation of the meninges in the brain or spinal cord, which requires immediate hospitalization with intravenous antibiotics and anticoagulants.

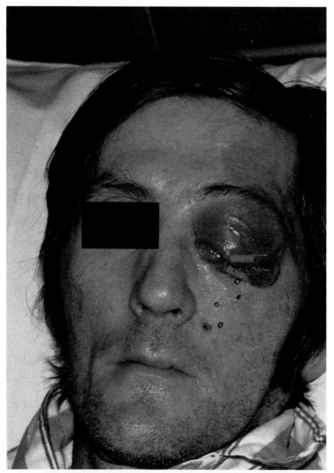

FIGURE 12-9 Cavernous sinus thrombosis, an infection of the venous sinus, with edema of the eyelids and conjunctivae, tearing, and extruded eyeballs. (From Reynolds PA, Abrahams PH: *McMinn's interactive clinical anatomy: head and neck*, ed 2, London, 2001, Mosby Ltd.)

Spread by Lymphatics

The lymphatics of the head and neck can allow the spread of infection from the teeth and associated oral tissues. This occurs because the pathogens can travel in the lymph through the lymphatic vessels that connect the series of nodes from the oral cavity to other tissues or organs. Thus these pathogens can move from a **primary node** near the infected site to a **secondary node** at a distant site.

The route of dental infection traveling through the nodes varies according to the teeth involved. The submental nodes drain the mandibular incisors and their associated tissues. Then the submental nodes empty into the submandibular nodes or directly into the deep cervical nodes. The submandibular nodes are the primary nodes for all the teeth and associated tissues, except the mandibular incisors and maxillary third molars (Figure 12-10). The submandibular nodes then empty into the superior deep cervical nodes.

The superior deep cervical nodes are the primary nodes for the maxillary third molars and their associated tissues, and they empty into either the inferior deep cervical nodes or directly into the jugular trunk and then into the vascular system. Once the infection is in the vascular system, it can be spread to other tissues and organs, as previously discussed.

LYMPHADENOPATHY

A lymph node involved in infection undergoes **lymphadenopathy,** which results in a size increase and a change in the consistency of the lymph node so that it becomes palpable. This change in the lymph node allows it to better fight the infectious process. Evaluation of the involved nodes can determine the degree of regional involvement in the infectious process, which is instrumental in the diagnosis and management of the infectious process.

Spread by Spaces

The fascial spaces of the head and neck can allow the spread of infection from the teeth and associated oral tissues because the pathogens can travel within the fascial planes, from one space near the infected site to another, more distant space by means of the spread of the related inflammatory exudate (Figure 12-11; see Figure 12-10). When involved in infections, the space can undergo cellulitis (see Table 12-2), which can cause a change in the normal proportions of the face (see Chapter 2).

If the maxillary teeth and associated tissues are infected, the infection can spread into the maxillary vestibular space, buccal space, or canine space. If the mandibular teeth and associated tissues are infected, the infection can spread into the mandibular vestibular space, buccal space, submental space, sublingual

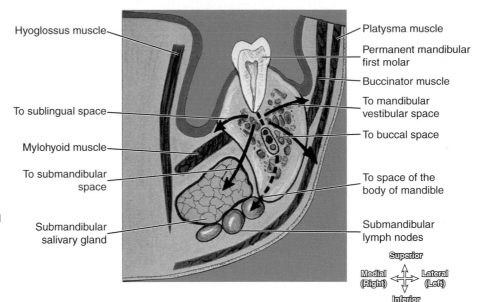

Hyoglossus muscle

Platysma muscle

Permanent mandibular first molar

Buccinator muscle

To sublingual space

To mandibular vestibular space

To buccal space

Mylohyoid muscle

To submandibular space

To space of the body of mandible

Submandibular salivary gland

Submandibular lymph nodes

Superior

Medial (Right) — Lateral (Left)

Inferior

FIGURE 12-10 The spread of dental infection from a permanent mandibular first molar in a coronal section. (From Reynolds PA, Abrahams PH: *McMinn's interactive clinical anatomy: head and neck*, ed 2, St Louis, 2001, Mosby.)

space, submandibular space, masticator spaces, or the space of the body of the mandible, depending on the location of the tooth and extent of infection.

The insertion of the mylohyoid muscle along the mandible dictates which mandibular subspace is initially affected by an odontogenic infection. The apex

of the first molar is above the mylohyoid muscle, so involvement of this tooth, or teeth anterior to this, will first involve the sublingual space. In contrast, the apices of the second and third molars are below the mylohyoid muscle, and infection here will first spread to the submylohyoid space. However, these spaces

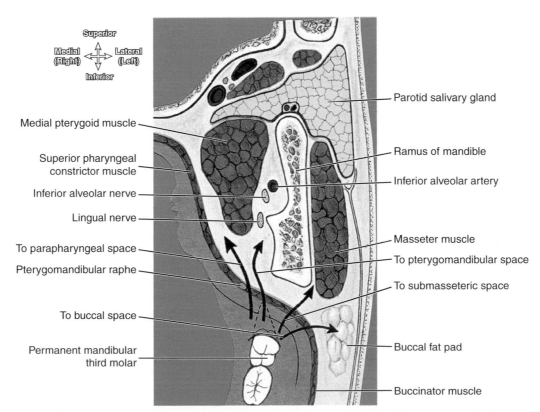

Superior

Medial (Right) — Lateral (Left)

Inferior

Parotid salivary gland

Medial pterygoid muscle

Superior pharyngeal constrictor muscle

Ramus of mandible

Inferior alveolar artery

Inferior alveolar nerve

Lingual nerve

To parapharyngeal space

Masseter muscle

Pterygomandibular raphe

To pterygomandibular space

To submasseteric space

To buccal space

Permanent mandibular third molar

Buccal fat pad

Buccinator muscle

FIGURE 12-11 The spread of dental infection from a permanent mandibular third molar in a horizontal section. (From Reynolds PA, Abrahams PH: *McMinn's interactive clinical anatomy: head and neck*, ed 2, London, 2001, Mosby Ltd.)

freely communicate around the posterior border of the mylohyoid muscle, and so both subspaces typically become involved.

From these spaces, the infection can spread into other spaces of the jaws and neck such as the parapharyngeal and retropharyngeal spaces, causing serious complications (discussed next).

LUDWIG'S ANGINA

One of the most serious lesions of the jaw region is **Ludwig's angina,** cellulitis of the submandibular space (Figure 12-12). It involves the spread of infection from any of the mandibular teeth or associated tissues to one space initially, the submental, the sublingual, or even the submandibular space itself.

The infection then involves the submandibular space bilaterally, with a risk of spreading to the parapharyngeal space and then onto the retropharyngeal space of the neck. With this lesion, there is massive bilateral submandibular regional swelling, which extends down the anterior cervical triangle to the clavicles. Swallowing, speaking, and breathing may be difficult, and high fever and drooling are evident. Respiratory obstruction may rapidly develop because the continued swelling elevates the tongue, displacing it backward, thus blocking the pharyngeal airway. Contrast-enhanced computed tomography scan has become the imaging modality of choice in the evaluation of the patient with a deep tissue cervical infection.

As the retropharyngeal space or "danger space" finally becomes involved, edema of the larynx may cause complete respiratory obstruction, asphyxiation,

and death. Thus Ludwig's angina is an acute medical emergency requiring immediate hospitalization, and it may necessitate an emergency cricothyrotomy to create a patent airway. With the advent of earlier care of abscessed teeth and routine antibiotic treatment, Ludwig's angina has become an uncommon dental emergency in healthy patients. However, symptoms may be masked in partially treated cases, and risk is increased in medically compromised patients. Also, with the recent popularity of piercing of oral sites such as the tongue, there has been an increase in infections of these sites (Figure 12-13).

PREVENTION OF THE SPREAD OF DENTAL INFECTIONS

Early diagnosis and treatment of dental infections must occur in all patients. Particular care must be taken not to contaminate surgical sites such as those resulting from extraction, implant placement, or periodontal treatment. There must also be strict adherence to standard precautions of infection control during nonsurgical dental treatment so as to prevent the spread of infection during, for example, restorative and periodontal débridement therapy such as the removal of heavy plaque accumulations. Using an antiseptic rinse before treatment, a rubber dam, or an antimicrobial-laced external water supply during treatment when ultrasonics or irrigators are used may be of help in preventing the spread of infection. Also important is not administering a local anesthetic through an area of dental infection so as to avoid moving the pathogens deeper into the tissues by needle track contamination. After treatment, an antiseptic home rinse or antibiotic coverage might be prescribed if a risk of infection exists.

A thorough medical history with periodic updates will allow the dental professional to perform safe treatment of medically compromised patients and

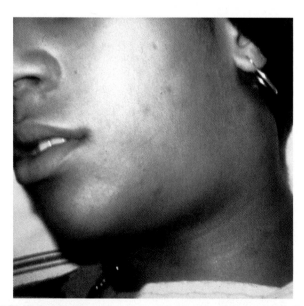

FIGURE 12-12 Ludwig's angina showing involvement of the submandibular and submental spaces resulting from an abscess of the permanent mandibular third molar. (Courtesy Dr. Mark Gabrielson.)

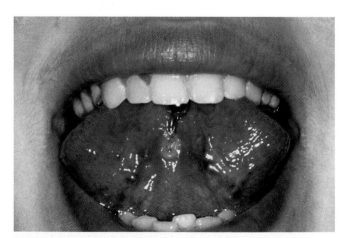

FIGURE 12-13 Localized infection on the ventral surface of the tongue due to a tongue piercing.

avoid serious complications due to dental diseases. These patients may require antibiotic premedication before dental treatment or other changes in the dental treatment plan so as to prevent serious sequelae. A medical consultation is indicated when there is uncertainty as to the risk of opportunistic infection for an individual patient.

Dental infections can have significant medical ramifications including death. As the healthcare professional most familiar with a patient's oral health, the dental professional must be knowledgeable about the appearances, causes, and symptoms of the lesions of dental infections, as well as being expert in the means of their prevention. In addition, the dental professional must keep up with recent guidelines for standard precautions for infection control such as those reported by the Centers for Disease Control.

Finally, scientific evidence has linked severe dental infections with increased susceptibility to certain important systemic diseases and conditions such as cardiovascular disease, diabetes mellitus, adverse pregnancy outcomes, pulmonary infections, and possibly rheumatoid arthritis. This is because the gram-negative bacteria that cause dental infections such as periodontal disease and endodontic infections trigger production of lipopolysaccharides, heat-shock proteins, and proinflammatory cytokines. Due to these associations, it is imperative that dental infections be prevented when possible or promptly recognized and adequately treated.

■ REVIEW QUESTIONS

1. Which of the following complications is likely with untreated Ludwig's angina?
   A. Abducens nerve paralysis
   B. Meningitis
   C. Respiratory obstruction
   D. Sinus perforation
   E. Double vision

2. Which of the following cranial nerves may be involved with cavernous sinus thrombosis?
   A. Oculomotor and trochlear nerves
   B. Vagus and glossopharyngeal nerves
   C. Hypoglossal and accessory nerves
   D. Optic and olfactory nerves

3. Which of the following statements correctly describes an oral abscess?
   A. Inflammation of the bone
   B. Inflammation of the meninges
   C. Infection confined in oral mucosal space
   D. Diffuse inflammation of soft tissue

4. Which of the following statements concerning cavernous sinus thrombosis is correct?
   A. Associated major veins have valves.
   B. Only dental infections can spread to the sinus.
   C. Eye tissues are not affected.
   D. Needle track contamination may be involved.

5. If an infection involves the lingual surface of the mandibular third molar, where is a swelling most likely to be observed?
   A. In the mandibular vestibule
   B. Beneath the tongue
   C. In the submandibular region
   D. In the buccal and submental regions

6. Which of the following types of infectious processes presents as a diffuse inflammation of soft tissue spaces?
   A. Meningitis
   B. Cellulitis
   C. Osteomyelitis
   D. Sinusitis

7. Which of the following is an infection-resistance factor of gram-negative anaerobic bacteria?
   A. Ability to be killed by penicillin
   B. Production of antimicrobial biofilm
   C. Ability to survive in an oxygen-heavy environment
   D. Production of beta-lactamase enzyme

8. Which of the following anatomical structures do not have functional valves, thus aiding in the spread of dental infections by blood backflow?
   A. Paranasal sinuses
   B. Head and neck arteries
   C. Dural sinuses
   D. Skeletal fossae

9. Which of the following lymph nodes are primary nodes for all the teeth (except the mandibular incisors and maxillary third molars) and thus can be involved in the spread of dental infections?
   A. Submental nodes
   B. Submandibular nodes
   C. Superior deep cervical nodes
   D. Inferior deep cervical nodes

10. Which of the following can only present as bacteria traveling in the vascular system?
    A. Thrombus
    B. Embolus
    C. Sequestra
    D. Bacteremia

Bibliography

American Academy of Periodontology: Parameter on acute periodontal diseases, *J Periodontol* 71:863-866, 2000.

American Academy of Periodontology: Parameter on occlusal traumatism in patients with chronic periodontitis, *J Periodontol* 71:873-875, 2000.

American Academy of Periodontology: Parameter on systemic conditions affected by periodontal diseases, *J Periodontol* 71:880-883, 2000.

Bath-Balogh M, Fehrenbach MJ: *Illustrated dental embryology, histology, and anatomy,* ed 2, St. Louis, 2006, Saunders.

Budenz AW: Local anesthetics and medically complex patients, *J Calif Dent Assoc* 28(8):611-619, 2000.

Cawson RA: *Essentials of oral pathology and oral medicine,* ed 7, Edinburgh, 2002, Churchill Livingstone.

Clemente CD: *Anatomy,* ed 4, Philadelphia, 1997, Lippincott, Williams & Wilkins.

Darby ML, Walsh MM: *Dental hygiene theory and practice,* ed 2, Philadelphia, 2003, Saunders.

Djurdjanovic D et al: Computerized classification of temporomandibular joint sounds, *IEEE Trans Biomed Eng* 47(8):977-984, 2000.

Dorland's medical dictionary, ed 30, Philadelphia, 2003, WB Saunders.

Drake R, Vogl W, Mitchell A: *Gray's anatomy for students,* Edinburgh, 2005, Churchill and Livingstone.

Fu YS et al: *Head and neck pathology: with clinical correlations,* Edinburgh, 2001, Churchill Livingstone.

Fukayama H et al: Efficacy of anterior and middle superior alveolar (AMSA) anesthesia using a new injection system: the wand, *Quintessence Int* 34(7):537-541, 2003.

Glick M: Exploring our role as health care providers: the oral-medical connection, *J Am Dent Assoc* 136(6):716-720, 2005.

Hayt MW, Abrahams JJ, Blair J: Magnetic resonance imaging of the temporomandibular joint, *Top Magn Reson Imaging* 11(2):138-146, 2000.

Herrera D, Roldan S, Sanz M: The periodontal abscess: a review, *J Clin Periodontol* 27(6):377-386, 2000.

Ibsen AC, Phelan JA: *Oral pathology for the dental hygienist,* ed 4, St. Louis, 2004, Saunders.

Lee S et al: Anesthetic efficacy of the anterior middle superior alveolar (AMSA) injection, *Anesth Prog* 51(3):80-89, 2004.

Logan BM, Reynolds PA, Hutchings RT: *Color atlas of head and neck anatomy,* ed 3, London, 2003, Mosby Ltd.

Malamed SF: *Handbook of local anesthesia,* ed 5, St Louis, 2004, Mosby.

McQuone SJ, Eisele DW: *Emergencies of the head and neck,* St Louis, 2000, Mosby.

Michalowicz BS et al: No heritability of temporomandibular joint signs and symptoms, *J Dent Res* 79(8):1573-1578, 2000.

Antibacterial prophylaxis for dental, GI, and GU procedures, *Med Lett Drugs Ther* July 18;47(1213):59-60, 2005.

Mosby's dental dictionary, St Louis, 2004, Mosby.

Nakai Y et al: Effectiveness of local anesthesia in pediatric dental practice, *J Am Dent Assoc* 131(12):1699-1705, 2000.

Niwa H, Satoh Y, Matsuura H: Cardiovascular responses to epinephrine-containing local anesthetics for dental use: a comparison of hemodynamic responses to infiltration anesthesia and ergometer-stress testing, *Oral Surg Oral Med Oral Pathol Oral Radiol Endod* 90(2):171-181, 2000.

Nomina anatomica, ed 6, Edinburgh, 1989, Churchill Livingstone.

Papapanou PN: Population studies of microbial ecology in periodontal health and disease, *Ann Periodontol* 7(1):54-61, 2002.

Peretz B, Bimstein E: The use of imagery suggestions during administration of local anesthetic in pediatric dental patients, *ASDC J Dent Child* 67(4):231, 263-267, 2000.

Pogrel MA, Thamby S: Permanent nerve involvement resulting from inferior alveolar nerve blocks, *J Am Dent Assoc* 131(7):901-907, 2000.

Reynolds PA, Abrahams PH: *McMinn's interactive clinical anatomy: head and neck,* ed 2, London, 2001, Mosby Ltd.

Toyama M et al: Magnetic resonance arthrography of the temporomandibular joint, *J Oral Maxillofac Surg* 58(9):978-984, 2000.

Werner JA et al: The sentinel node concept in head and neck cancer: solution for the controversies in the N0 neck? *Head Neck* 26(7):603-611, 2004.

Procedure for Performing Extraoral and Intraoral Examinations

NOTE: Ask patient to remove glasses, dentures, or appliances. Inquire about the history of the lesion if it presents during general evaluation and whether any discomfort occurs during the examinations.

REGIONS	STEPS
Extraoral regions	
Overall evaluation of the face, head, and neck including skin	With patient sitting upright and relaxed, visually observe symmetry and coloration.
Parietal and occipital regions including scalp, hair, and occipital nodes	Standing near the patient, visually inspect the entire scalp by moving the hair, especially around the hairline, starting from one ear and proceeding to the other ear. Standing behind the patient, have the patient lean the head forward and bilaterally palpate the base of the head.
Temporal region including auricular nodes and ears	Standing near the patient on each side, visually inspect and bilaterally palpate the well as the scalp and face around each ear. Visually inspect and manually palpate each ear.
Frontal region including forehead and frontal sinuses	Standing near the patient, visually inspect and bilaterally palpate the forehead including the frontal sinuses.
Orbital region including the eyes	Standing near the patient, visually inspect the eyes and their movements and responses.
Nasal region including the nose	Standing near the patient, visually inspect and bilaterally palpate the nasal region, starting at the root of the nose and proceeding to its apex.
Infraorbital and zygomatic regions including the muscles of facial expression, facial nodes, maxillary sinuses and bone, and temporomandibular joint	Standing near the patient, visually inspect inferior to the orbits, especially noting the use of the muscles of facial expression. Visually inspect and bilaterally palpate each side of the face, moving from the infraorbital region to the labial commissure and then to the surface of the mandible. Visually inspect and bilaterally palpate the maxillary sinuses. Digitally palpate the joint and its associated muscles. Ask the patient to open and close the mouth several times. Then ask the patient to move the opened jaw to the left, then the right, and then forward. Or using digital palpation of the mandible's movement, gently place a finger into the outer portion of the external acoustic meatus. Note any sounds made by the joint.

REGIONS	STEPS
Extraoral regions—cont'd	
Buccal region including the masseter muscle, parotid salivary gland, and mandible	Standing near the patient, visually inspect and bilaterally palpate the masseter muscle and parotid gland by starting in front of each ear and moving to the cheek area and down to the angle of the mandible. Place the fingers of each hand over the masseter muscle and ask the patient to clench the teeth together several times.
Mental region including the chin	Standing near the patient, visually inspect and bilaterally palpate the chin.
Anterior and posterior cervical triangle regions including sternocleidomastoid muscle and associated nodes	Have the patient look straight ahead. Then have the patient turn the head to the opposite side to make the sternocleidomastoid muscle more prominent. First on one side and then on the other side of the neck, manually palpate with one hand starting below the ear, and continue the whole length of the muscle surface to the clavicles. Then manually palpate deeper on the underside of the anterior and posterior aspects of the muscle in the same direction as before. Then have the patient raise the shoulders up and forward and manually palpate using one hand on each side, the most inferior portion of the neck in the area of the clavicles.
Submandibular and submental triangle regions including submandibular and sublingual salivary glands and associated nodes	Standing slightly behind the patient first on one side, then on the other, have the patient lower the chin and manually palpate directly underneath the chin and inside of the mandible. Then push the tissue in the area over the bony edge of the mandible on each side, where it is grasped and rolled.
Anterior midline cervical region including hyoid bone, thyroid gland, and cartilage	Examination of the thyroid gland is carried out by locating the thyroid cartilage and passing the fingers up and down, examining for abnormal masses or overall size. Then standing near the patient, place one hand on each side of the trachea and gently displace the thyroid tissue to the other side of the neck, while the other hand manually palpates the displaced glandular tissue. Then compare the two lobes of the thyroid using visual inspection and bimanual or manual palpation. Then ask the patient to swallow to check for mobility of the gland by visually inspecting it while it moves superiorly. The patient may need to drink a glass of water in order to swallow.
<u>**Intraoral regions**</u>	
Oral cavity including lips, buccal and labial mucosa, parotid glands and ducts, alveolar ridges, and attached gingiva	Visually inspect the lips including the commissures. Ask the patient to close the lips and then to smile. Bidigitally palpate the lower lip in a systematic manner from one commissure to the other. Use the same technique for the upper lip. Then have the patient open the mouth slightly, and gently pull the lower lip away from the teeth to observe the labial mucosa. Use the same technique for the upper lip. Then gently pull the buccal mucosa slightly away from the teeth to bidigitally palpate, using circular compression. Dry the area and observe the flow of saliva from each duct. Retract the mucosal tissues enough to visually inspect the vestibular area and bidigitally palpate, using circular compression including the gingival tissues.
Palate and pharynx including the hard and soft palates, tonsillar pillars, uvula, and portions of the oropharynx and nasopharynx	Have the patient tilt the head back slightly and extend the tongue. Visually inspect the soft palate. Use a mouth mirror to intensify the light source and view the palatal and pharyngeal regions. Then gently place the mouth mirror (mirror side down) on the middle of the tongue and ask the patient to say "ah." As this is done, visually observe the uvula and the visible portions of the pharynx. Compress the hard and soft palates with the first or second finger of one hand, avoiding circular compression to prevent initiating the gag reflex.

REGIONS	STEPS
Intraoral regions—cont'd **Tongue including all surfaces and swallowing pattern**	To examine the dorsal and lateral surfaces of the tongue, have the patient gently extend the tongue and wrap a gauze square around the anterior third of the tongue in order to obtain a firm grasp. Then turn the tongue slightly on its side and visually inspect and bidigitally palpate its base and lateral borders. Digitally palpate the dorsal surface. To examine the ventral surface, have the patient lift the tongue; visually inspect and digitally palpate the surface. While holding the lips apart, ask the patient to swallow and observe the swallowing pattern. Patient may need to drink a glass of water in order to swallow.
Floor of the mouth including the submandibular and sublingual salivary glands and ducts	While the patient lifts the tongue to the palate, visually inspect the mucosa of the floor of the mouth. Use the mouth mirror to assist in lighting. Bimanually palpate the sublingual region by placing one index finger intraorally and fingertips of the opposite hand extraorally under the chin, compressing the tissue between the fingers. Check the lingual frenum. Dry the sublingual caruncle with gauze and observe the saliva flow from the duct.

Glossary of Key Terms and Anatomical Structures

Abducens nerve (ab-**doo**-senz) Sixth cranial nerve (VI) that serves an eye muscle.

Abducens nerve paralysis (pah-**ral**-i-sis) Loss of function of the sixth cranial nerve.

Abscess (**ab**-ses) Infection with suppuration resulting from the entrapment of pathogens in a contained space.

Accessory lymph nodes (ak-**ses**-o-ree) Deep cervical nodes located along the accessory nerve.

Accessory nerve Eleventh cranial nerve (XI) that serves the trapezius and sternocleidomastoid muscles, as well as muscles of the soft palate and pharynx.

Action Movement accomplished by a muscle when the muscle fibers contract.

Action potential (po-**ten**-shal) Rapid depolarization of a cell membrane that results in propagation of the nerve impulse along the membrane.

Adenoids (**ad**-in-oidz) Another term for the pharyngeal tonsils.

Afferent nerve (**af**-er-ent) Sensory nerve that carries information from the periphery of the body to the brain or spinal cord.

Afferent nervous system Sensory nerve system that carries information from receptors to the brain or spinal cord.

Afferent vessels (**af**-er-ent) Type of lymphatic vessel in which lymph flows into the lymph node.

Ala, alae (**a**-lah, **a**-lay) Winglike cartilaginous structures that laterally bound the nares.

Alveolar mucosa (al-**ve**-o-lar) Mucosa that lines the vestibules of the oral region.

Alveolar process of the mandible Portion of the mandible that contains the roots of the maxillary teeth.

Alveolar process of the maxilla Ridge of maxillary bone that houses the roots of the maxillary teeth.

Anastomosis, anastomoses (ah-nas-tah-**moe**-sis, ah-nas-tah-**moe**-sees) Communication of a blood vessel with another by a connecting channel.

Anatomical nomenclature (an-ah-**tom**-ik-al **no**-men-kla-cher) System of names of anatomical structures.

Anatomical position Position in which the body is erect, arms at the sides, palms and toes directed forward, and eyes looking forward.

Anesthesia (ann-es-**thee**-zee-ah) The loss of feeling or sensation resulting from the use of certain drugs or gases that serve as inhibitory neurotransmitters.

Angle of the mandible Angle at the intersection of the posterior and inferior borders of the ramus.

Angular artery (**ang**-u-lar) Arterial branch that is a termination of the facial artery and supplies the tissues along the side of the nose.

Anterior Front of an area of the body.

Anterior arch Arch of the atlas or first cervical vertebra.

Anterior auricular lymph nodes (aw-**rik**-you-lar) Superficial nodes located anterior to the ear.

Anterior cervical triangle Anterior region of the neck.

Anterior ethmoidal nerve (eth-**moy**-dal) Nerve from the nasal cavity and paranasal sinuses that converges with other orbital branches to form the nasociliary nerve.

Anterior faucial pillar (**faw**-shawl **pil**-er) Vertical fold anterior to each palatine tonsil created by the palatoglossal muscle.

Anterior jugular lymph nodes (**jug**-you-lar) Superficial cervical nodes located along the anterior jugular vein.

Anterior jugular vein Vein that begins below the chin, descends near the midline, and drains into the external jugular vein.

Anterior middle superior alveolar (ASMA) block Local anesthetic block that achieves anesthesia of most of the maxillary teeth and associated tissues except those innervated by the posterior superior alveolar nerve.

Anterior superior alveolar artery Arterial branch from the infraorbital artery that gives off dental and alveolar branches that supply the pulp tissue and periodontium of the anterior maxillary teeth.

Anterior superior alveolar (ASA) block Local anesthetic block that achieves anesthesia of the pulp of the maxillary canine and incisor and their associated facial tissues.

Anterior superior alveolar (ASA) nerve Nerve that serves the maxillary anterior teeth and tissues and is formed from dental and interdental branches and later joins the infraorbital nerve.

Anterior suprahyoid muscle group (soo-prah-**hi**-oid) Suprahyoid muscles located anterior to the hyoid bone that include the anterior belly of the digastric, mylohyoid, and geniohyoid muscles.

Antitragus (an-tie-**tra**-gus) Flap of tissue opposite the tragus of the ear.

Aorta (ay-**ort**-ah) Major artery that gives rise to the common carotid and subclavian arteries on the left side of the body and to the brachiocephalic artery on the right side.

Aperture (**ap**-er-cher) Opening or orifice in bone.

Apex (**ay**-peks) Pointed end of a conical structure.

Apex of the nose Tip of the nose.

Apex of the tongue Tip of the tongue.

Arch Prominent bridgelike bony structure.

Arteriole (ar-**ter**-ee-ole) Smaller artery that branches off an artery and connects with a capillary.

Artery Type of blood vessel that carries blood away from the heart.

Articular eminence (ar-**tik**-you-ler) Eminence on the temporal bone that articulates with the mandible at the temporomandibular joint.

Articular fossa Fossa on the temporal bone that articulates with the mandible at the temporomandibular joint.

Articulating surface of the condyle (ar-**tik**-you-late-ing) Portion of the head of the condyle that articulates with the temporal bone at the temporomandibular joint.

Articulation (ar-tik-you-**lay**-shin) Area where the bones are joined to each other.

Ascending palatine artery (ah-**send**-ing **pal**-ah-tine) Arterial branch from the facial artery that supplies the palatine muscles and tonsils.

Ascending pharyngeal artery (ah-**send**-ing fah-**rin**-je-al) Medial arterial branch from the external carotid artery that supplies the pharyngeal walls, soft palate, and brain tissue.

Atherosclerosis (ath-uh-roh-skluh-**roh**-sis) The narrowing and blocking of the arteries by a buildup of plaque.

Atlas (**at**-lis) First cervical vertebra, which articulates with the occipital bone.

Attached gingiva (jin-**ji**-vah) Gingiva that tightly adheres to the bone over the roots of the teeth.

Auricle (**aw**-ri-kl) Oval flap of the external ear.

Auriculotemporal nerve (aw-**rik**-yule-lo-**tem**-poh-ral) Nerve that serves tissues of the ear and scalp and the parotid salivary gland and joins the posterior trunk of the mandibular division of the trigeminal nerve.

Autonomic nervous system (ANS) (awt-o-**nom**-ik) Subdivision of the efferent division of the peripheral nervous system that operates without conscious control and is further subdivided into the sympathetic and parasympathetic nervous systems.

Axis (**ak**-sis) Second cervical vertebra, which articulates with the first and third cervical vertebrae.

B

Bacteremia (bak-ter-ee-**me**-ah) Bacteria traveling within the vascular system.

Base of the tongue The posterior third or root of the tongue.

Bell's palsy (**pawl**-ze) Type of unilateral facial paralysis involving the facial nerve.

Body of the hyoid bone (**hi**-oid) Anterior midline portion of the hyoid bone.

Body of the mandible Horizontal portion of the mandible.

Body of the maxilla Portion of the maxilla that contains the maxillary sinus.

Body of the sphenoid bone (**sfe**-noid) Middle portion of the bone containing the sphenoidal sinuses.

Body of the tongue Anterior two thirds of the tongue.

Bones Mineralized structures of the body that protect internal soft tissues and serve as the biomechanical basis for movement.

Brachiocephalic artery (bray-kee-oo-sah-**fal**-ik) Artery that branches directly off the aorta on the right side of the body and gives rise to the right common carotid and subclavian arteries.

Brachiocephalic vein Vein that is formed from the merger of the internal jugular and subclavian veins with the right and left brachiocephalic veins, forming the superior vena cava.

Brain Division of the central nervous system subdivided into the cerebrum, the cerebellum, and the brainstem.

Brainstem Division of the brain that includes the medulla, pons, and midbrain.

Bridge of the nose Bony structure inferior to the nasion in the nasal region.

Buccal (**buk**-al) Structures closest to the inner cheek.

Buccal artery Arterial branch from the maxillary artery that supplies the buccinator muscle and cheek tissues.

Buccal block Local anesthetic block for anesthesia of the buccal periodontium of the mandibular molars including the gingiva, periodontal ligament, and alveolar bone.

Buccal fat pad Dense pad of tissue covered by the buccal mucosa.

Buccal lymph nodes Superficial nodes of the face located at the mouth angle and superficial to the buccinator muscle.

Buccal mucosa Mucosa that lines the inner cheek.

Buccal nerve Nerve that serves the skin of the cheek and buccal tissue of the mandibular molar teeth and joins with the muscular nerve branches to form the anterior trunk of the mandibular division of the trigeminal nerve.

Buccal region Region of the head that is composed of the soft tissues of the cheek of the face.

Buccal space Fascial space between buccinator and masseter muscles.

Buccinator muscle (buck-**sin**-nay-tor) Muscle of facial expression that forms a portion of the cheek.

Buccopharyngeal fascia (buk-o-fah-**rin**-je-al) Deep cervical fascia that encloses the entire upper portion of the alimentary canal.

C

Canal Opening in bone that is long, narrow, and tubelike.

Canines (**kay**-nines) Anterior teeth that also are the third teeth from the midline in each quadrant.

Canine eminence Facial ridge of bone over the maxillary canine.

Canine fossa Fossa at the roots of the maxillary canine teeth.

Canine space Fascial space located lateral to the apex of the maxillary canine.

Capillary (kap-i-lare-ee) Smaller blood vessel that branches off an arteriole to supply blood directly to tissue.

Carotid canal (kah-rot-id) Canal in the temporal bone that carries the internal carotid artery.

Carotid pulse Reliable pulse palpated from the common carotid artery.

Carotid sheath Deep cervical fascia forming a tube running down the side of the neck.

Carotid sinus Swelling in the artery just before the common carotid artery bifurcates into the internal and external carotid arteries.

Carotid triangle Smaller triangular region of the neck superior to the omohyoid muscle and a portion of the anterior cervical triangle.

Cavernous sinus thrombosis (kav-er-nus sy-nus throm-bo-sus) Infection of the cavernous venous sinus.

Cavernous venous sinus Venous sinus located on the side of the sphenoid bone that communicates with the pterygoid plexus and superior ophthalmic vein.

Cellulitis (sel-you-lie-tis) Diffuse inflammation of soft tissue.

Central nervous system (CNS) Division of the nervous system that consists of the spinal cord and brain.

Cerebellum (ser-e-bel-um) Second largest division of the brain; it coordinates muscles and maintains normal muscle tone and posture, as well as coordinating balance.

Cerebrum (ser-e-brum) Largest division of the brain; it coordinates sensory data and motor functions, as well as governing many aspects of intelligence and reasoning, learning, and memory.

Cervical muscles Muscles of the neck that include the sternocleidomastoid and trapezius muscles.

Cervical vertebrae (ver-teh-bray) Vertebrae in the vertebral column between the skull and thoracic vertebrae.

Chorda tympani nerve (kor-dah tim-pan-ee) Branch of the facial nerve that serves the submandibular and sublingual salivary glands and tongue.

Ciliary nerves (sil-ee-a-re) Nerves to or from the eyeball, with some ciliary nerves converging with branches from the nose to form the nasociliary nerve.

Circumvallate lingual papillae (serk-um-val-ate) Large lingual papillae anterior to the sulcus terminalis.

Common carotid artery (kah-rot-id) Artery that travels in the carotid sheath up the neck to branch into the internal and external carotid arteries.

Condyle (kon-dyl) Oval bony prominence typically found at articulations.

Condyle of the mandible Projection of bone from the ramus of the mandible that participates in the temporomandibular joint.

Conjunctiva (kon-junk-ti-vah) Membrane lining the inside of the eyelids and front of the eyeball.

Contralateral (kon-trah-lat-er-il) Structures on the opposite side of the body.

Cornu (kor-nu) Small, hornlike prominence.

Coronal suture (kor-oh-nahl) Suture between the frontal and parietal bones.

Coronoid notch Notch in the anterior border of the ramus.

Coronoid process Anterior superior projection of the ramus of the mandible.

Corrugator supercilii muscle (cor-rew-gay-tor soo-per-sili-eye) Muscle of facial expression in the eye region that is used when frowning.

Cranial bones (kray-nee-al) Skull bones that form the cranium and include the occipital, frontal, parietal, temporal, sphenoid, and ethmoid bones.

Cranial nerves Portion of the peripheral nervous system that is connected to the brain and carries information to and from the brain.

Cranium (kray-nee-um) Structure that is formed by the cranial skull bones and includes the occipital, frontal, parietal, temporal, sphenoid, and ethmoid bones.

Crest Roughened border or ridge on the bone surface.

Cribriform plate (krib-ri-form) Horizontal plate of the ethmoid bone that is perforated with foramina for the olfactory nerves.

Crista galli (kris-tah gal-lee) Vertical midline continuation of the perpendicular plate of the ethmoid bone into the cranial cavity.

D

Deep Structures located inward, away from the body surface.

Deep cervical lymph nodes Nodes located along the internal jugular vein that are divided into two groups, superior and inferior, based on the point where the omohyoid muscle crosses the vein.

Deep parotid lymph nodes (pah-rot-id) Nodes located deep to the parotid salivary gland.

Deep temporal arteries (tem-poh-ral) Arterial branches from the maxillary artery that supply the temporalis muscle.

Deep temporal nerves Muscular nerve branches that form the anterior trunk of the mandibular division of the trigeminal nerve and innervate the deep surface of the temporalis muscle.

Dens (denz) Odontoid process of the second cervical vertebra.

Depression of the mandible (de-presh-in) Lowering of the lower jaw.

Depressor anguli oris muscle (de-pres-er an-gu-lie or-is) Muscle of facial expression in the mouth region that depresses the angle of the mouth.

Depressor labii inferioris muscle (lay-be-eye in-fere-ee-o-ris) Muscle of facial expression in the mouth region that depresses the lower lip.

Descending palatine artery (de-send-ing pal-ah-tine) Branch of the maxillary artery which terminates in both the greater palatine artery and lesser palatine artery.

Diencephalon (di-en-sef-a-lon) Division of the brain that consists of the thalamus and hypothalamus.

Digastric muscle (di-gas-trik) Suprahyoid muscle with an anterior and a posterior belly.

Disc of the temporomandibular joint Fibrous disc located between the temporal bone and condyle of the mandible.

Distal (dis-tl) Area that is farther away from the median plane of the body.

Dorsal (dor-sal) Back of an area of the body.

Dorsal surface of the tongue Top surface of the tongue.

Duct Passageway to carry the secretion from the exocrine gland to the location where it will be used.

E

Efferent nerve (ef-er-ent) Motor nerve that carries information away from the brain or spinal cord to the periphery of the body.

Efferent nervous system Motor nerve system that carries information from the brain or spinal cord to muscles or glands.

Efferent vessel Type of lymphatic vessel in which lymph flows out of the lymph node in the area of the node's hilus.

Elevation of the mandible (el-eh-**vay**-shun) Raising of the lower jaw.

Embolus, emboli (**em**-bol-us, **em**-bol-eye) Foreign material, or thrombus, traveling in the blood that can block the vessel.

Eminence (**em**-i-nins) Tubercle or rounded elevation on the bony surface.

Endocrine gland (**en**-dah-krin) Type of gland without a duct, with the secretion being poured directly into the blood, which then carries the secretion to the region being used.

Epicranial aponeurosis (ep-ee-**kray**-nee-all ap-o-new-**row**-sis) Scalpal tendon from which the frontal belly of the epicranial muscle arises.

Epicranial muscle Muscle of facial expression in the scalp region that has a frontal and an occipital belly.

Epiglottis (ep-ih-**glah**-tis) A flap of cartilage that, during swallowing, folds back to cover the entrance to the larynx, preventing food and liquid from entering the trachea and then the lungs.

Ethmoid bone (**eth**-moid) Single midline cranial bone of the skull.

Ethmoidal sinuses Paired paranasal sinuses located in the ethmoid bone, which are also called *ethmoid air cells*.

Exocrine gland (**ek**-sah-krin) Type of gland with an associated duct that serves as a passageway for the secretion to be emptied directly into the location where the secretion is to be used.

External Outer side of the wall of a hollow structure.

External acoustic meatus (ah-**koos**-tik me-**ate**-us) Canal leading to the tympanic cavity.

External carotid artery (kah-**rot**-id) Artery that arises from the common carotid artery and supplies the extracranial tissues of the head and neck including the oral cavity.

External jugular lymph nodes (**jug**-you-lar) Superficial cervical nodes located along the external jugular vein.

External jugular vein Vein that forms from the posterior division of the retromandibular vein.

External nasal nerve (**nay**-zil) Nerve from portions of the nose skin that converges with other branches to form the nasociliary nerve.

External oblique line (ob-**leek**) Crest on the lateral side of the mandible, where the ramus joins the body.

Extrinsic tongue muscles (eks-**trin**-sik) Tongue muscles with different origins outside the tongue.

Eyelids Movable upper and lower tissues that cover and protect each eyeball.

F

Facial (**fay**-shal) Structures closest to the facial surface.

Facial artery Anterior arterial branch from the external carotid artery with a complicated path as it gives off the ascending palatine, submental, inferior and superior labial, and angular arteries.

Facial bones Skull bones that create the face and include the lacrimal bone, nasal bone, vomer, inferior nasal concha, zygomatic bone, maxilla, and mandible.

Facial lymph nodes Superficial nodes located along the facial vein that include the malar, nasolabial, buccal, and mandibular nodes.

Facial nerve Seventh cranial nerve (VII) that serves the muscles of facial expression, posterior suprahyoid muscles, lacrimal gland, sublingual and submandibular salivary glands, tongue portion, and portion of skin through its greater petrosal, chorda tympani, and posterior auricular nerves and muscular branches.

Facial paralysis (pay-**ral**-i-sis) Loss of action of the facial muscles.

Facial vein Vein that drains into the internal jugular vein after draining the facial areas.

Fascia, fasciae (**fash**-e-ah, **fash**-e-ay) Layers of fibrous connective tissue that underlie the skin and surround the muscles, bones, vessels, nerves, organs, and other structures of the body.

Fascial spaces (**fash**-e-al) Potential spaces between the layers of fascia in the body.

Fauces (**faw**-seez) Faucial isthmus or junction between the oral region and oropharynx.

Filiform lingual papillae (**fil**-i-form) Papillae that give the tongue its velvety texture.

Fissure (**fish**-er) Opening in bone that is narrow and cleftlike.

Fistula, fistulae (**fis**-chool-ah, **fis**-chool-ay) Passageway in the skin, mucosa, or even bone allowing drainage of an abscess at the surface.

Foliate lingual papillae (**fo**-le-ate) Ridges of papillae on lateral tongue surface.

Foramen, foramina (for-**ay**-men, for-**am**-i-nah) Short, windowlike opening in bone.

Foramen cecum (**se**-kum) Depression on the dorsal surface of the tongue where the sulcus terminalis points backward toward the pharynx.

Foramen lacerum (lah-**ser**-um) Foramen among the sphenoid, occipital, and temporal bones that is filled with cartilage.

Foramen magnum (**mag**-num) Foramen in the occipital bone that carries the spinal cord, vertebral arteries, and eleventh cranial nerve.

Foramen ovale (o-**val**-ee) Foramen in the sphenoid bone for the mandibular division of the trigeminal or fifth cranial nerve.

Foramen rotundum (row-**tun**-dum) Foramen in the sphenoid bone that carries the trigeminal or fifth cranial nerve.

Foramen spinosum (**spine**-o-sum) Foramen in the sphenoid bone for the middle meningeal artery.

Fossa, fossae (**fos**-ah, **fos**-ay) Depression on a bony surface.

Frontal bone Single cranial bone that forms the forehead and a portion of the orbits.

Frontal eminence (**em**-i-nins) Prominence of the forehead.

Frontal nerve Nerve from the merger of the supraorbital and supratrochlear nerves that continues into the ophthalmic nerve when joined by the lacrimal and nasociliary nerves.

Frontal plane Plane created by an imaginary line that divides the body at any level into anterior and posterior portions.

Frontal process of the maxilla   Process that forms a portion of the orbital rim.

Frontal process of the zygomatic bone   Process that forms a portion of the orbital wall.

Frontal region   Region of the head that includes the forehead and supraorbital area.

Frontal section   Section of the body through any frontal plane.

Frontal sinuses   Paired paranasal sinuses located internally in the frontal bone.

Frontonasal duct (frunt-o-**na**-zil)   Drainage canal of each frontal sinus to the nasal cavity.

Fungiform lingual papillae (**fung**-i-form)   Papillae with a mushroom-shaped appearance.

G

Ganglion, ganglia (**gang**-gle-on, **gang**-gle-ah)   Accumulation of neuron cell bodies outside the central nervous system.

Genial tubercles (ji-**ni**-il)   Midline bony projections or the mental spines on the inner aspect of the mandible.

Genioglossus muscle (ji-nee-o-**gloss**-us)   Extrinsic tongue muscle that arises from the genial tubercles.

Geniohyoid muscle (ji-nee-o-**hi**-oid)   Anterior suprahyoid muscle that is deep to the mylohyoid muscle.

Gingiva, gingivae (jin-**ji**-vah, jin-**ji**-vay)   Mucosa surrounding the maxillary and mandibular teeth.

Glabella (glah-**bell**-ah)   Smooth, elevated area on the frontal bone between the supraorbital ridges.

Gland   Structure that produces a chemical secretion necessary for normal body functioning.

Glossopharyngeal nerve (**gloss**-oh-fah-**rin**-je-al)   Ninth cranial nerve (IX) that serves the parotid salivary gland, a pharyngeal muscle, and a tongue portion.

Goiter (**goit**-er)   Enlarged thyroid gland due to a disease process.

Golden Proportions   Guidelines that can be used to consider the facial view of the anterior teeth or the vertical dimensions of the face to create a pleasing proportion.

Gow-Gates mandibular nerve block   Block that anesthetizes the inferior alveolar, mental, incisive, lingual, mylohyoid, auriculotemporal, and buccal (long) nerves.

Greater cornu   Pair of projections from the sides of the body of the hyoid bone.

Greater palatine artery (**pal**-ah-tine)   Arterial branch from the maxillary artery that travels to the palate.

Greater palatine (GP) block   Local anesthetic block that achieves anesthesia for the lingual tissues of the maxillary posterior teeth and posterior palatal tissues.

Greater palatine foramen   Foramen in the palatine bone that carries the greater palatine nerve and blood vessels.

Greater palatine (GP) nerve   Nerve that serves the posterior hard palate and posterior lingual gingiva and then joins the maxillary nerve.

Greater petrosal nerve (peh-**troh**-sil)   Branch of the facial nerve that serves the lacrimal gland, nasal cavity, and minor salivary glands of the hard and soft palates.

Greater wing of the sphenoid bone (**sfe**-noid)   Posterolateral process of the body of the sphenoid bone.

H

Hamulus (**ha**-mu-lis)   Process of the medial pterygoid plate of the sphenoid bone.

Hard palate (**pal**-it)   Anterior portion of the palate formed by the palatine processes of the maxilla and the horizontal plates of the palatine bones.

Head   Rounded surface projecting from a bone by a neck.

Helix (**heel**-iks)   The superior and posterior free margin of the auricle.

Hematoma (hee-mah-**toe**-mah)   Vascular lesions or bruise that results when a blood vessel is injured and a small amount of blood escapes into the surrounding tissue and clots.

Hemorrhage (**hem**-ah-rij)   Vascular lesions that allows large amounts of blood to escape into the surrounding tissue without clotting when a blood vessel is seriously injured.

Hilus (**hi**-lus)   Depression on one side of a lymph node where lymph flows out by way of an efferent lymphatic vessel.

Horizontal plane   Plane created by an imaginary line that divides the body at any level into superior and inferior portions.

Horizontal plates of the palatine bones   Plates that form the posterior portion of the hard palate.

Hyoglossus muscle (hi-o-**gloss**-us)   Extrinsic tongue muscle that originates from the hyoid bone.

Hyoid bone (**hi**-oid)   Bone suspended in the neck that allows the attachment of many muscles.

Hyoid muscles   Muscles that attach to the hyoid bone and can be classified by whether they are superior or inferior to the hyoid bone.

Hypoglossal canal (hi-poh-**gloss**-al)   Canal in the occipital bone that carries the twelfth cranial nerve.

Hypoglossal nerve   Twelfth cranial nerve (XII) that serves the muscles of the tongue.

Hypothalamus (hi-po-**thal**-a-mus)   Portion of the diencephalus that regulates homeostasis.

I

Incisive artery (in-**sy**-ziv)   Arterial branch from the inferior alveolar artery that divides into dental and alveolar branches to supply the pulp tissue and periodontium of the mandibular anterior teeth.

Incisive block   Local anesthetic block that achieves anesthesia of the pulp and facial tissues of the mandibular anterior and premolar teeth.

Incisive foramen   Foramen in the maxilla that carries branches of the right and left nasopalatine nerves and blood vessels and is marked by the incisive papilla.

Incisive nerve   Nerve that is formed from dental and interdental branches of the mandibular anterior teeth and merges with the mental nerve to form the inferior alveolar nerve.

Incisive papilla (pah-**pil**-ah)   Bulge of tissue on the hard palate over the incisive foramen.

Incisors (in-**sigh**-zers)   Anterior teeth that are the first and second from the midline and consist of both centrals and laterals, respectively.

Incisura (in-si-**su**-rah)   Indentation or notch at the edge of the bone.

Inferior   Area that faces away from the head and toward the feet of the body.

Inferior alveolar artery (al-**ve**-o-lar)   Arterial branch from the maxillary artery that supplies the mandibular posterior teeth and branches into the mental and incisive arteries.

Inferior alveolar (IA) block (al-**ve**-o-lar)   Local anesthetic block that achieves anesthesia of the pulp and lingual tissues of the mandibular teeth, as well as facial tissues of the mandibular anterior and premolar teeth.

Inferior alveolar (IA) nerve   Nerve formed from the merger of the incisive and mental nerves that serves the tissues of the chin, lower lip, and labial mucosa of the mandibular anterior and premolar teeth and later joins the posterior trunk of the mandibular division of the trigeminal nerve.

Inferior alveolar vein   Vein formed by the merger of the dental, alveolar, and mental branches that drains the pulp tissue and periodontium of the mandibular teeth, as well as the tissues of the chin.

Inferior articular processes (ar-**tik**-you-lar)   Processes of the first and second cervical vertebrae that allow articulation with the vertebrae below.

Inferior labial artery   Arterial branch from the facial artery that supplies the lower lip tissues.

Inferior labial vein   Vein that drains the lower lip and then drains into the facial vein.

Inferior nasal conchae (**nay**-zil **kong**-kay)   Paired facial bones that project inwardly from the maxilla to form walls of the nasal cavity.

Inferior orbital fissure (or-bit-al)   Fissure between the greater wing of the sphenoid bone and maxilla that carries the infraorbital and zygomatic nerves, as well as the infraorbital artery and inferior ophthalmic vein.

Infrahyoid muscles (in-frah-**hi**-oid)   Hyoid muscles that are inferior to the hyoid bone.

Infraorbital artery   Arterial branch from the maxillary artery that gives off the anterior superior alveolar artery and branches to the orbit.

Infraorbital (IO) block   Local anesthetic block that achieves anesthesia in the tissues supplied by the middle and anterior superior alveolar nerves including the pulp and facial tissues of the maxillary anterior and premolar teeth.

Infraorbital canal   Canal off the infraorbital sulcus that terminates on the surface of the maxilla as the infraorbital foramen.

Infraorbital foramen   Foramen of the maxilla that transmits the infraorbital nerve and blood vessels.

Infraorbital (IO) nerve   Nerve that is involved in forming the maxillary nerve and is formed from branches of the upper lip, cheek portion, lower eyelid, and side of the nose.

Infraorbital region   Region of the head that is located below the orbital region and lateral to the nasal region.

Infraorbital rim   Inferior rim of the orbit.

Infraorbital sulcus   Groove in the floor of the orbital surface.

Infratemporal crest (in-frah-**tem**-poh-ral)   Crest that divides each greater wing of the sphenoid bone into temporal and infratemporal surfaces.

Infratemporal fossa   Fossa inferior to the temporal fossa and infratemporal crest on the greater wing of the sphenoid bone.

Infratemporal space   Space that occupies the infratemporal fossa.

Infratrochlear nerve (in-frah-**trok**-lere)   Nerve from the medial eyelid and side of the nose that converges with other branches to form the nasociliary nerve.

Innervation (in-er-**vay**-shin)   Supply of nerves to tissues or organs.

Insertion   End of the muscle that is attached to the more movable structure.

Interdental gingiva (in-ter-**den**-tal)   Attached gingiva between the teeth.

Intermediate tendon (in-ter-**me**-dee-it **ten**-don)   Tendon between two muscle bellies such as the anterior and posterior bellies of the digastric muscle.

Internal   Inner side of the wall of a hollow structure.

Internal acoustic meatus (ah-**koos**-tik)   Bony meatus in the temporal bone that carries the seventh and eighth cranial nerves.

Internal carotid artery (kah-**rot**-id)   Artery off the common carotid artery that gives rise to the ophthalmic artery and supplies intracranial structures.

Internal jugular vein (**jug**-you-lar)   Vein that travels in the carotid sheath from the jugular foramen and drains the tissues of the head and neck.

Internal nasal nerves (**nay**-zil)   Nerves from the nasal cavity that converge with other branches to form the nasociliary nerve.

Intertragic notch (in-ter-**tra**-gic)   Deep notch between the tragus and antitragus on the surface of the ear.

Intrinsic tongue muscles (in-**trin**-sik)   Muscles located entirely inside the tongue.

Investing fascia   Most external layer of the deep cervical fascia.

Ipsilateral (ip-see-**lat**-er-il)   Structures on the same side of the body.

Iris (**eye**-ris)   Central area of coloration of the eyeball.

J

Joint   Site of a junction or union between two or more bones.

Joint capsule of the temporomandibular joint   Fibrous capsule that encloses the temporomandibular joint.

Jugular foramen (**jug**-you-lar)   Foramen between the occipital and temporal bones that carries the internal jugular vein and ninth, tenth, and eleventh cranial nerves.

Jugular notch of the occipital bone   Occipital or medial portion of the jugular foramen.

Jugular notch of the temporal bone   Temporal or lateral portion of the jugular foramen.

Jugular trunk   Lymphatic vessel that drains one side of the head and neck and then empties into that side's lymphatic duct.

Jugulodigastric lymph node (jug-you-lo-di-**gas**-trik)   Superior deep cervical node located below the posterior belly of the digastric muscle.

Jugulo-omohyoid lymph node (jug-you-lo-o-mo-**hi**-oid) Inferior deep cervical node located at the crossing of the omohyoid muscle and internal jugular vein.

L

Labial (**lay**-be-al) Structures closest to the lips.

Labial commissure (**kom**-i-shoor) Corner of the mouth where the upper and lower lips meet.

Labial frenum (**free**-num) Fold of tissue or frenulum located at the midline between the labial mucosa and alveolar mucosa of the maxilla and mandible.

Labial mucosa Lining of the inner portions of the lips.

Labiomental groove (lay-bee-o-**ment**-il) A groove that separates the lower lip from the chin.

Lacrimal bones (**lak**-ri-mal) Paired facial bones that help form the medial wall of the orbit.

Lacrimal fluid Tears or watery fluid excreted by the lacrimal gland.

Lacrimal fossa Fossa of the frontal bone that contains the lacrimal gland.

Lacrimal gland Gland in the lacrimal fossa of the frontal bone that produces lacrimal fluid or tears.

Lacrimal nerve Nerve that serves the lateral portion of the eyelid and other eye tissues and joins the frontal and nasociliary nerves to form the ophthalmic nerve.

Lambdoidal suture (lam-**doid**-al) Suture between the occipital bone and both parietal bones.

Laryngopharynx (lah-ring-gah-**far**-inks) Inferior portion of pharynx close to the laryngeal opening.

Lateral Area that is farther away from the median plane of the body or structure.

Lateral canthus, canthi (**kan**-this, **kan**-thy) Outer corner of the eye or outer canthus where the upper and lower eyelids meet.

Lateral deviation of the mandible (de-vee-**ay**-shun) Shifting of the lower jaw to one side.

Lateral masses Lateral portions of the first cervical vertebra where it articulates with the occipital bone above and the axis below.

Lateral pterygoid muscle (**teh**-ri-goid) Muscle of mastication that lies in the infratemporal fossa.

Lateral pterygoid nerve Muscular branch from the anterior trunk of the mandibular division of the trigeminal nerve that serves the lateral pterygoid muscle.

Lateral pterygoid plate Portion of the pterygoid process.

Lateral surface of the tongue Side of the tongue.

Lesser cornu Pair of projections of the hyoid bone.

Lesser palatine artery (**pal**-ah-tine) Arterial branch from the maxillary artery that travels to the soft palate.

Lesser palatine foramen Foramen in the palatine bone that transmits the lesser palatine nerve and blood vessels.

Lesser palatine nerve Nerve that serves the soft palate and palatine tonsillar tissues along with the posterior nasal cavity and then joins the maxillary nerve.

Lesser petrosal nerve (peh-**troh**-sil) Parasympathetic fibers from the ninth cranial nerve that exit the skull through the foramen ovale of the sphenoid bone.

Lesser wing of the sphenoid bone (**sfe**-noid) Anterior process of the body of the sphenoid bone.

Levator anguli oris muscle (le-**vate**-er **an**-gu-lie **or**-is) Muscle of facial expression in the mouth region that elevates the angle of the mouth.

Levator labii superioris alaeque nasi muscle (**lay**-be-eye soo-per-ee-**or**-is **a**-lah-cue **naz**-eye) Muscle of facial expression in the mouth region that elevates the upper lip and ala of the nose.

Levator labii superioris muscle Muscle of facial expression in the mouth region that elevates the upper lip.

Levator veli palatini muscle (**vee**-lie pal-ah-**teen**-ee) Muscle of the soft palate that raises the soft palate to close off the nasopharynx.

Ligament (**lig**-ah-mint) Band of fibrous tissue connecting bones.

Line Straight, small ridge of bone.

Lingual (**ling**-gwal) Structures closest to the tongue.

Lingual artery Anterior arterial branch from the external carotid artery that supplies tissues superior to the hyoid bone, as well as the tongue and floor of the mouth.

Lingual frenum (**free**-num) Midline fold of tissue or frenulum between the ventral surface of the tongue and floor of the mouth.

Lingual nerve Nerve that serves the tongue, floor of the mouth, and lingual gingiva of the mandibular teeth and joins the posterior trunk of the mandibular division of the trigeminal nerve.

Lingual papillae (pah-**pil**-ay) Small elevated structures covering the dorsal surface of the body of the tongue.

Lingual tonsil (**ton**-sil) Indistinct layer of lymphoid tissue located on the dorsal surface of the tongue's base.

Lingual veins Veins that include the deep lingual, dorsal lingual, and sublingual veins.

Lingula (**lin**-gu-lah) Bony spine overhanging the mandibular foramen.

Lobule (**lob**-yule) Inferior fleshy protuberance from the helix of the auricle.

Local infiltration (lo-kal in-fil-**tray**-shun) Type of injection that anesthetizes a small area, including one or two teeth and associated structures, when the local anesthetic agent is deposited near terminal nerve endings.

Ludwig's angina (**lood**-vigz an-**ji**-nah) Serious infection of the submandibular space, with a risk of spread to the neck and chest.

Lymph (limf) Tissue fluid that drains from the surrounding region and into the lymphatic vessels.

Lymphadenopathy (lim-fad-in-**op**-ah-thee) Process in which there is an increase in the size and a change in the consistency of lymphoid tissue.

Lymphatic ducts (lim-**fat**-ik) Larger lymphatic vessels that drain smaller vessels and then empty into the venous system.

Lymphatics Portion of the immune system with nodes, ducts, tonsils, and vessels.

Lymphatic vessels System of channels that drain tissue fluid from the surrounding regions.

Lymph nodes Organized, bean-shaped lymphoid tissue that filters the lymph by way of lymphocytes to fight disease and is grouped into clusters along the connecting lymphatic vessels.

M

Major salivary glands Large, paired glands with associated named ducts that include the parotid, submandibular, and sublingual glands.

Malar lymph nodes (may-lar) Superficial nodes of the face located in the infraorbital region.

Mandible (man-di-bl) Single facial bone that articulates bilaterally with the temporal bones at the temporomandibular joints.

Mandibular canal (man-**dib**-you-lar) Canal in the mandible where the inferior alveolar nerve and blood vessels travel.

Mandibular foramen Foramen of the mandible that allows the inferior alveolar nerve and blood vessels to exit or enter the mandibular canal.

Mandibular lymph nodes Superficial nodes of the face located over the surface of the mandible.

Mandibular nerve Third division of the trigeminal nerve that is formed by the merger of posterior and anterior trunks and joins with the ophthalmic and maxillary nerves to form the trigeminal ganglion of the trigeminal nerve.

Mandibular notch Notch located on the mandible between the condyle and coronoid process.

Mandibular teeth Teeth of the mandible.

Marginal gingiva (mar-ji-nal) Nonattached gingiva at the gingival margin of each tooth.

Masseter muscle (mass-et-er) Most obvious and strongest muscle of mastication.

Masseteric artery (mass-et-**tehr**-ik) Arterial branch from the maxillary artery that supplies the masseter muscle.

Masseteric nerve Muscular nerve branch from the anterior trunk of the mandibular division of the trigeminal nerve that serves the masseter muscle and temporomandibular joint.

Masseteric-parotid fascia (mass-et-**tehr**-ik-pah-**rot**-id) Deep fascia that is located inferior to the zygomatic arch and over the masseter muscle.

Masticator space (mass-ti-**kay**-tor) Fascial space that includes the entire area of the mandible and muscles of mastication.

Mastoid air cells (mass-toid) Air spaces in the mastoid process of the temporal bone that communicate with the middle ear cavity.

Mastoid notch Notch on the mastoid process of the temporal bone.

Mastoid process Area on the petrous portion of the temporal bone that contains the air cells and on which the cervical muscles attach.

Maxilla, maxillae (mak-**sil**-ah, mak-**sil**-lay) Upper jaw that consists of two maxillary bones.

Maxillary artery (mak-sil-lare-ee) Terminal arterial branch from the external carotid artery.

Maxillary nerve Second division of the sensory root of the trigeminal nerve that is formed by the convergence of many nerves including the infraorbital nerve and serves many maxillary tissues such as the maxillary sinus, palate, nasopharynx, and overlying skin.

Maxillary process of the zygomatic bone Process that forms a portion of the infraorbital rim and orbital wall.

Maxillary sinuses Paranasal sinuses in each body of the maxilla.

Maxillary sinusitis (si-nu-**si**-tis) Infection of the maxillary sinus.

Maxillary teeth (mak-sil-lare-ee) Teeth of the maxilla.

Maxillary tuberosity (too-beh-**ros**-i-tee) Elevation on the posterior aspect of the maxilla that is perforated by the posterior superior alveolar foramina.

Maxillary vein Vein that after collecting from the pterygoid plexus merges with the superficial temporal vein to form the retromandibular vein.

Meatus (me-**ate**-us) Opening or canal in the bone.

Medial (me-dee-il) Area that is closer to the median plane of the body or structure.

Medial canthus, canthi (kan-this, **kan**-thy) Inner angle or canthus of the eye.

Medial pterygoid muscle (teh-ri-goid) Muscle of mastication that inserts on the medial surface of the mandible.

Medial pterygoid plate Portion of the pterygoid process.

Median (me-dee-an) Structure at the median plane.

Median lingual sulcus (ling-wal **sul**-kus) Midline depression on the dorsal surface of the tongue that corresponds to the deeper median septum.

Median palatine raphe (pal-ah-tine **ra**-fe) Midline fibrous band of the palate.

Median palatine suture Midline suture between the palatine processes of the maxillae and between the horizontal plates of the palatine bones.

Median pharyngeal raphe (fah-**rin**-je-al **ra**-fe) Midline fibrous band on the posterior wall of the pharynx.

Median plane (me-dee-an) Plane created by an imaginary line dividing the body into right and left halves.

Median septum (sep-tum) Midline fibrous structure that divides the tongue and corresponds to a midline depression, the median lingual sulcus, on the dorsal surface of the tongue.

Medulla (me-**dul**-ah) Division of the brainstem that is involved with the regulation of heartbeat, breathing, vasoconstriction, and reflex centers.

Meningitis (men-in-**jite**-is) Inflammation of the meninges of the brain or spinal cord.

Mental artery (ment-il) Arterial branch from the inferior alveolar artery that exits the mental foramen and supplies the tissues of the chin.

Mental block Local anesthetic block that achieves anesthesia of the facial tissues of the mandibular premolars and anterior teeth.

Mental foramen Foramen between the apices of the mandibular first and second premolars that transmits the mental nerve and blood vessels.

Mental nerve Nerve that joins the incisive nerve to form the inferior alveolar nerve and serves the tissues of the chin and lower lip and the labial mucosa of the mandibular anterior teeth.

Mental protuberance (pro-**too**-ber-ins) Mandibular bony prominence of the chin.

Mental region Region of the head where the major feature is the chin.

Mentalis muscle (ment-**ta**-lis) Muscle of facial expression in the mouth region that raises the chin.

Metastasis (meh-**tas**-tah-sis) Spread of cancer from the original or primary site to another or secondary site.

Midbrain   Division of the brainstem that includes relay stations for hearing, vision, and motor pathways.

Middle meningeal artery (meh-**nin**-je-al)   Arterial branch from the maxillary artery that supplies the meninges of the brain by the way of the foramen spinosum.

Middle meningeal vein   Vein that drains blood from the meninges of the brain into the pterygoid plexus of veins.

Middle nasal conchae (**nay**-zil **kong**-kay)   Lateral portions of the ethmoid bone in the nasal cavity.

Middle superior alveolar (MSA) block (al-**ve**-o-lar)   Local anesthetic block that achieves anesthesia of the pulp and buccal tissues of the maxillary premolars and the mesiobuccal root of the maxillary first molar.

Middle superior alveolar (MSA) nerve   Nerve that serves the maxillary premolar teeth and tissues, as well as the mesiobuccal root of the maxillary first molar; is formed from dental, interdental, and interradicular branches, and later joins the infraorbital nerve.

Middle temporal artery (**tem**-poh-ral)   Arterial branch from the superficial temporal artery that supplies the temporalis muscle.

Midsagittal section (mid-**saj**-i-tl)   Section of the body through the median plane.

Minor salivary glands   Small glands scattered in the tissues of the buccal, labial, and lingual mucosa; soft and hard palates; and floor of the mouth, as well as associated with the circumvallate lingual papillae.

Molars (**mo**-lers)   Most posterior teeth including firsts, seconds, and thirds.

Motor root of the trigeminal nerve   Root of the trigeminal nerve.

Mucobuccal fold (mu-ko-**buk**-al)   Fold in the vestibule where the labial or buccal mucosa meets the alveolar mucosa.

Mucogingival junction (mu-ko-**jin**-ji-val)   Border between the alveolar mucosa and attached gingiva.

Mucosa (mu-**ko**-sah)   Mucous membrane such as that lining the oral cavity.

Muscle   Type of body tissue that shortens under neural control, causing soft tissue and bony structures to move.

Muscle of the uvula (**u**-vu-lah)   Muscle of the soft palate that is within the uvula.

Muscles of facial expression   Paired muscles that give the face expression and are located in the superficial fascia of the facial tissues.

Muscles of mastication (mass-ti-**kay**-shun)   Pairs of muscles attached to and moving the mandible including the temporalis, masseter, and medial and lateral pterygoid muscles.

Muscles of the pharynx (**far**-inks)   Muscles that include the stylopharyngeus, pharyngeal constrictor, and soft palate muscles.

Muscles of the soft palate (**pal**-it)   Muscles that include the palatoglossal, palatopharyngeus, levator veli palatini, and tensor veli palatini muscles and muscle of the uvula.

Muscles of the tongue   Muscles of the tongue that can be further grouped according to whether they are intrinsic or extrinsic.

Muscular triangle   Smaller triangular region of the neck inferior to the omohyoid muscle and a portion of the anterior cervical triangle.

Mylohyoid artery (my-lo-**hi**-oid)   Arterial branch from the inferior alveolar artery that supplies the floor of the mouth and the mylohyoid muscle.

Mylohyoid groove   Groove on the mandible where the mylohyoid nerve and blood vessels travel.

Mylohyoid line   Line on the inner aspect of the mandible.

Mylohyoid muscle   Anterior suprahyoid muscle that forms the floor of the mouth.

Mylohyoid nerve   Nerve branch from the inferior alveolar nerve that serves the mylohyoid muscle and the anterior belly of the digastric muscle.

N

Naris, nares (**nay**-ris, **nay**-rees)   Nostril of the nose.

Nasal bones (**nay**-zil)   Paired facial bones that form the bridge of the nose.

Nasal cavity   Cavity of the nose.

Nasal conchae (**kong**-kay)   Projecting structures that extend inward from the lateral walls of the nasal cavity.

Nasal meatus   Groove beneath each nasal concha that contains openings for communication with the paranasal sinuses or nasolacrimal duct.

Nasal region   Region of the head where the main feature is the external nose.

Nasal septum (**sep**-tum)   Vertical partition of the nasal cavity.

Nasion (**nay**-ze-on)   Midline junction between the nasal and frontal bones.

Nasociliary nerve (nay-zo-**sil**-ee-a-re)   Nerve that joins the frontal and lacrimal nerves to form the ophthalmic nerve.

Nasolabial lymph nodes (nay-zo-**lay**-be-al)   Superficial nodes of the face located near the nose.

Nasolabial sulcus (**sul**-kus)   Groove running upward between the labial commissure and ala of the nose.

Nasolacrimal duct (nay-zo-**lak**-rim-al)   Duct formed at the junction of the lacrimal and maxillary bones that drains the lacrimal fluid or tears.

Nasolacrimal sac   The lacrimal fluid ends up in this structure after passing over the eyeball.

Nasopalatine (NP) block (nay-zo-**pal**-ah-tine)   Local anesthetic block that achieves anesthesia of the anterior portion of the hard palate.

Nasopalatine (NP) nerve   Nerve that serves the anterior hard palate and lingual gingiva of the maxillary anterior teeth and then joins the maxillary nerve.

Nasopharynx (nay-zo-**far**-inks)   Portion of the pharynx that is superior to the level of soft palate.

Nerve   Bundle of neural processes outside the central nervous system; portion of the peripheral nervous system.

Nerve block   Type of injection that anesthetizes a larger area than the local infiltration and usually more teeth because the local anesthetic agent is deposited near large nerve trunks.

Nervous system   The extensive, intricate network of structures that activates, coordinates, and controls all functions of the body.

Neuron (**noor**-on)   Cellular component of the nervous system that is individually composed of a cell body and neural processes.

Neurotransmitter (**nu**-ro-**tranz**-mitt-er)   Chemical agent of the neuron that is discharged with the arrival of the action potential, diffuses across the synapse, and binds to receptors on the other cell's membrane.

Normal flora (flor-ah)   Resident microorganisms that usually do not cause infections.

Notch   Indentation at the edge of a bone.

O

Occipital artery (ok-sip-it-tal)   Posterior arterial branch from the external carotid artery that supplies the suprahyoid and sternocleidomastoid muscles and posterior scalp tissues.

Occipital bone   Single cranial bone in the most posterior portion of the skull.

Occipital condyles   Projections of the occipital bone that articulate with lateral masses of the first cervical vertebra.

Occipital lymph nodes   Superficial nodes located on the posterior base of the head.

Occipital region   Region of the head overlying the occipital bone and covered by the scalp.

Occipital triangle   Smaller triangular region of the neck superior to the omohyoid muscle and a portion of the posterior cervical triangle.

Oculomotor nerve (ok-yule-oh-mote-er)   Third cranial nerve (III) that serves some of the eye muscles.

Odontogenic infections (o-dont-o-jen-ic)   Dental infections involving the teeth or associated tissues.

Olfactory nerve (ol-fak-ter-ee)   First cranial nerve (I) that transmits smell from the nose to the brain.

Omohyoid muscle (o-mo-hi-oid)   Infrahyoid muscle with superior and inferior bellies.

Ophthalmic artery (of-thal-mic)   Arterial branch that supplies the eye, orbit, and lacrimal gland.

Ophthalmic nerve   First division of the sensory root of the trigeminal nerve that arises from the frontal, lacrimal, and nasociliary nerves.

Ophthalmic veins   Veins that drain the tissues of the orbit.

Opportunistic infections (op-or-tu-nis-tik)   Normal flora creating an infectious process because the body's defenses are compromised.

Optic canal (op-tik)   Canal in the orbital apex between the roots of the lesser wing of the sphenoid bone.

Optic nerve   Second cranial nerve (II) that transmits sight from the eye to the brain.

Oral cavity   Inside of the mouth.

Oral region   Region of the head that contains the lips, oral cavity, palate, tongue, and floor of the mouth and portions of the pharynx.

Orbicularis oculi muscle (or-bik-you-laa-ris **oc**-yule-eye)   Muscle of facial expression that encircles the eye.

Orbicularis oris muscle   Muscle of facial expression that encircles the mouth.

Orbit (or-bit)   Eye cavity that contains the eyeballs.

Orbital apex (or-bit-al)   Deepest portion of the orbit composed of portions of the sphenoid and palatine bones.

Orbital plate of the ethmoid bone   Plate that forms most of the medial orbital wall.

Orbital region   Region of the head with the eyeball and all its supporting structures.

Orbital walls   Walls of the orbit composed of portions of the frontal, ethmoid, lacrimal, maxillary, zygomatic, and sphenoid bones.

Origin   End of the muscle that is attached to the least movable structure.

Oropharynx (or-o-far-inks)   Portion of the pharynx that is between the soft palate and opening of the larynx.

Osteomyelitis (os-tee-o-my-il-ite-is)   Inflammation of bone marrow.

Ostium, ostia (os-tee-um, **os**-tee-ah)   Small opening in bone.

Otic ganglion (ot-ik)   Ganglion associated with the lesser petrosal nerve and branches of the mandibular nerve.

P

Palatal (pal-ah-tal)   Structures closest to the palate.

Palate (pal-it)   Roof of the mouth.

Palatine bones (pal-ah-tine)   Paired bones of the skull that consist of two plates, a vertical and a horizontal plate.

Palatine process of the maxilla   Paired processes that articulate with each other and form the anterior portion of the hard palate.

Palatine rugae (ru-gay)   Irregular ridges of tissues surrounding the incisive papilla on the hard palate.

Palatine tonsils   Tonsils located between the anterior and posterior faucial pillars.

Palatoglossal muscle (pal-ah-to-gloss-el)   Muscle of the soft palate that forms the anterior faucial pillar.

Palatopharyngeus muscle (pal-ah-to-fah-rin-je-us)   Muscle of the soft palate that forms the posterior faucial pillar.

Paranasal sinuses (pare-ah-na-zil)   Paired, air-filled cavities in bone that include the frontal, sphenoidal, ethmoidal, and maxillary sinuses.

Parapharyngeal space (pare-ah-fah-rin-je-al)   Fascial space located lateral to the pharynx.

Parasympathetic nervous system (pare-ah-sim-pah-thet-ik)   Division of the autonomic nervous system that is involved in "rest or digest."

Parathyroid glands (par-ah-thy-roid)   Small endocrine glands located close to or even inside the thyroid gland.

Parathyroid hormone   Hormone produced and secreted by the parathyroid glands directly into the blood to regulate calcium and phosphorus levels.

Paresthesia (par-es-the-ze-ah)   Abnormal sensation from an area, such as burning or prickling.

Parietal bones (pah-ri-it-al)   Paired cranial bones of the skull that articulate with each other and other skull bones.

Parietal region   Region of the head that overlies the parietal bones and is covered by the scalp.

Parotid duct (pah-rot-id)   Duct associated with the parotid salivary gland that opens into the oral cavity at the parotid papilla.

Parotid papilla (pah-pil-ah)   Small elevation of tissue that marks the opening of the parotid salivary gland and is located opposite the second maxillary molar on the inner cheek.

Parotid salivary gland   Major gland located over the mandibular ramus that is divided into superficial and deep lobes.

Parotid space   Fascial space created inside the investing fascial layer of the deep cervical fascia as it envelops the parotid salivary gland.

Pathogens (path-ah-jens)   Flora that are not normal body residents and can cause an infection.

Perforation (per-fo-ray-shun)   Abnormal hole in a hollow organ such as in the wall of a sinus.

Peripheral nervous system (PNS) (per-**if**-er-al) Division of the nervous system that consists of the afferent and efferent nervous systems.

Perpendicular plate (per-pen-**dik**-you-lar) Midline vertical plate of the ethmoid bone.

Petrotympanic fissure (pe-troh-tim-**pan**-ik) Fissure between the tympanic and petrosal portions of the temporal bone, just posterior to the articular fossa, through which the chorda tympani nerve emerges.

Petrous portion of the temporal bone (**pet**-rus) Inferior portion of the bone that contains the mastoid process and air cells.

Pharyngeal constrictor muscles (fah-**rin**-je-il kon-**strik**-tor) Three paired muscles that form the lateral and posterior walls of the pharynx.

Pharyngeal tonsil Tonsil located on the posterior wall of the nasopharynx.

Pharynx (**far**-inks) Portion of both the respiratory and digestive tracts that is divided into the nasopharynx, oropharynx, and laryngopharynx.

Philtrum (**fil**-trum) Vertical groove in the midline of the upper lip.

Piriform aperture (**pir**-i-form) Anterior opening of the nasal cavity.

Plaque Substance that consists of mainly cholesterol, calcium, clotting proteins, and other substances that can be found lining arteries.

Plate Flat structure of bone.

Platysma muscle (plah-**tiz**-mah) Muscle of facial expression that runs from the neck to the mouth.

Plexus (**plek**-sis) Network of blood vessels, usually veins.

Plica fimbriata, plicae fimbriatae (**pli**-kah fim-bree-**ay**-tah, **pli**-kay fim-bree-**ay**-tay) Fold with fringelike projections on the ventral surface of the tongue.

Pons (ponz) Division of the brainstem that connects the medulla with the cerebellum.

Posterior Back of an area of the body.

Posterior arch Arch on the first cervical vertebra.

Posterior auricular artery (aw-**rik**-yule-lar) Posterior arterial branch from the external carotid artery that supplies the tissues around the ear.

Posterior auricular nerve Branch of the facial nerve that serves the occipital belly of the epicranial muscle, the stylohyoid muscle, and the posterior belly of the digastric muscle.

Posterior cervical triangle Lateral region of the neck.

Posterior digastric nerve (di-**gas**-trik) Nerve that supplies the posterior belly of the digastric muscle.

Posterior faucial pillar (**faw**-shawl **pil**-er) Vertical fold posterior to each palatine tonsil created by the palatopharyngeus muscle.

Posterior nasal apertures (**nay**-zil) Posterior openings of the nasal cavity.

Posterior superior alveolar artery (al-**ve**-o-lar) Arterial branches from the maxillary artery that supply the pulp tissue and periodontium of the maxillary posterior teeth and maxillary sinus.

Posterior superior alveolar (PSA) block Local anesthetic block that is used to achieve pulpal and buccal tissue anesthesia of the maxillary molars.

Posterior superior alveolar foramina Foramina on the maxillary tuberosity that carry the posterior superior alveolar nerve and blood vessels.

Posterior superior alveolar (PSA) nerve Nerve that directly joins the maxillary nerve after serving maxillary molars and tissues.

Posterior superior alveolar vein Vein that is formed from the merger of dental and alveolar branches that drain the pulp tissue and periodontium of the maxillary teeth.

Posterior suprahyoid muscle group (soo-prah-**hi**-oid) Suprahyoid muscles posterior to the hyoid bone that include the posterior belly of the digastric and stylohyoid muscles.

Postglenoid process (post-**gle**-noid) Process of the temporal bone.

Premolars (pre-**mo**-lers) Posterior teeth that are the fourth and fifth teeth from the midline in the permanent dentition and that include firsts and seconds, respectively.

Previsceral space (pre-**vis**-er-al) Fascial space located between the visceral and investing fasciae.

Primary node Lymph node that drains lymph from a particular region.

Primary sinusitis (sy-nu-**si**-tis) Inflammation of the sinus.

Process General term for any prominence on a bony surface.

Protrusion of the mandible (pro-**troo**-shun) Bringing of the lower jaw forward.

Proximal (**prok**-si-mil) Area closer to the median plane of the body.

Pterygoid arteries (**teh**-ri-goid) Arterial branches from the maxillary artery that supply the pterygoid muscles.

Pterygoid canal Small canal at the superior border of each posterior nasal aperture.

Pterygoid fascia Deep fascia located on the medial surface of the medial pterygoid muscle.

Pterygoid fossa Fossa between the medial and lateral pterygoid plates of the sphenoid bone.

Pterygoid fovea (fo-**vee**-ah) Depression on the anterior surface of the condyle of the mandible.

Pterygoid plexus of veins Collection of veins around the pterygoid muscles and maxillary arteries that drain the deep face and alveolar veins into the maxillary vein.

Pterygoid process Portion of the sphenoid bone that forms the lateral borders of the posterior nasal apertures.

Pterygomandibular fold (teh-ri-go-man-**dib**-yule-lar) Fold of tissue in the oral cavity that covers the pterygomandibular raphe.

Pterygomandibular raphe (**ra**-fe) Fibrous structure that extends from the hamulus to the posterior end of the mylohyoid line.

Pterygomandibular space Fascial space that is a portion of the infratemporal space.

Pterygopalatine fossa (teh-ri-go-**pal**-ah-tine) Fossa deep to the infratemporal fossa and between the pterygoid process and maxillary tuberosity.

Pterygopalatine ganglion Ganglion associated with the greater petrosal nerve and branches of the maxillary nerve.

Pupil (**pew**-pil) Black area in the center of the iris that responds to changing light conditions.

Pustule (**pus**-tule) Small, elevated, circumscribed, suppuration-containing lesion of either the skin or the oral mucosa.

R

Ramus (**ray**-mus) Plate of the mandible that extends superiorly from the body of the mandible.

Regions of the head Regions that include the frontal, parietal, occipital, temporal, orbital, nasal, infraorbital, zygomatic, buccal, oral, and mental regions.

Regions of the neck Regions that include the anterior and posterior cervical triangles.

Resting potential (po-**ten**-shal) Charge difference between the fluid outside and inside a cell that results in differences in the distribution of ions.

Retraction of the mandible (re-**trak**-shun) Bringing of the lower jaw backward.

Retroauricular lymph nodes (reh-tro-aw-**rik**-you-lar) Superficial nodes located posterior to the ear.

Retromandibular vein (reh-tro-man-**dib**-you-lar) Vein that is formed by the merger of the superficial temporal and maxillary veins and divides into anterior and posterior divisions below the parotid salivary gland.

Retromolar pad (re-tro-**moh**-lar) Dense pad of tissue distal to the last tooth of the mandible that covers the retromolar triangle.

Retromolar triangle Portion of the mandibular alveolar process just posterior to the most distal mandibular molar that is covered by the retromolar pad.

Retropharyngeal lymph nodes (ret-ro-far-**rin**-je-al) Deep nodes located near the deep parotid nodes and at the level of the first cervical vertebra.

Retropharyngeal space Fascial space located immediately posterior to the pharynx.

Right lymphatic duct Duct formed from the convergence of the lymphatics of the right arm and thorax and the right jugular trunk that drains this side of the head and neck.

Risorius muscle (ri-**soh**-ree-us) Muscle of facial expression in the mouth region that is used when smiling widely.

Root of the nose Area of the nasal region between the eyes.

S

Sagittal plane (**saj**-i-tel) Any plane of the body created by an imaginary plane parallel to the median plane.

Sagittal suture Suture between the paired parietal bones.

Saliva (sah-**li**-vah) Product produced by the salivary glands.

Salivary gland (**sal**-i-ver-ee) Gland that produces saliva that lubricates and cleanses the oral cavity and helps in digestion.

Scalp Layers of soft tissue overlying the bones of the cranium.

Sclera (**skler**-ah) White area of the eyeball.

Secondary node Lymph node that drains lymph from a primary node.

Secondary sinusitis (sy-nu-**si**-tis) Inflammation of the sinus related to another source.

Sensory root of the trigeminal nerve Root of the trigeminal nerve that has ophthalmic, maxillary, and mandibular divisions.

Skull Structure composed of both the cranial bones or cranium and facial bones.

Soft palate (**pal**-it) Posterior nonbony portion of the palate.

Somatic nervous system (SNS) Subdivision of the efferent division peripheral nervous system that includes all nerves controlling the muscular system and external sensory receptors.

Space of the body of the mandible (**man**-di-bl) Fascial space formed by the periosteum covering the body of the mandible.

Sphenoid bone (**sfe**-noid) Single midline cranial bone with a body and several pairs of processes.

Sphenoidal sinuses Paired sinuses located in the body of the sphenoid bone.

Sphenomandibular ligament (sfe-no-man-**dib**-you-lar) Ligament that connects the spine of the sphenoid bone with the lingula of the mandible.

Sphenopalatine artery (sfe-no-**pal**-ah-tine) Terminal arterial branch from the maxillary artery that supplies the nose including a branch through the incisive foramen.

Spine Abrupt small prominence of bone.

Spinal cord Division of the central nervous system that runs along the dorsal side of the body and links the brain to the rest of the body.

Spine of the sphenoid bone Spine located at the posterior extremity of the sphenoid bone.

Squamosal suture (**skway**-mus-al) Suture between the temporal and parietal bones.

Squamous portion of the temporal bone (**skway**-mus) Portion that forms the braincase and portions of the zygomatic arch and temporomandibular joint.

Sternocleidomastoid muscle (SCM) (stir-no-klii-do-**mass**-toid) Paired cervical muscle that serves as a primary landmark of the neck.

Sternohyoid muscle (ster-no-**hi**-oid) Infrahyoid muscle that is located superficial to the thyroid gland and cartilage.

Sternothyroid muscle (ster-no-**thy**-roid) Infrahyoid muscle that inserts on the thyroid cartilage.

Stoma (**stow**-mah) Opening such as a fistula.

Styloglossus muscle (sty-lo-**gloss**-us) Extrinsic tongue muscle that originates from the styloid process of the temporal bone.

Stylohyoid muscle (sty-lo-**hi**-oid) Posterior suprahyoid muscle that originates from the styloid process of the temporal bone.

Stylohyoid nerve Branch of the facial nerve that supplies the stylohyoid muscle.

Styloid process (**sty**-loid) Bony projection of the temporal bone that serves as an attachment for muscles and ligaments.

Stylomandibular ligament (sty-lo-man-**dib**-you-lar) Ligament that connects the styloid process with the angle of the mandible.

Stylomastoid artery (sty-lo-**mass**-toid) Artery that is a branch from the posterior auricular artery and supplies the mastoid air cells.

Stylomastoid foramen Foramen in the temporal bone that carries the facial or seventh cranial nerve.

Stylopharyngeus muscle (sty-lo-fah-**rin**-je-us) Paired longitudinal muscle of the pharynx arising from the styloid process.

Subclavian artery (sub-**klay**-vee-an) Artery that arises from the aorta on the left and the brachiocephalic artery on the right and gives off branches to supply both intracranial and extracranial structures, as well as the arm.

Subclavian triangle Smaller triangular region of the neck inferior to the omohyoid muscle and a portion of the posterior cervical triangle.

Subclavian vein Vein from the arm that drains the external jugular vein and then joins with the internal jugular vein to form the brachiocephalic vein.

Sublingual artery (sub-**ling**-gwal) Arterial branch from the lingual artery that supplies the sublingual salivary gland, floor of the mouth, and mylohyoid muscle.

Sublingual caruncle (**kar**-unk-el) Papilla near the midline of the floor of the mouth where the sublingual and submandibular ducts open into the oral cavity.

Sublingual duct Duct associated with the sublingual salivary gland that opens at the sublingual caruncle.

Sublingual fold Fold of tissue on the floor of the mouth where other smaller ducts of the sublingual salivary gland open into the oral cavity.

Sublingual fossa Fossa on the medial surface of the mandible, above the mylohyoid line, that contains the sublingual salivary gland.

Sublingual salivary gland Major gland located in the sublingual fossa.

Sublingual space Fascial space located below the oral mucosa, thus making this tissue its roof.

Subluxation (sub-luk-**ay**-shun) Acute episode of temporomandibular joint disorder in which both joints become dislocated, often due to excessive mandibular protrusion and depression.

Submandibular fossa (sub-man-**dib**-you-lar) Fossa on the medial surface of the mandible, below the mylohyoid line, that contains the submandibular salivary gland.

Submandibular ganglion Ganglion superior to the deep lobe of the submandibular salivary gland that communicates with the chorda tympani and lingual nerves.

Submandibular lymph nodes Superficial cervical nodes located at the inferior border of the ramus of the mandible.

Submandibular salivary gland Major gland that is located in the submandibular fossa.

Submandibular space Fascial space located lateral and posterior to the submental space on each side of the jaws.

Submandibular triangle Portion of the anterior cervical triangle formed by the mandible and anterior and posterior bellies of the digastric muscle.

Submasseteric space (sub-mas-et-**tehr**-ik) Fascial space located between the masseter muscle and external surface of the vertical ramus.

Submental artery (sub-**men**-tal) Arterial branch from the facial artery that supplies the submandibular lymph nodes, submandibular salivary glands, and mylohyoid and digastric muscles.

Submental lymph nodes Superficial cervical nodes located inferior to the chin.

Submental space Fascial space located midline between the symphysis and hyoid bone.

Submental triangle Unpaired midline portion of the anterior cervical triangle created by the right and left anterior bellies of the digastric muscle and the hyoid bone.

Submental vein Vein that drains the tissues of the chin and then drains into the facial vein.

Sulcus, sulci (**sul**-kus, **sul**-ky) Shallow depression or groove such as that on a bony surface or between a tooth and the inner surface of the marginal gingiva.

Sulcus terminalis (ter-mi-**nal**-is) V-shaped groove on the dorsal surface of the tongue.

Superficial Structures located toward the surface of the body.

Superficial parotid lymph nodes (pah-**rot**-id) Nodes located just superficial to the parotid salivary gland.

Superficial temporal artery (**tem**-poh-ral) Terminal arterial branch from the external carotid artery that arises in the parotid salivary gland and gives off the transverse facial and middle temporal arteries, as well as frontal and parietal branches.

Superficial temporal vein Vein that drains the side of the scalp and goes on to form the retromandibular vein along with the maxillary vein.

Superior Area that faces toward the head of the body, away from the feet.

Superior articular processes (ar-**tik**-you-lar) Processes from a vertebra that allow articulation with the vertebra above.

Superior labial artery Arterial branch from the facial artery that supplies the upper lip tissues.

Superior labial vein Vein that drains the upper lip and then drains into the facial vein.

Superior nasal conchae (**nay**-zil **kong**-kay) Lateral portions of the ethmoid bone in the nasal cavity.

Superior orbital fissure (**or**-bit-al) Fissure between the greater and lesser wings of the sphenoid bone that transmits structures from the cranial cavity to the orbit.

Superior thyroid artery (**thy**-roid) Anterior arterial branch from the external carotid artery that supplies the tissues inferior to the hyoid bone including the thyroid gland.

Superior vena cava (**vee**-na **kay**-va) Vein formed from the union of the brachiocephalic veins that empties into the heart.

Suppuration (sup-u-**ray**-shun) Pus containing pathogenic bacteria, white blood cells, tissue fluid, and debris.

Supraclavicular lymph nodes (soo-prah-klah-**vik**-you-ler) Deep cervical nodes located along the clavicle.

Suprahyoid muscles (soo-prah-**hi**-oid) Hyoid muscles located superior to the hyoid bone that can be further divided by their anterior or posterior relationship to the hyoid bone.

Supraorbital nerve (soo-prah-**or**-bit-al) Nerve from the forehead and anterior scalp that merges with the supratrochlear nerve to form the frontal nerve.

Supraorbital notch Notch on the frontal bone located on the supraorbital ridge.

Supraorbital ridge Ridge on the frontal bone located over the orbit.

Supraorbital vein Vein that joins the supratrochlear vein to form the facial vein in the frontal region.

Supratrochlear nerve (soo-prah-**trok**-lere) Nerve from the nose bridge and medial portions of the upper eyelid and forehead that merges with the supraorbital nerve to form the frontal nerve.

Supratrochlear vein   Vein that joins the supraorbital vein to form the facial vein in the frontal region.

Suture (**su**-cher)   Generally immovable articulation in which bones are joined by fibrous tissue.

Sympathetic nervous system (sim-pah-**thet**-ik)   Division of the autonomic nervous system that is involved in "fight or flight."

Symphysis (**sim**-fi-sis)   Midline articulation where bones are joined by fibrocartilage such as the midline ridge on the mandible that fuses together in early childhood.

Synapse (**sin**-aps)   Junction between two neurons or between a neuron and an effector organ where neural impulses are transmitted by electrical or chemical means.

Synovial cavities of the temporomandibular joint (sy-**no**-vee-al)   Upper and lower spaces created by the division of the joint by the disc.

Synovial fluid of the temporomandibular joint   Fluid secreted by the membranes lining the synovial cavities.

T

T-cell lymphocytes (**lim**-fo-sites)   White blood cells of the immune system that mature in the thymus gland in response to stimulation by thymus hormones.

Temporal bones (**tem**-poh-ral)   Paired cranial bones that form the lateral walls and articulate with the mandible at the temporomandibular joint.

Temporal fascia   Deep fascia covering the temporalis muscle down to the zygomatic arch.

Temporal fossa   Fossa on the lateral surface of the skull that contains the body of the temporalis muscle.

Temporalis muscle (tem-poh-**ral**-is)   Muscle of mastication that fills the temporal fossa.

Temporal lines (**tem**-poh-ral)   Two separate parallel ridges, superior and inferior, on the lateral surface of the skull.

Temporal process of the zygomatic bone   Process that forms a portion of the zygomatic arch.

Temporal region   Region of the head where the external ear is a prominent feature.

Temporal space   Fascial space formed by the temporal fascia covering the temporalis muscle.

Temporomandibular disorder (TMD) (tem-poh-ro-man-**dib**-you-lar)   Disorder involving one or both temporomandibular joints.

Temporomandibular joint (TMJ)   Articulation between the temporal bone and mandible that allows for movement of the mandible.

Temporomandibular joint ligament   Ligament associated with the temporomandibular joint.

Temporozygomatic suture (tem-por-oh-zi-go-**mat**-ik)   Suture between the temporal and zygomatic bones.

Tensor veli palatini muscle (**ten**-ser **vee**-lie pal-ah-**teen**-ee)   Muscle of the soft palate that stiffens it.

Thalamus (**thal**-a-mus)   Portion of the diencephalon that serves as a central relay point for incoming nervous impulses.

Thoracic duct (tho-**ras**-ik)   Lymphatic duct draining the lower half of the body and left side of the thorax and draining the left side of the head and neck through the left jugular trunk.

Thrombus, thrombi (**throm**-bus, **throm**-by)   Clot that forms on the inner blood vessel wall.

Thymus gland (**thy**-mus)   Endocrine gland located inferior to the thyroid gland and deep to the sternum.

Thyrohyoid muscle (thy-ro-**hi**-oid)   Infrahyoid muscle that appears as a continuation of the sternothyroid muscle.

Thyroid gland (**thy**-roid)   Endocrine gland having two lobes and located inferior to the thyroid cartilage.

Thyroxine (thy-**rok**-sin)   Hormone produced and secreted by the thyroid gland directly into the blood.

Tonsillar tissue (**ton**-sil-lar)   Masses of lymphoid tissue located in the oral cavity and pharynx to protect the body against disease processes.

Tonsils (**ton**-sils)   Tonsillar tissue that includes the palatine, lingual, pharyngeal, and tubal tonsils.

Tragus (**tra**-gus)   Flap of tissue that is a portion of the auricle and anterior to the external acoustic meatus.

Transverse facial artery (trans-**vers**)   Arterial branch from the superficial temporal artery that supplies the parotid salivary gland.

Transverse foramen   Foramen on the transverse processes of each cervical vertebra that carries the vertebral artery.

Transverse palatine suture (**pal**-ah-tine)   Suture between the palatine processes of the maxillae and horizontal plates of the palatine bones.

Transverse process   Lateral projections of the cervical vertebrae.

Transverse section   Section of the body through any horizontal plane.

Trapezius muscle (trah-**pee**-zee-us)   Cervical muscle that covers the lateral and posterior surfaces of the neck.

Trigeminal ganglion (try-**jem**-i-nal **gang**-gle-on)   Sensory ganglion located intracranially on the petrous portion of the temporal bone.

Trigeminal nerve (try-**jem**-i-nal)   Fifth cranial nerve (V) that serves the muscles of mastication and cranial muscles through its motor root and serves the teeth, tongue, and oral cavity and most of the facial skin through its sensory root.

Trigeminal neuralgia (noor-**al**-je-ah)   Type of lesion of the trigeminal nerve involving facial pain.

Trochlear nerve (**trok**-lere)   Fourth cranial nerve (IV) that serves an eye muscle.

Tubal tonsil (**tube**-al)   Tonsil located in the nasopharynx near the auditory tube.

Tubercle (**too**-ber-kl)   Eminence or small rounded elevation on the bony surface.

Tubercle of the upper lip   Thicker area in the upper lip where the philtrum terminates.

Tuberosity (too-beh-**ros**-i-tee)   Large, often rough prominence on the surface of bone.

Tympanic portion of the temporal bone (tim-**pan**-ik)   Portion that forms most of the external acoustic meatus.

U

Uvula of the palate (**u**-vu-lah)   Midline muscular structure that hangs from the posterior margin of the soft palate.

V

Vagus nerve (**vay**-gus)   Tenth cranial nerve (X) that serves the muscles of the soft palate, pharynx, and larynx, a portion of the ear skin, and many organs of the thorax and abdomen.

Vein   Type of blood vessel that travels to the heart, carrying blood.

Venous sinuses (**vee**-nus)   Blood-filled space between two layers of tissue.

Ventral (**ven**-tral)   Front of an area of the body.

Ventral surface of the tongue   Underside of the tongue.

Venule (**ven**-yule)   Smaller vein that drains the capillaries of the tissue area and then joins larger veins.

Vermilion border (ver-**mil**-yon)   Outline of the entire lip from the surrounding skin.

Vermilion zone   Darker appearance of the lips.

Vertebral fascia (**ver**-teh-brahl)   Deep cervical fascia that covers the vertebrae, spinal column, and associated muscles.

Vertebral foramen   Central foramen in the vertebrae for the spinal cord and associated tissues.

Vertical dimension of the face   The face divided into thirds.

Vertical plates of the palatine bones   Plates that form a portion of the lateral wall of the nasal cavity and orbital apex.

Vestibular space of the mandible (**man**-di-bl)   Space of the lower jaw.

Vestibular space of the maxilla (mak-**sil**-ah)   Space of the upper jaw.

Vestibules (**ves**-ti-bules)   Upper and lower spaces among the cheeks, lips, and gingival tissues in the oral region.

Vestibulocochlear nerve (ves-tib-you-lo-**kok**-lear)   Eighth cranial nerve (VIII) that serves to convey signals from the inner ear to the brain.

Visceral fascia (**vis**-er-al)   Deep cervical fascia that is a single midline tube running down the neck.

Vomer (**vo**-mer)   Single facial bone that forms the posterior portion of the nasal septum.

von Ebner's glands (**eeb**-ners)   Minor salivary glands associated with the circumvallate lingual papilla.

Z

Zygomatic arch (zy-go-**mat**-ik)   Arch formed by the union of the temporal process of the zygomatic bone and zygomatic process of the temporal bone.

Zygomatic bones   Paired facial bones that form the cheek bones.

Zygomatic nerve   Nerve that is formed from the merger of the zygomaticofacial and zygomaticotemporal nerves and joins the maxillary nerve.

Zygomatic process of the frontal bone   Process lateral to the orbit.

Zygomatic process of the maxilla   Process that forms a portion of the infraorbital rim.

Zygomatic region   Region of the head that overlies the cheek bone.

Zygomaticofacial nerve (zy-go-**mat**-i-ko-**fay**-shal)   Nerve that serves the skin of the cheek and joins with the zygomaticotemporal nerve to form the zygomatic nerve.

Zygomaticotemporal nerve (zy-go-**mat**-i-ko-**tem**-poh-ral)   Nerve that serves the skin of the temporal region and joins with the zygomaticofacial nerve to form the zygomatic nerve.

Zygomaticus major muscle (zy-go-**mat**-i-kus)   Muscle of facial expression in the mouth region that is used when smiling.

Zygomaticus minor muscle   Muscle of facial expression in the mouth region that elevates the upper lip.

Index

Note: Page numbers followed by f indicate figures; those followed by t indicate tables